THE SOUTH LONDON AND MAUDSLEY NHS TRUST

OXLEAS NHS TRUST

PRESCRIBING GUIDELINES
2003

The Maudsley

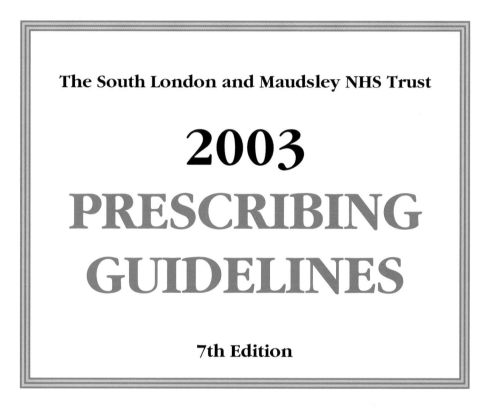

The South London and Maudsley NHS Trust

2003

PRESCRIBING

GUIDELINES

7th Edition

David Taylor
Carol Paton
Robert Kerwin

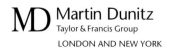

Martin Dunitz
Taylor & Francis Group
LONDON AND NEW YORK

© Taylor, Paton, Kerwin 2003

First published in the United Kingdom in 2003
by Martin Dunitz, an imprint of the Taylor & Francis Group,
11 New Fetter Lane, London EC4P 4EE

Tel.:   +44 (0) 20 7583 9855
Fax.:   +44 (0) 20 7842 2298
E-mail: info@dunitz.co.uk
Website: http://www.dunitz.co.uk

Although every effort has been made to ensure that all owners of copyright material have been
acknowledged in this publication, we would be glad to acknowledge in subsequent reprints or
editions any omissions brought to our attention.

A CIP record for this book is available from the British Library.

ISBN 1 84184 176 5

Distributed in the USA by
Fulfilment Center
Taylor & Francis
10650 Toebben Drive
Independence, KY 41051, USA
Toll Free Tel.:   +1 800 634 7064
E-mail: taylorandfrancis@thomsonlearning.com

Distributed in Canada by
Taylor & Francis
74 Rolark Drive
Scarborough, Ontario M1R 4G2, Canada
Toll Free Tel.:   +1 877 226 2237
E-mail: tal_fran@istar.ca

Distributed in the rest of the world by
Thomson Publishing Services
Cheriton House
North Way
Andover, Hampshire SP10 5BE, UK
Tel.:   +44 (0)1264 332424
E-mail: salesorder.tandf@thomsonpublishingservices.co.uk

Printed and bound in Great Britain by The Cromwell Press Ltd, Trowbridge

Contents

Authors and editors

David Taylor, Senior Editor and Lead Author
Chief Pharmacist, South London and Maudsley NHS Trust
Honorary Senior Lecturer, Institute of Psychiatry

Carol Paton, Author
Chief Pharmacist, Oxleas NHS Trust

Robert Kerwin, Founding Editor
Professor of Clinical Neuropharmacology, Institute of Psychiatry
Consultant Psychiatrist, South London and Maudsley NHS Trust

Preface

This 7ᵗʰ edition of *The Maudsley Prescribing Guidelines* differs importantly from previous editions. The most obvious difference is the change of authors: we have said farewell to Harry McConnell and Denise McConnell and now welcome Carol Paton. Harry and Denise contributed importantly to previous editions of *The Prescribing Guidelines* and their input is keenly missed. Carol Paton is the chief pharmacist of Oxleas NHS Trust, our neighbouring mental health trust. Because of Carol's widely recognised expertise in psychopharmacology and because the same strategic health authority now oversees both of our trusts, it was considered desirable or even necessary to invite Carol to contribute as an author. This issue of *The Guidelines* is intended to be official prescribing policy for both the South London & Maudsley and Oxleas NHS trusts.

The second major change in this new edition is the use of a standardised method in the construction of guidance. We have studied literature reports identified from searches of EMBASE, Medline and PsychLIT performed during late 2002 and early 2003. We have also collected posters and abstracts from major conferences taking place throughout the world in 2001 and 2002. Collected reports have then been ranked according to their scientific validity in the usual way (meta-analyses first, then individual controlled, randomised controlled trials, and so on) and guidance constructed largely according to the ranking. We have also made use of the excellent Cochrane reviews of medication used in psychiatry. This method has allowed us to be more precise about what is behind individual statements and guidance but it does mean that the number of references listed has increased several-fold. We hope that this approach is seen as more robust and transparent. A very few sections have yet to be fully researched in this way, but in these cases, recent review articles have been cited. Rather more sections are poorly informed by published literature and so we have relied more heavily on clinical experience and clinical guidance. Some may argue against this practice, but we feel that it is better to provide recommendations and guidance based on expert opinion, experience and limited data than not to provide it at all.

The third major change is the inclusion of guidance issued in the UK by the National Institute of Clinical Excellence (NICE). In therapeutic areas where NICE guidance is available we have summarised it and supported it by ensuring that our guidance, in its detail, follows the same broad aim as that of NICE.

We hope that this new edition of *The Prescribing Guidelines* is seen as an improvement on previous editions but hope too that the 7th edition retains these essential features which make *The Prescribing Guidelines* so useful to clinicians working in mental health.

David Taylor
May 2003

Acknowledgements

The Maudsley Prescribing Guidelines are a product of the authors' knowledge and expertise and the helpful contributions of a large number of specialists and experts. The input from these experts not only allows a greater range of subjects to be covered but also provides crucial, if informal, peer review of many sections. We are, therefore, deeply indebted to previous contributors and to the following contributors to the present edition of *The Guidelines*.

Steve Bazire
Ayesha Begum
Anthony Cleare
Anne Connolly
Vivienne Curtis
Sarah Elliot
Raadiyya Esop
Sean Hood
Maria Isaac
Mike Isaac
Noreen Jakeman
Nick Lintzeris
Simon Lovestone
Shubhra Mace
Shameem Mir
Robin Murray
Peter Pratt
Kathy Reed
Lucy Reeves
Larry Rifkin
Paramala Santosh
Railton Scott
Melinda Sweeting
Mike Travis

Notes on using *The Maudsley Prescribing Guidelines*

The main aim of *The Guidelines* is to provide clinicians with practically useful advice on the prescribing of psychotropic agents in commonly-encountered clinical situations. The advice contained in this handbook is based on a combination of literature review, clinical experience and expert contribution. We do not claim that this advice is necessarily 'correct' or that it deserves greater prominence than guidance provided by other professional bodies or special interest groups. We hope, however, to have provided guidance that helps to assure the safe, effective and economic use of medicines in mental health. We hope also to have made clear the sources of information used to inform guidance given.

Please note that many of the recommendations provided here go beyond the licensed or labelled indications of many drugs, both in the UK and elsewhere. Note also that, while we have endeavoured to make sure all quoted doses are correct, clinicians should always consult statutory texts before prescribing. Users of *The Guidelines* should also bear in mind that the contents of this handbook are based on information available to us up to April 2003. Much of the advice contained here will become outdated as more research is conducted and published.

No liability is accepted for any injury, loss or damage, however caused.

Notes on inclusion of drugs

The Guidelines are used in many other countries outside the UK. With this in mind, we have included in this edition those drugs in widespread use throughout the western world in April 2003. Thus, we have included, for example, ziprasidone and aripiprazole, even though neither drug is marketed in the UK at this time. Their inclusion gives *The Guidelines* relevance in those countries where such drugs are marketed and may also be of benefit to UK readers, since many of these drugs can be obtained through formal pharmaceutical importers. We have also included nefazodone (despite its imminent withdrawal from many European countries) because it is likely to be fairly widely used for the next year or so. Conversely, duloxetine and milnacipran have not been included, because our clinical experience with them and that of our advisers, is negligible. Many older drugs (methotrimeprazine, pericyazine, maprotiline, etc.) are either only briefly mentioned or not included on the basis that these drugs are not in widespread use at the time of writing.

Notes on commonly used abbreviations

Throughout this text we have abbreviated *British National Formulary* to *BNF* and extrapyramidal side-effects to EPSEs. All other abbreviations are explained in the text itself.

chapter 1

Plasma level monitoring of psychotropics and anticonvulsants

Introduction

Plasma level monitoring is a process subject to considerable confusion and misunderstanding. In psychiatry, as in other areas of medicine, plasma level determinations are frequently undertaken without good cause and acted upon inappropriately. In other instances, plasma levels are underused.

Before taking a blood sample for plasma level assay, make sure that the following criteria are satisfied:

- **Is there an assay method available?**
  Only a minority of drugs have available assays.

- **Is the drug at 'steady state'?**
  Plasma levels are usually only meaningful when samples are taken after steady-state levels have been achieved. This takes 4–5 drug half-lives.

- **Is the timing of the sample correct?**
  Sampling time is vitally important. If the recommended sampling time is 12 hours post-dose, then the sample should be taken 11–13 hours post-dose if possible; 10–14 hours post-dose, if absolutely necessary. For trough samples, take the blood sample immediately before the next dose is due. Do not, under any circumstances, withhold the next dose for more than 1 or (possibly) 2 hours until a sample is taken. Withholding for longer than this will inevitably give a misleading result (it will give a lower result than that ever seen in the usual, regular dosing), and this may lead to an inappropriate dose increase.

  If a sample is not taken within 1–2 hours of the required time, then it is more likely to mislead than inform. The only exception is if toxicity is suspected – sampling at the time of suspected toxicity is appropriate.

- **Will the level have any inherent meaning?**
  Is there a target range of plasma levels? If so, then plasma levels (from samples taken at the right time) will usefully guide dosing. If there is not an accepted target range, plasma levels can only indicate adherence or toxicity. However, if the sample is being used to check compliance, then

1

bear in mind that a plasma level of zero indicates only that the drug has not been taken in the past several days. Plasma levels above zero may indicate erratic compliance, full compliance or even long-standing non-compliance disguised by recent taking of prescribed doses.

- **Is there a clear reason for plasma level determination?**
  Only the following reasons are valid:
  - to confirm compliance (but see above)
  - if toxicity is suspected
  - if drug interaction is suspected
  - if clinical response is difficult to assess directly (and where a target range of plasma levels has been established)
  - if the drug has a narrow therapeutic index and toxicity concerns are considerable.

Interpreting sample results

The basic rule for sample level interpretation is to act upon assay results only in the absence of reliable clinical observation (*'treat the patient, not the level'*). For example, if a patient is responding to a drug but has a plasma level below the accepted target range, then the dose should not normally be increased. If a patient has intolerable adverse effects but a plasma level within the target range, then a dose decrease may be appropriate.

Where a plasma level result is substantially different from previous results, a repeat sample is usually advised. Check dose, timing of dose and recent compliance but ensure, in particular, the correct timing of sample. Many anomalous results are a consequence of changes in sample timing.

References for table opposite

1. Taylor D, Duncan D. Doses of carbamazepine and valproate in bipolar affective disorder. *Psychiatric Bulletin* 1997; **21**: 221–223.
2. Eadie MJ. Anticonvulsant drugs. *Drugs* 1984; **27**: 328–363.
3. Cohen AF, Land GS, Breimer DD *et al.* Lamotrigine, a new anticonvulsant: pharmacokinetics in normal humours. *Clinical Pharmacology and Therapeutics* 1987; **42**: 535–541.
4. Kilpatrick ES, Forrest G, Brodie MJ. Concentration-effect and concentration-toxicity relations with lamotrigine: a prospective study. *Epilepsia* 1996; **37**: 534–538.
5. Taylor D, Duncan D. Plasma levels of tricyclics and related antidepressants: are they necessary or useful? *Psychiatric Bulletin* 1995; **19**: 548–550.
6. Davis R, Peters DH, McTavish D. Valproic acid – a reappraisal of its pharmacological properties and clinical efficacy in epilepsy. *Drugs* 1994; **47**: 332–372.
7. Perucca E. Pharmacological and therapeutic properties of valproate. *CNS Drugs* 2002; **16**: 695–714.

Table Interpreting sample results

Drug	Target range	Sample timing	Time to steady state	Comments	References*
Carbamazepine	>7 mg/l bipolar disorder 4–12 mg/l epilepsy	Trough	2 weeks	Carbamazepine induces its own metabolism. Time to steady state dependent on autoinduction	1,2
Clozapine	350–500 µg/l	Trough	2–3 days	See page 4	See page 4
Lamotrigine	Not established	Trough	5 days	Useful for compliance monitoring only	3,4
Lithium	0.6–1.0 mmol/l *(may be > 1.0 mmol/l in mania)*	12 hours post-dose	5 days	Well-established target range	–
Olanzapine	20–40 µg/l	12 hours post-dose	1 week	See page 5	See page 5
Phenytoin	10–20 mg/l	Trough	Variable	Follows zero-order kinetics. Free levels may be useful	2
Tricyclics	Nortriptyline 50–150 µg/l Amitriptyline 100–200 µg/l	Trough	2–3 days	Rarely used and of dubious benefit. Use ECG to assess toxicity	5
Valproate	50–100 mg/l Epilepsy and bipolar disorder	Trough	2–3 days	Some doubt over value of levels in epilepsy and bipolar disorder. Dosing should therefore be governed by clinical response and tolerability. Target range is a useful guide in the absence of clinical indicators	1,2,6,7

Note: Plasma level monitoring of other drugs is not recommended (unless to confirm compliance).
* For references see foot of page 2 opposite.

3

Clozapine plasma levels

Clozapine plasma levels are broadly related to daily dose[1] but there is sufficient variation to make impossible any precise prediction of plasma level. Plasma levels are generally lower in younger patients, males[2] and smokers[3].

The plasma level threshold for response to clozapine has been suggested to be 200 µg/l[4], 350 µg/l[5-7], 370 µg/l[8], 420 µg/l[9] and 504 µg/l[10].

Despite these varied estimates of response threshold, plasma levels can be useful in optimising treatment. In those not responding to clozapine, dose should be adjusted to give plasma levels in the range **350–500 µg/l**. Those not tolerating clozapine may benefit from a reduction to a dose giving plasma levels in this range.

References

1. Haring C, Fleischhacker WW, Schett P et al. Influence of patient-related variables on clozapine levels. *American Journal of Psychiatry* 1990; **147**: 1471–1475.
2. Haring C, Meise M, Humpel C et al. Dose-related plasma levels of clozapine: influence of smoking behaviour, sex and age. *Psychopharmacology* 1989; **99**: S38–S40.
3. Taylor D. Pharmacokinetic interactions involving clozapine. *British Journal of Psychiatry* 1997; **171**: 109–112.
4. Vanderzwaag C, McGee M, McEvoy JP et al. Response of patients with treatment-refractory schizophrenia to clozapine within three serum level ranges. *American Journal of Psychiatry* 1996; **153**: 1579–1583.
5. Perry PJ, Miller DD, Arndt SV, Cadoret RJ. Clozapine and norclozapine plasma concentrations and clinical response of treatment refractory schizophrenic patients. *American Journal of Psychiatry* 1991; **148**: 231–235.
6. Miller DD. Effect of phenytoin on plasma clozapine concentrations in two patients. *Journal of Clinical Psychiatry* 1991; **52**: 23–25.
7. Spina E, Avenoso A, Facciola G et al. Relationship between plasma concentrations of clozapine and norclozapine and therapeutic response in patients with schizophrenia resistant to conventional neuroleptics. *Psychopharmacology* 2000; **148**: 83–89.
8. Hasegawa M, Gutierrez-Esteinou R, Way L et al. Relationship between clinical efficacy and clozapine concentrations in plasma in schizophrenia: effect of smoking. *Journal of Clinical Psychopharmacology* 1993; **13**: 383–390.
9. Potkin SG, Bera R, Gulasekaram B et al. Plasma clozapine concentrations predict clinical response in treatment-resistant schizophrenia. *Journal of Clinical Psychiatry* 1994; **55**(Suppl. B): 133–136.
10. Perry PJ. Therapeutic drug monitoring of atypical antipsychotics. *CNS Drugs* 2000; **13**: 167–171

Olanzapine plasma levels

Plasma levels of olanzapine are linearly related to daily dose but there is substantial variation[1], with higher levels seen in women[2]. The threshold level for response has been suggested to be 9.3 µg/l (trough sample)[3] and 23.2 µg/l (12-hour post-dose sample)[2]. Severe toxicity may be associated with levels above 100 µg/l and death seen at levels above 160 µg/l[4]. A target range for therapeutic use of **20–40 µg/l** has been proposed[5].

In practice, the dose of olanzapine should be governed by response and tolerability. Plasma level determinations should be reserved for those suspected of non-compliance or those not responding to the maximum licensed dose. In the latter case, dose may then be adjusted to give 12-hour plasma levels of 20–40 µg/l.

References

1. Aravagiri M, Ames D, Wirshing WC *et al.* Plasma level monitoring of olanzapine in patients with schizophrenia: determination by high-performance liquid chromatography with electrochemical detection. *Therapeutic Drug Monitoring* 1997; **19**: 307–313.
2. Perry PJ. Therapeutic drug monitoring of atypical antipsychotics. *CNS Drugs* 2000; **13**: 167–171
3. Perry PJ, Miller DD, Arndt SV, Cadoret RJ. Clozapine and norclozapine plasma concentrations and clinical response of treatment refractory schizophrenic patients. *American Journal of Psychiatry* 1999; **148**: 231–235.
4. Rao ML, Hiemke C, Grasma der K, Bauman P. Olanzapine: pharmacology, pharmacokinetics and therapeutic drug monitoring. *Fortschrite der Neurologie-Psychiatrie* 2001; **69**: 510–570.
5. Robertson MD, McMullin MM. Olanzapine concentrations in clinical serum and postmortem blood specimens – when does therapeutic become toxic? *Journal of Forensic Science* 2000; **42**: 418–421.

chapter 2

Schizophrenia

General introduction to antipsychotics[*]

The class of drugs used to treat schizophrenia and other psychotic illnesses is known as 'antipsy-chotics' (the terms 'neuroleptics' and 'major tranquillisers' are also sometimes used although neither is strictly correct).

The antipsychotic potency of most antipsychotics is directly proportional to their ability to block dopamine receptors in the brain, although the exact mechanism by which they exert their antipsychotic effect is probably more complicated than this. They vary greatly in their selectivity for dopamine receptors, many also having significant effects on acetylcholine, noradrenaline, histamine and 5HT pathways. A wide range of side-effects is therefore to be expected, the most common of which are listed below.

Extra-pyramidal side-effects

- **Dystonic reactions** (such as oculogyric crises and torticollis) may be treated with oral, im or iv anticholinergics, depending on their severity. Approximately 10% of patients exposed to the older typical drugs develop an acute dystonic reaction[1]. This is more likely in the early stages of treatment or after an increase in dose and can be both painful and very frightening. Adverse early experiences are likely to reduce long-term willingness to take medication.
- **Parkinsonian tremor** is seen in approximately 20% of patients prescribed typical drugs[2]. It can be treated with anticholinergic drugs, but *not* dopamine agonists, as these would obviously diminish the dopamine antagonistic action of the antipsychotics. Anticholinergics should not be prescribed routinely with antipsychotics. The majority of patients appear to cope without them in the long term. It is also worth noting that anticholinergics have their own side-effects (dry mouth, blurred vision, constipation, cognitive impairment, etc.) and are thought to exacerbate tardive dyskinesia. They can also be misused for their euphoric effects and have a 'street value'.
- **Akathisia** (a subjectively unpleasant state of motor restlessness) responds poorly to anticholiner-gics. It is decidedly unpleasant and contributes to anxiety and dysphoria. Approximately 20–25% of patients prescribed the older drugs are affected[3]. If this is severe, it is often best to try a different antipsychotic drug (ideally an atypical). Alternatively a non-selective beta-blocker such as propranolol (10–20 mg tds)[4] or the antihistamine cyproheptadine (4–8 mg bd)[5,6] may be

[*] *This section contains a brief overview of antipsychotic properties. Many issues are covered in greater depth in later sections.*

worth a try. These approaches are probably equally effective[7]. It is important that akathisia is distinguished from agitation secondary to psychosis, as it may have serious consequences if left untreated (akathisia has been linked to violence and suicide)[8]. For further guidance see page 66.

- **Tardive dyskinesia** (TD) has traditionally been thought to be caused by super-sensitivity of dopamine receptors, which develops because of prolonged therapy with dopamine-blocking drugs. This theory has been supported by the observation that TD is temporarily improved by increasing the dose of the offending drug (this is the wrong approach clinically as it can only perpetuate the problem). Undoubtedly, the aetiology of TD is more complex, probably involving GABA pathways to a significant extent. In the present state of our knowledge, TD is best dealt with by:
  - reducing and discontinuing anticholinergics
  - reducing the antipsychotic dose to the minimum that is effective
  - substituting older drugs with atypical antipsychotics[9]
  - trying clozapine if appropriate (may actually treat TD as well as psychosis)[10].

If the above fail to control the abnormal movements, various other options (e.g. tetrabenazine, sodium valproate, etc.) may be worth pursuing depending on the circumstances of each individual case[11]. See pages 62, 66–67 for further guidance.

It is worth noting that TD was seen in psychiatric patients long before the introduction of antipsychotic drugs[12,13] (and indeed occurs independently of psychiatric illness in around 2% of the normal elderly population)[14]. There was a recorded prevalence of 5% in patients with schizophrenia before the introduction of antipsychotics, rising to up to 20% thereafter[14]. Recent studies of older patients with schizophrenia who have never been treated with antipsychotic drugs show a prevalence rate similar to populations treated with antipsychotics. All patients treated with antipsychotics are at risk of developing TD, although patients with affective illness, diabetes, learning disabilities, females and the elderly seem to be more likely to be affected[14]. Those with mood disorders may also be more at risk of developing tardive dystonia. The presence of EPSEs during treatment with antipsychotics is associated with a three-fold increase in risk of TD, and it is likely that the newer atypical antipsychotics (which produce less frequent EPSEs) will be associated with a lower incidence of TD[9].

Hyperprolactinaemia

This is an expected phenomenon as prolactin is under the inhibitory control of dopamine. It can lead to galactorrhoea, amenorrhoea, gynaecomastia, hypogonadism, sexual dysfunction and an increased risk of osteoporosis[15–17]. Long-stay psychiatric female inpatients have been noted to have a nine-fold increase in the risk of breast cancer when compared to the normal population[18]. Although other risk factors are undoubtedly important in this group of patients, prolonged hyperprolactinaemia is likely to be a contributing factor.

A measurement of serum prolactin can be a useful indicator that the (older, typical) antipsychotic drug is being taken and is reaching CNS dopamine receptors. Prolactin levels of several thousand microgram/litre may be seen when very high doses of antipsychotics are prescribed.

Of the newer, atypical antipsychotics, sertindole, quetiapine, ziprasidone, aripiprazole and clozapine, have no important effect on prolactin. Olanzapine has a transient minimal effect. Risperidone, amisulpride and zotepine have potent prolactin elevating effects, similar to conventional drugs. For further guidance on hyperprolactinaemia, see page 65.

Reduced seizure threshold

Grand-mal seizures are a recognised side-effect of antipsychotic therapy (the higher the dose, the greater the risk). As a very general rule of thumb, the more sedative and less potent drugs carry a higher risk than the more potent, less sedative drugs. Clozapine carries the greatest risk[19]. Some antipsychotics have little or no effect on seizure threshold. See page 198 for further information on treating patients with pre-existing epilepsy.

Postural hypotension

Postural hypotension is mediated through adrenergic α_1 blockade, and so can usually be predicted for any drug with significant affinity for this receptor. It is a particular risk when phenothiazines are prescribed for the elderly, but can also occur with higher doses of other antipsychotics in much younger patients. The atypical antipsychotics clozapine, risperidone, quetiapine and sertindole all have important affinity for α_1 receptors, making dosage titration necessary.

Anticholinergic side-effects

Anticholinergic side-effects include dry mouth (which may contribute to dental decay, ill-fitting dentures), blurred vision (which can contribute to falls in the elderly), and constipation (impaction can occur). Clozapine in particular has been associated with severe constipation resulting in GI obstruction[20]. Anticholinergic effects may also have a detrimental impact on cognitive functioning.

Antipsychotics with potent anticholinergic effects (notably chlorpromazine and clozapine) should never be given to patients who have closed-angle glaucoma. Drugs with less potent anti-cholinergic side-effects (e.g. haloperidol) can be used with caution in open-angle glaucoma that is being treated and monitored, as long as the dosage used does not produce mydriasis. Drugs such as haloperidol, trifluoroperazine and sulpiride may be used in prostatic hypertrophy.

Neuroleptic malignant syndrome[21-23]

Neuroleptic malignant syndrome is thought to occur in 0.5% of newly treated patients and to be greatly under-diagnosed. It is a potentially life threatening complication of neuroleptic treatment with mortality estimated as being up to 20%. The main symptoms of NMS are mild hyperthermia, fluctuating consciousness, muscular rigidity, autonomic instability and severe EPSEs (primarily rigidity). Serum CPK is always raised. Leucocytosis (with a left shift) and abnormal LFTs are common. The enormous load of muscle breakdown products can lead to severe renal damage. The syndrome is believed to be caused by the rapid blockade of hypothalamic and striatal dopamine receptors, leading to a 'resetting' of the thermo-regulatory systems and severe skeletal muscle spasm, which contributes to a considerable heat load that cannot be dissipated. The risk is greater the higher the starting dose of the antipsychotic and the more rapidly it is increased. All antipsychotics and other psychotropics, lithium and SSRIs have been implicated in NMS, with the majority of cases attributable to haloperidol. It is difficult to know if this is an inherent characteristic of haloperidol or if it is better explained by the fact that haloperidol is very widely prescribed in situations where initial high-dose antipsychotic therapy may be indicated.

Although primarily associated with antipsychotics, other drugs that interfere with dopaminergic neurotransmission have also been implicated in NMS[21] (e.g. MAOIs, TCAs, metoclopramide and tetrabenazine). Levodopa withdrawal has also been implicated.

Weight gain

In comparison with the general population, people with schizophrenia are more likely to be over-weight and have increased quantities of visceral fat[24,25]. They are also at greater risk of developing hypertension, cardiovascular disease, type 2 diabetes and dyslipidaemias. In addition, antipsychotic-induced weight gain, particularly with atypicals, can be significant.

A substantial proportion of patients will gain 7% of their baseline body weight, which increases the risk of obesity-related morbidity (e.g. type 2 diabetes, heart disease, some cancers, etc). Relative weight gain is difficult to determine, as there is no standard way of measuring it (e.g. 5% gain, 7% gain, BMI, etc). In general, clozapine has the greatest potential to cause weight gain, followed by olanzapine and then quetiapine and risperidone and then amisulpride. Ziprasidone may be relatively weight-neutral[26,27]. See page 72 for further information. Several case reports/case series associate clozapine and olanzapine with the development of hyperglycaemia, diabetes mellitus and ketoacidosis. Being male, non-Caucasian, aged around 40 years and possibly being obese/recent weight gain would appear to be risk factors. The maximum period of risk may be in the first 6 months of treatment. The likely mechanism is insulin resistance and this does not seem to be clearly dose-related. In approximately one-third of cases, ongoing treatment with oral hypoglycaemics or insulin is required, despite treatment with clozapine or olanzapine being discontinued[28]. See page 80 for further guidance on weight gain and diabetes.

Others

Some antipsychotic drugs are sedative, some cardio-toxic and many are associated with idiosyncratic side-effects. Further information can be found under the individual drug headings. Antipsychotic treatment is a risk factor for venous thromboembolism[29].

References

1. American Psychiatric Association. Practice guideline for the treatment of patients with schizophrenia. *American Journal of Psychiatry* 1997; **154**(Suppl. 1): 1–63.
2. Bollini P, Pampallona S, Orza MJ *et al.* Antipsychotic drugs: is more worse? A meta-analysis of the published randomised controlled trials. *Psychological Medicine* 1994; **24**: 307–316.
3. Halstead SM, Barnes TRE, Speller JC. Akathisia: prevalence and associated dysphoria in an in-patient population with chronic schizophrenia. *British Journal of Psychiatry* 1994; **164**: 177–183.
4. Miller CH, Fleischhaker WW. Managing antipsychotic-induced acute and chronic akathisia. *Drug Safety* 2000; **22**: 73–81.
5. Weiss D, Aizenberg D, Hermesh H *et al.* Cyproheptadine treatment in neuroleptic-induced akathisia. *British Journal of Psychiatry* 1995; **167**: 483–486.
6. Poyurovsky M & Weizman A. Serotonin-based pharmacotherapy for acute neuroleptic-induced akathisia: a new approach to an old problem. *British Journal of Psychiatry* 2001; **179**: 4–8.
7. Tsvi F, Haggai H, Aizenberg D *et al.* Cyproheptadine versus propranolol for the treatment of acute neuroleptic-induced akathisia: A comparative double-blind study. *Journal of Clinical Psychopharmacology* 2001; **21**: 612–615.
8. Van Putten T, Marder SR. Behavioral toxicity of antipsychotic drugs. *Journal of Clinical Psychiatry* 1987; **48**(Suppl. 9): 13–19.
9. Glazer W. Expected incidence of tardive dyskinesia associated with atypical antipsychotics. *Journal of Clinical Psychiatry* 2000; **61**(Suppl. 4): 21–26.
10. Simpson GM. The treatment of tardive dyskinesia and tardive dystonia. *Journal of Clinical Psychiatry* 2000; **61**(Suppl. 4): 39–44.
11. Duncan D, McConnell H, Taylor D. Tardive dyskinesia: how is it prevented and treated? *Psychiatric Bulletin* 1997; **21**: 422–425.
12. Fenton WS. Prevalence of spontaneous dyskinesia in schizophrenia. *Journal of Clinical Psychiatry* 2000; **61**(Suppl. 4): 10–14.
13. McCreadie RG, Padmavali R, Thara R *et al.* Spontaneous dyskinesia and parkinsonism in never-medicated, chronically ill patients with schizophrenia: 18 month follow-up. *British Journal of Psychiatry* **181**:135–137.
14. American Psychiatric Association. *Tardive Dyskinesia: A task force report of the American Psychiatric Association.* Washington, DC: American Psychiatric Association, 1992.
15. Dickson RA, Seeman MV, Corenblum B. Hormonal side effects in women: typical versus atypical antipsychotic treatment. *Journal of Clinical Psychiatry* 2000; **61**(Suppl. 4): 10–15.
16. Halbreich U, Paller S. Accelerated osteoporosis in psychiatric patients: possible pathophysiological processes. *Schizophrenia Bulletin* 1996; **22**: 447–454.
17. Smith SM, O'Keane V, Murray R. Sexual dysfunction in patients taking conventional antipsychotic medication. *British Journal of Psychiatry* 2002; **181**: 49–55.
18. Halbreich U, Shen J, Panorov V. Are chronic psychiatric patients at increased risk for developing breast cancer? *American Journal of Psychiatry* 1996; **153**: 559–560.
19. Devinsky O, Honigfeld G, Patin J. Clozapine-related seizures. *Neurology* 1991; **41**: 369–371.
20. Anon. Clozapine (Clozaril) and gastrointestinal obstruction. *Current Problems in Pharmacovigilance* 1999; **25**: 5.
21. Velamoor VR. Neuroleptic malignant syndrome: recognition, prevention and management. *Drug Safety* 1998; **19**: 73–82.
22. Pelonero AL, Levenson JL, Pandurangi AK. Neuroleptic malignant syndrome: a review. *Psychiatric Services* 1999; **49**: 1163–1172.
23. Adityanjee A, Aderibigbe YA, Mathews T. Epidemiology of neuroleptic malignant syndrome. *Clinical Neuropharmacology* 1999; **22**: 151–158.
24. Mayer JM. Effects of atypical antipsychotics on weight and serum lipid levels. *Journal of Clinical Psychiatry* 2001; **62**: 27–34.
25. Thakore JH, Mann JN, Vlahos I, Martin A, Reznek R. Increased visceral fat distribution in drug-naive and drug-free patients with schizophrenia. *International Journal of Obesity and Related Metabolic Disorders* 2002; **26**: 137–141.
26. Taylor DM, McAskill R. Atypical antipsychotics and weight gain – a systematic review. *Acta Psychiatrica Scandinavica* 2000; **101**: 416–432.
27. Allison DB, Mentore JL, Moonseong H *et al.* Antipsychotic induced weight gain: a comprehensive research synthesis. *American Journal of Psychiatry* 1999; **156**: 1686–1696.
28. Mir S, Taylor D. Atypical antipsychotics and hyperglycaemia. *International Clinical Psychopharmacology* 2001; **16**: 63–74.
29. Zornberg GL, Jick H. Antipsychotic drug use and risk of first-time idiopathic venous thromboembolism: a case control study. *Lancet* 2000; **356**: 1219–1223.

Antipsychotics – equivalent doses

Antipsychotic drugs vary greatly in potency and this is usually expressed as differences in 'neuroleptic equivalents'. Most of the data relating to neuroleptic equivalents originate from early central dopamine binding studies (antipsychotic efficacy is, of course, undoubtedly far more complex than simple D_2 blockade), and atypical antipsychotics such as clozapine fare poorly in such comparative studies. *BNF* maximum doses for antipsychotic drugs bear little relationship to their 'neuroleptic equivalents'. Bearing these major limitations in mind and using the comparisons as a rough guide for the purpose of transferring a patient from one typical drug to another, followed by an early review, the table below represents the best guide from the information presently available[1,2].

Table Equivalent doses

Drug	Equivalent dose (consensus) (mg/day)	Range of values in literature (mg/day)
Chlorpromazine	100	–
Thioridazine	100	75–100
Fluphenazine	2	2–5
Trifluoperazine	5	2.5–5
Flupenthixol	3	2–3
Zuclopenthixol	25	25–60
Haloperidol	3	1.5–5
Sulpiride	200	200–270
Pimozide	2	2
Loxapine	10	10–25
Fluphenazine *depot*	5/week	1–12.5/week
Pipothiazine *depot*	10/week	10–12.5/week
Flupenthixol *depot*	10/week	10–20/week
Zuclopenthixol *depot*	100/week	40–100/week
Haloperidol *depot*	15/week	5–25/week

It is illogical to convert atypical antipsychotics into 'equivalents' and dosage guidelines are discussed under each individual drug. See pages 12–13 for further discussion.

References

1. Foster P. Neuroleptic equivalence. *Pharmaceutical Journal* 1989; **243**: 431–432.
2. Atkins M, Burgess A, Bottomley C *et al.* Chlorpromazine equivalents: a consensus of opinion for both clinical and research applications. *Psychiatric Bulletin* 1997; **21**: 224–226.

Antipsychotics – minimum effective doses

The table below suggests the minimum dose of antipsychotic likely to be effective in schizophrenia (first episode or relapse). At least some patients will respond to the dose suggested, although others may require higher doses. Given the variation in individual response, all doses should be considered approximate. Primary references are provided where available but consensus opinion has also been used (as have standard texts such as the *BNF* and *Summaries of Product Characteristics*). Only oral treatment with commonly used drugs is covered.

Table Minimum effective dose/day – antipsychotics

Drug	1st episode	Relapse	References
Chlorpromazine	200 mg*	300 mg	–
Haloperidol	2 mg	>4 mg	1–3
Sulpiride	400 mg*	800 mg	4
Trifluoperazine	10 mg*	15 mg	–
Amisulpride	400 mg*	800 mg	5–7
Aripiprazole	15 mg*	15 mg	8
Olanzapine	5 mg	10 mg	9–10
Quetiapine	150 mg*	300 mg	11–13
Risperidone	2 mg	4 mg	14–15
Ziprasidone	80 mg*	80 mg	16–17
Zotepine	75 mg*	150 mg	18–19

*Estimate – too few data available

References

1. Oosthuizen P, Emsley R, Turner J *et al.* Determining the optimal dose of haloperidol in first-episode psychosis. *Journal of Psychopharmacology* 2001; **15**: 251–255.
2. McGorry P. Recommended haloperidol and risperidone doses in first-episode psychosis. *Journal of Clinical Psychiatry* 1999; **60**: 794–795.
3. Waraich P, Adams C, Roque M, Hamill KM, Marti J. Haloperidol dose for the acute phase of schizophrenia (Cochrane Review). In: The Cochrane Library, Issue 4, 2002. Oxford: Update Software
4. Soares BGO, Fenton M, Chue P. Sulpiride for schizophrenia (Cochrane Review). In: The Cochrane Library, Issue 4, 2002. Oxford: Update Software.
5. Mota Neto JIS, Lima MS, Soares BGO. Amisulpiride for schizophrenia (Cochrane Review). In: The Cochrane Library, Issue 4, 2002. Oxford: Update Software.
6. Puech A, Fleurot O, Rein W. Amisulpride, an atypical antispsychotic, in the treatment of acute episodes of schizophrenia: a dose-ranging study vs. haloperidol. *Acta Psychiatrica Scandinavica* 1998; **98**: 65–72.
7. Moller H, Boyer P, Fleurot O *et al.* Improvement of acute exacerbations of schizophrenia with amisulpride: a comparison with haloperidol. *Psychopharmacology* 1997; **132**: 396–401.
8. Taylor D. Aripiprazole: a review of its pharmacology and clinical utility. *International Journal of Clinical Practice* 2003; **57**: 49–54.
9. Sanger T, Lieberman J, Tohen, M *et al.* Olanzapine versus haloperidol treatment in first-episode psychosis. *American Journal of Psychiatry* 1999; **156**: 79–87.
10. Kasper S. Risperidone and olanzapine: optimal dosing for efficacy and tolerability in patients with schizophrenia. *International Clinical Psychopharmacology* 1998; **13**: 253–262.
11. Small J, Hirsch S, Arvanitis L. Quetiapine in patients with schizophrenia. *Archives of General Psychiatry* 1997; **54**: 549–557
12. Peuskens J, Link C. A comparison of quetiapine and chlorpromazine in the treatment of schizophrenia. *Acta Psychiatrica Scandinavica* 1997; **96**: 265–273.

13. Arvantis LA, Miller BG. Multiple fixed doses of 'Seroquel' (quetiapine) in patients with acute exacerbation of schizophrenia: a comparison with haloperidol and placebo. The Seroquel Trial 13 Study Group. *Biological Psychiatry* 1997; **42**: 233–46.
14. Lane H-Y, Chiu W-C, Chou J *et al.* Risperidone in acutely exacerbated schizophrenia: dosing strategies and plasma levels. *Journal of Clinical Psychiatry* 2000; **61**: 209–214.
15. Williams R. Optimal dosing with risperidone: updated recommendations. *Journal of Clinical Psychiatry* 2001; **62**: 282–289.
16. Bagnall A-M, Lewis R, Leitner M. Ziprasidone for schizophrenia and severe mental illness (Cochrane Review). In: The Cochrane Library, Issue 4, 2002. Oxford: Update Software.
17. Taylor D. Ziprasidone – an atypical antipsychotic. *Pharmaceutical Journal* 2001; **266**: 396–401.
18. Petit M, Raniwalla J, Tweed J. A comparison of an atypical and typical antipsychotic, zotepine versus haloperidol, in patients with acute exacerbation of schizophrenia: a parallel-group double-blind trial. *Psychopharmacology Bulletin* 1996; **32**: 81–87.
19. Palmgren K, Wighton A, Reynolds C *et al.* The safety and efficacy of zotepine in the treatment of schizophrenia: results of a one-year naturalistic clinical trial. *International Journal of Psychiatry in Clinical Practice* 2000; **4**: 299–306.

Antipsychotics – licensed maximum doses

The table below lists the UK licensed maximum doses of antipsychotics.

Drug	Maximum dose (mg/day)
Chlorpromazine	1000
Thioridazine	600 (see *BNF*)
Fluphenazine	20
Trifluoperazine	None (suggest 50)
Flupentixol	18
Zuclopenthixol	150
Haloperidol	30 (see *BNF*)
Sulpiride	2400
Pimozide	20
Loxapine	250
Amisulpride	1200
Aripiprazole*	30
Clozapine	900
Risperidone	16
Olanzapine	20
Quetiapine	750
Ziprasidone*	160
Zotepine	450
Fluphenazine depot	50/week
Pipothiazine depot	50/week
Haloperidol depot	300 every 4 weeks
Flupenthixol depot	400/week
Zuclopenthixol depot	600/week

Note: Doses above these maxima should only be used in extreme circumstances: there is no evidence for improved efficacy.

* Not available in the UK at time of publication. US labelling used.

New antipsychotics – costs

Newer antipsychotics are relatively costly medicines, although their benefits may make them cost-effective in practice. Cost minimisation is a practical option that reduces drug expenditure without compromising patient care or patient quality of life. It involves using the right drug for the most appropriate condition (see Protocols) and using the minimum effective dose in each patient. The table below gives the cost (£/patient/30 days) as of March 2003 of atypicals at their estimated lowest effective dose, their approximate average clinical dose and their licensed maximum dose. The table allows comparison of different doses of the same drug and of different drugs at any of the three doses. It is hoped that the table will encourage the use of lower doses of less expensive drugs, given equality in other respects and allowing for clinical requirements.

Table Monthly costs of new antipsychotics

Drug	Minimum effective dose cost (see page 12)	Approximate average clinical dose cost	Maximum dose cost
Amisulpride	400 mg/day (depends on indication – see BNF) £66.00	800 mg/day £132.00	1200 mg/day £198.00
Olanzapine	10 mg/day £104.52	15 mg/day £156.78	20 mg/day £209.05
Risperidone (oral)	4 mg/day £77.22	6 mg/day £117.00	16 mg/day £308.80
Risperidone (injection)	25 mg/2 weeks £165.86	37.5 mg/2 weeks £231.68	50 mg/2 weeks £297.10
Quetiapine	300 mg/day £113.10	500 mg/day £169.65	750 mg/day £282.75
Zotepine	150 mg £50.62	300 mg/day £94.55	450 mg/day £145.18

Notes:
- Costs for UK adults (30 days) MIMS February 2003
- Average clinical doses are for inpatients receiving maintenance therapy
- Clozapine costs not included because it has different indications

Choice of antipsychotic

The *BNF* states 'the various antipsychotic drugs differ somewhat in predominant actions and side-effects. Selection is influenced by the degree of sedation required and the patient's susceptibility to EPSEs. However, the differences between antipsychotic drugs are less important than the greater variability in patient response'.

Phenothiazines

These are often divided into a further 3 subgroups, depending on their basic chemistry and, coincidentally, the degree of sedation they produce.

Chlorpromazine and **promazine** are the most sedative, and chlorpromazine the most widely prescribed phenothiazine. The pharmacology of chlorpromazine is complex but well documented. As well as the side-effects common to all antipsychotics, chlorpromazine causes photosensitivity reactions (hence the need for liberal amounts of high-factor sun screen and straw hats in the summer), and occasionally a hypersensitivity reaction resembling obstructive jaundice (the block being biochemical and not mechanical). Chlorpromazine is epileptogenic in a dose-dependent fashion and can cause significant weight gain. Promazine has a relatively good side-effect profile and so is suitable for the elderly, if it is sufficient to control symptoms. It is not effective in schizophrenia.

Thioridazine, pericyazine and **pipothiazine** are relatively less likely to produce EPSEs. Because of concerns over QTc prolongation[1], the product licence for thioridazine has been restricted to the second-line treatment of schizophrenia in patients who are under the direct care of a consultant psychiatrist[2]. There are further restrictions on its use in patients with cardiovascular disease or those receiving a wide range of other drugs[1]. It is essentially impossible to prescribe thioridazine within its product licence. Long-term therapy with high doses of thioridazine is not recommended because of its ability to cause pigmentary retinopathy. Pericyazine has achieved some success in curbing acts of spontaneous aggression/antisocial behaviour in younger people, most probably because of its potent sedative effect.

Fluphenazine and **trifluoperazine** are the least sedative phenothiazines but are more likely to cause EPSEs. Trifluoperazine is available as tablets and liquid and controlled-release capsules. There is little rationale in prescribing the more expensive controlled-release preparation, as sedation aside, most antipsychotics can be administered once-daily in their conventional form.

Butyrophenones

Haloperidol is the most widely prescribed drug in this group. It is a very potent D_2 blocker. It has been suggested that plasma levels of 5–12 µg/l are associated with optimal response and that such levels are achievable with daily doses of no more than 20 mg. Studies have shown that optimal response is achieved from daily doses of no more than 10 mg although much higher doses are commonly seen (and are associated with a high prevalence of EPSEs)[3]. Some studies suggest a non-linear relationship between dose and response, with a paradoxical response being possible when high doses are used. It has been suggested that the observed paradoxical response may be due to an increased incidence of EPSEs i.e. akathisia and akinesia being interpreted as increased agitation and an increase in negative symptoms, respectively. The *BNF* maximum dose for oral haloperidol has decreased from 120 mg to 15 mg/day (or 30 mg in treatment-resistant schizophrenia: September 2002 edition). **Droperidol** is no longer available in the UK (because of an association with QTc prolongation).

Thioxanthines

Flupentixol is the most widely prescribed member of this group and is used mostly in depot form. Low doses of flupentixol are claimed to have an antidepressant effect and, although there is a small hint (by no means proven) in some very old literature that this may be the case in psychosis, it is not a suitable treatment for depression in schizophrenia.

Diphenylbutylpiperidines

Pimozide is the only member of this group that is still prescribed. It is relatively specific for dopamine receptors and therefore has a narrower side-effect profile. It is claimed to be particularly useful in the treatment of monosymptomatic hypochondriacal psychoses (marketing hype originating from a small open case series – a very poor evidence base). In August 1990, the Committee on Safety of Medicines (CSM) reported that 13 reports of sudden unexpected death associated with the use of pimozide had been received, which led them to recommend a maximum daily dose of 20 mg, and also that anyone receiving more than 16 mg daily should have periodic ECGs carried out. The Committee go on to request reports of ventricular arrhythmias and sudden unexpected death associated with any antipsychotic[4].

Atypical antipsychotics

The term 'atypical' was originally associated with the inability of a compound to produce catalepsy in laboratory animals (a screening model thought to have good predictive validity in identifying potential antipsychotic agents). Atypical antipsychotics were also defined as having no effect on serum prolactin. More recently, the term has been used to describe antipsychotics that are highly selective D_2 blockers, those that are relatively selective for D_2 receptors in mesolimbic areas, those that have a high $5HT_2:D_2$ receptor blocking ratio and those that are claimed to have an effect on negative symptomatology. The definition of this term is likely to become even more confused in the future, should any of the more novel compounds presently being developed reach the market (dopamine partial and autoreceptor agonists, NMDA agonists, $5HT_3$ antagonists, sigma antagonists, etc.). Atypical antipsychotics do cause fewer EPSEs than most of the older drugs, but are not devoid of other side-effects. These effects are discussed for individual drugs below.

Clozapine

Clozapine is the archetypal atypical antipsychotic. Clozapine has been around since the 1960s and was withdrawn from use after an association with neutropenia (incidence 3%) and agranulocytosis (0.8%) was made. The pivotal study by Kane *et al.*[5] in the late 1980s proved that clozapine was more effective than conventional antipsychotics and it was reintroduced in the UK with compulsory haematological monitoring. Patients must be registered with the CPMS and have a full blood count performed weekly for the first 18 weeks (when the risk of neutropenia/agranulocytosis is greatest)[6], fortnightly until 52 weeks of treatment, and then monthly thereafter if haematologically stable (the incidence of agranulocytosis after one year is similar to that associated with the phenothiazines[6]). Studies have shown that 30% of patients who have previously been refractory to treatment improve significantly after 6 weeks' treatment with clozapine, and up to 60% respond after 1 year. Local experience has shown that even patients who have not been identified as 'responders' by staff feel subjectively better on clozapine and that levels of aggression and violence in this population have fallen[7]. Clozapine is perhaps most useful in patients who are actively and floridly psychotic. Although claims are made for its efficacy in negative symptomatology, clinical gains in this area are much less marked[8,9]. Clozapine treatment has been linked to a reduction in suicidality[10], although this has been disputed[11]. (See page 52.)

The pharmacology of clozapine is unusual compared with other antipsychotics in that it only binds weakly to D_1 and D_2 receptors, while having an affinity for D_4, $5HT_2$, $5HT_3$, α_1 and α_2 adrenergic, ACh M_1 and H_1 receptors. Which one/combination if any of these effects is responsible for the superior clinical profile of clozapine is a subject of extensive speculation, but as of yet, no firm conclusion.

Clozapine also has a unique side-effect profile in that it has been associated with an extremely low incidence of EPSEs, and is thought not to cause/precipitate TD (it has even been suggested that clozapine can be an effective treatment for existing TD – see page 68. Clozapine does not raise prolactin levels and so is not associated with amenorrhoea. Menstruation will return and effective contraception is essential in sexually active females.

Clozapine is associated with a greater incidence of seizures than other antipsychotics and this is probably related to high plasma levels in susceptible individuals. The incidence of seizures increases markedly at doses of 600 mg/day or above and is probably related to plasma level. Grand mal seizures may be prevented with sodium valproate.

Clozapine also has other troublesome side-effects in that sialorrhoea can be a significant problem. The mechanism of this effect is not completely understood – it has been suggested that it is mediated through cholinergic, adrenergic and 5HT pathways. It is best dealt with practically (by encouraging the patient to sleep with their head propped up on several pillows or with a towel over their pillow). Several pharmacological strategies have been tried such as anticholinergics (procyclidine, hyoscine, pirenzepine, atropine), amitriptyline, propranolol, clonidine and desmopressin[12]. All of these approaches are associated with their own side-effects, both physical and psychiatric, and should be tried with caution. See page 54 for further details.

Raised body temperature can also be a problem in the early days of clozapine treatment. Although this problem is described in the literature as benign hyperthermia, temperatures of over 40°C have been described. Unless the temperature becomes very elevated (above 38.5°C with paracetamol cover), there is no reason for stopping clozapine, as this effect is transient (it must, of course, be differentiated from fever secondary to neutropenia). Fever may also be associated with myocarditis (see page 50).

Clozapine has also been linked to the development of hypersensitivity myocarditis[13] (risk estimated to be increased 1000-fold in the first month of treatment) and cardiomyopathy[13] (risk estimated to be increased 5-fold). It is unclear at present whether this risk is higher than that associated with other antipsychotics. See page 50 for further information about the side-effects of clozapine and how to manage them.

A therapeutic range may exist for clozapine where serum concentrations of >350 µg/l are required for efficacy. There are many limitations to these data and serum levels should be interpreted with caution[14]. See page 4 for further discussion and guidelines.

A 'withdrawal syndrome' has been described when clozapine treatment is withdrawn abruptly[15] (as it must be when the blood profile dictates). Whether this represents rapid return of the original psychopathology, supersensitivity psychosis, a true withdrawal syndrome, or a mixture of all three is unclear.

Other atypical antipsychotics[16]

The other 'atypical antipsychotics', sulpiride, amisulpride, risperidone, sertindole, olanzapine, quetiapine, ziprasidone and zotepine have not been proven to be effective in treating resistant illness. They are advocated as better tolerated first-line treatments[17].

Sulpiride was arguably the first member of this group to be marketed. Conventional antipsychotics are all effective in treating positive symptoms (i.e. formal thought disorder, passivity feelings, delusions and hallucinations) and, given prophylactically, they substantially reduce the relapse rate for many patients (see page 42). None of these compounds however, directly or significantly, improves the manifestations of negative symptomatology (i.e. anergia, apathy, flattening of affect and poverty of speech), all of which are a major cause of long-term deterioration, withdrawal and isolation amongst patients with schizophrenia.

Sulpiride was the first antipsychotic for which claims were made regarding its effect upon negative symptomatology (although it must be noted that this effect is not striking). It has a dose-related selectivity for pre-synaptic D_4 and post-synaptic D_2 receptors. In low doses (less than 800 mg/day) the main affinity is for D_4 receptors, which are auto-inhibitory. The inhibitory control of dopamine release is therefore decreased and more dopamine is available in the synaptic cleft. Above 800 mg/day the affinity for D_2 receptors dominates, resulting in the postsynaptic blockade of D_2 receptors. Sulpiride is associated with fewer EPSEs than the older drugs and, as such, may also be associated with less potential for causing TD.

Amisulpride is similar to sulpiride in that lower doses (300 mg/day or less) selectively block presynaptic dopamine receptors, leading to an increase in dopamine transmission in the prefrontal cortex (the site supposedly responsible for the genesis of negative symptoms). At higher doses, it blocks postsynaptic dopamine receptors and is relatively selective for limbic rather than striatal areas, which translates clinically into a low potential for EPSEs. Amisulpride is relatively free from sedation, anticholinergic side-effects and postural hypotension, but, like sulpiride, is a particularly potent elevator of serum prolactin. The difference clinically between amisulpride and sulpiride is unclear. Amisulpride is significantly more expensive.

Risperidone is a potent $5HT_2$:D_2 antagonist. It was developed in line with the observation that ritanserin (a potent $5HT_2$ receptor antagonist), when given in combination with conventional antipsychotics, was effective in treating the negative and affective symptoms of schizophrenia[18]. In doses of 6 mg or less per day, risperidone is associated with a low incidence of EPSEs and sedation. It is associated with hyperprolactinaemia. Risperidone has a first-dose hypotensive effect (due to α_1 blockade), and in order to minimise this, an increasing-dosage regime is used over the first few days. There have been reports of nausea, dyspepsia, abdominal pain, dyspnoea and chest pain associated with its use.

Prescribing surveys have shown that risperidone was and is frequently prescribed in both doses greater than 8 mg/day (so that EPSE are produced), and in combination with other antipsychotics (where treatment resistance is the real issue)[19]. This is illogical.

Sertindole is also associated with significant α_1 blockade and therefore dosage titration is required. Its major advantages are that it produces virtually no EPSEs within the licensed dosage range and has no effect on prolactin. Its major disadvantage is that it is associated with QTc prolongation and it is recommended that an ECG is obtained before initiating therapy. (A recent survey of junior doctors in psychiatry demonstrated that less than 20% were able to identify a prolonged QTc interval on an ECG[20].) Sertindole has been tentatively linked with a number of cases of 'antipsychotic-associated sudden death'[21], and in November 1998 its licence was suspended by several European countries. Sertindole was subsequently voluntarily withdrawn from general use by the manufacturers, but has now been reintroduced, following studies demonstrating its apparent safety.

Olanzapine is also a $5HT_2$:D_2 blocker. It is sedative, produces some postural hypotension and has anticholinergic side-effects. Although chemically and pharmacologically very similar to clozapine, olanzapine has been licensed as a first-line antipsychotic and there is currently no compelling evidence to support its efficacy in treatment-resistant illness. Olanzapine has minimal effects on serum prolactin and may be associated with a lower incidence of sexual dysfunction than other antipsychotics. Clinical trials have shown that 10–20 mg olanzapine/day is the most effective dose. Because it is so well tolerated, prescribers may feel tempted to increase the dose above 20 mg (the licensed maximum) in partial or non-responders. There is little objective evidence to support this treatment strategy and it cannot currently be recommended. Such patients would be more appropriately treated with clozapine. Olanzapine serum levels can be measured and this may be useful when non-compliance is suspected. A blood sample taken at 12 or 24 hours after the last dose is required (see page 5). The majority of patients who take 10–20 mg of olanzapine daily will have a serum level of 10–23 µg/l. It must be emphasised that this is a guide to compliance only and is not a proven therapeutic range. Olanzapine is expected to be available as an aqueous IM injection. See pages 3–6 for further guidance on plasma level monitoring.

Quetiapine has a low affinity for D_1, D_2 and $5HT_2$ receptors and moderate affinity for adrenergic α_1 and α_2 receptors. It is relatively mesolimbic-specific and does not raise serum prolactin; however, it does require dosage titration (like risperidone and sertindole). There are very few data to suggest that it may be effective in treatment-resistant illness. The published efficacy data for quetiapine have been said to be relatively poor compared with the other atypicals. This mainly relates to the high drop-out rates reported in short-term trials[22]. Quetiapine has been associated with the development of cataracts in laboratory animals. There are also some reports in humans[22] but a direct causal relationship has not been firmly established. Quetiapine has also been associated with raised plasma lipids; (this is true for clozapine and olanzapine as well – there are fewer data for the other atypical antipsychotics).

Zotepine is an antagonist at $5HT_{2a}$, $5HT_{2c}$, D_1, D_2, D_3 and D_4 receptors, a potent inhibitor of noradrenaline reuptake, a potent H_1 antagonist (sedative), with some α_1 adrenergic blocking activity (postural hypotension) and possibly some activity at NMDA receptors. It raises serum prolactin and is associated with a high incidence of seizures. Doses above 300 mg/day (frequently used according to the available literature) and antipsychotic polypharmacy increase this risk. There are very few trial data comparing zotepine with other atypical antipsychotics. There is no study of any quality in refractory illness reported in the English language literature.

References

1. Reilly JG, Ayis SA, Ferrier IN *et al.* QTc-interval abnormalities and psychotropic drug therapy in psychiatric patients. *Lancet* 2000; 355: 1048–1052.
2. Melleril SPC. Datasheet compendium, 2002.
3. Hilton T, Taylor D, Abel K. Which dose of haloperidol? *Psychiatric Bulletin* 1996; 20: 359–362.
4. Committee on Safety of Medicines. Cardiotoxic effects of pimozide. *Current Problems* 1990; 29: 1.
5. Kane J, Honifeld G, Singer J *et al.* Clozapine for the treatment resistant schizophrenic. *Archives of General Psychiatry* 1988; 45: 789–796.
6. Atkin F, Kendall F, Gould D *et al.* Neutropenia and angranulocytosis in patients receiving clozapine in the UK and Ireland. *British Journal of Psychiatry* 1996; 169: 483–488.
7. Wolfson PM, Paton C. Clozapine audit: what do patients and relatives think? *Journal of Mental Health* 1996; 5: 267–273.
8. Rosenheck R, Dunn L, Peszke M *et al.* Impact of clozapine on negative symptoms and on the deficit syndrome in refractory schizophrenia. *American Journal of Psychiatry* 1996; 156: 88–93.
9. Breier AF, Malhotra AK, Su T *et al.* Clozapine and risperidone in chronic schizophrenia: effects on symptoms, parkinsonian side effects and neuroendocrine response. *American Journal of Psychiatry* 1999; 156: 294–298.
10. Meltzer HY, Okayli G. Reduction of suicidality during clozapine treatment of neuroleptic resistant schizophrenia: impact on risk-benefit assessment. *American Journal of Psychiatry* 1995; 152: 183–190.
11. Sernyak MJ, Desia R, Stolar M *et al.* Impact of clozapine on completed suicide. *American Journal of Psychiatry* 2001; 158: 931–937.
12. Cree A, Mir S, Fahy T. A review of the treatment options for clozapine-induced hypersalivation. *Psychiatric Bulletin* 2001; 25: 114–116.
13. Killan JG, Kerr K, Lawrence C *et al.* Myocarditis and cardiomyopathy associated with clozapine. *Lancet* 1999; 354: 1841–1845.
14. Taylor D, Duncan D. The use of clozapine plasma levels in optimising therapy. *Psychiatric Bulletin* 1995; 19: 753–755.
15. Ekblom B, Eriksson K, Lindstrom LH. Supersensitivity psychosis in schizophrenic patients after sudden clozapine withdrawal. *Psychopharmacology* 1984; 83: 293–294.
16. Leysen JE, Janssen PMF, Heylen L *et al.* Receptor interactions of new antipsychotics: relation to pharmacodynamic and clinical effects. *International Journal of Psychiatry in Clinical Practice* 1998; 2(Suppl.1): 3–17.
17. Taylor DM, Duncan-McConnell D. Refractory schizophrenia and atypical antipsychotics. *Journal of Psychopharmacology* 2000; 14: 409–418.
18. Duinkerke SJ, Botter PA, Jansen AA. Ritanserin, a selective 5HT2/1C antagonist, and negative symptoms in schizophrenia. *British Journal of Psychiatry* 1993; 164: 451–455.
19. Taylor D, Holmes R, Hilton T *et al.* Evaluating and improving the quality of risperidone prescribing. *Psychiatric Bulletin* 1997; 21: 680–683.
20. Warner JP, Gledhill JA, Connell F *et al.* How well do psychiatric trainees interpret electrocardiographs? *Psychiatric Bulletin* 1996; 20: 651–652.
21. Pritze J, Bandelow B. The QT interval and the atypical antipsychotic sertindole. *International Journal of Psychiatry in Clinical Practice* 1998; 2: 265–273.
22. Srisurapsanont M, Disayavanish C, Taimkaewk K. Quetiapine for schizophrenia (Cochrane review). In: The Cochrane Library, Issue 3. Oxford: Update Software, 2000.
23. Valibhai F, Phan NB, Still DJ. Cataracts and quetiapine. *American Journal of Psychiatry* 2001; 158: 966.

Newer antipsychotics

Ziprasidone

Ziprasidone has been available in the USA and some European countries for several years. It is a D_2:5HT$_2$ antagonist with significant agonist activity at 5HT$_{1A}$ receptors and moderately potent inhibition of monoamine reuptake[1,2]. Efficacy is similar to haloperidol[3] and tolerability is good; most adverse effects occur at the same frequency as placebo and EPSEs, hyperprolactinaemia and weight gain are uncommon[4,5]. More recent studies suggest that ziprasidone is more effective in the treatment of negative symptoms than haloperidol[6] and as effective as amisulpride[7]. Ziprasidone has a moderate effect on the QT interval which may, at least in theory, make it relatively more likely than other antipsychotics to cause ventricular arrhythmia (see page 75)[8]. This potential problem should be set against the clear advantages of ziprasidone in relation to weight gain[9] and impaired glucose tolerance[10].

References

1. Taylor D. Ziprasidone – an atypical antipsychotic. *Pharmaceutical Journal* 2001; **266**: 396–401.
2. Davis R, Markham A. Ziprasidone. *CNS Drugs* 1997; **8**: 153–159.
3. Goff D C, Posever T, Herz L *et al.* An exploratory haloperidol-controlled dose-finding study of ziprasidone in hospitalized patients with schizophrenia or schizoaffective disorder. *Journal of Clinical Pyschopharmacology* 1998; **18**: 296–304.
4. Keck P, Buffenstein A, Ferguson J *et al.* Ziprasidone 40 and 120 mg/day in the acute exacerbation of schizophrenia and schizoaffective disorder: a 4-week placebo-controlled trial. *Pyschopharmacology* 1998; **140**: 173–184.
5. Keck P, Reeves K, Harrigan E. Ziprasidone in the short-term treatment of patients with schizoaffective disorder: results from two double-blind, placebo-controlled, multicenter studies. *Journal of Clinical Psychopharmacology* 2001; **21**: 27–35.
6. Hirsch S, Werner K, Bauml J *et al.* A 28-week comparison of Ziprasidone and Haloperidol in outpatients with stable schizophrenia. *Journal of Clinical Psychiatry* 2002; **63**: 6 516–522.
7. Olie J-P, Spina E, Benattia I. Ziprasidone vs amisulpride for negative symptoms of schizophrenia. Poster presented at ECNP annual conference. Barcelona, Spain October 2002.
8. Taylor D. Ziprasidone in the management of schizophrenia: the QT interval issue in context. *CNS Drugs* 2003; **17**(6): 423–430.
9. Taylor DM, McAskill R. Atypical antipsychotics and weight gain – a systematic review. *Acta Psychiatrica Scandinavica* 2000; **101**: 416–432.
10. Kingsbury SJ, Fayek M, Trufasiu D *et al.* The apparent effects of ziprasidone on plasma lipids and glucose. *Journal of Clinical Psychiatry* 2001; **62**: 347–349.

Aripiprazole

Aripiprazole is a partial agonist at D_2 receptors: full binding to D_2 receptors reduces dopaminergic neuronal activity by about 30% (in the absence of dopamine, aripiprazole acts as a weak agonist)[1]. It is a potent antagonist at 5HT$_{2A}$ receptors and a partial agonist at 5HT$_{1A}$ receptors[2].

Aripiprazole appears to be at least as effective as haloperidol[3] and risperidone[4] and is well tolerated with a low incidence (placebo level) of extrapyramidal symptoms[5]. It seems not to be associated with symptomatic hyperprolactinaemia, QTc prolongation, impaired glucose tolerance or substantial weight gain[6–9]. More published data are awaited.

References

1. Burris KD, Molski TF, Ryan E *et al.* Aripiprazole is a high affinity partial agonist at human D_2 dopamine receptors. *International Journal of Neuropsychopharmacology* 2000; **3**(Suppl. 1): S129.
2. Jordan S, Koprivica V, Chen R *et al.* The antipsychotic aripiprazole is a potent, partial agonist at the human 5HT$_{1A}$ receptor. *European Journal of Pharmacology* 2002; **441**: 137–140.
3. Kane JM, Carson WH, Saha AR *et al.* Efficacy and safety of aripiprazole and haloperidol versus placebo in patients with schizophrenia and schizoaffective disorder. *Journal of Clinical Psychiatry* 2002; **63**: 763–771.
4. Saha AR, Carson WH, Ali MW *et al.* Efficacy and safety of aripiprazole and risperidone vs placebo in patients with schizophrenia and schizoaffective disorder. *Journal of Biological Psychiatry* 2(Suppl. 1): 305S.

5. Petrie JL, Saha AR, McEvoy JP. Aripiprazole, a new atypical antipsychotic: phase 2 clinical trial results. *European Neuropsychopharmacology* 2002; 7(Suppl. 1): S157.
6. Pigott TA, Saha AR, Ali MW *et al.* Aripiprazole vs placebo in the treatment of stable, chronic schizophrenia. Poster presented at American Psychiatric Association 155th Annual meeting 2002 May 18–23rd, Philadelphia, PA, USA.
7. Stock E, Marder SR, Saha AR *et al.* Safety and tolerability meta-analysis of aripiprazole in schizophrenia. *International Journal of Neuropsychopharmacology* 2002; 5(Suppl. 1): S185.
8. Jody D, Saha AR, Iwamoto T *et al.* Meta-analysis of weight effects with aripiprazole. Poster presented at American Psychiatric Association 155th Annual Meeting 2002 May 18–23 Philadelphia, PA, USA.
9. Data on file, BMS.

Further reading

Taylor DM. Aripiprazole: A review of its pharmacology and clinical use. *International Journal of Clinical Practice* 2003; 57: 49–53.

Antipsychotics – general principles of prescribing

- The **lowest possible dose** should be used. For each patient, the dose should be titrated to the lowest known to be effective; dose increases should then only take place after two weeks of assessment during which the patient is clearly showing poor or no response. With depot medication, plasma levels rise for 6–12 weeks after initiation, even without a change in dose. Dose increases during this time are therefore inappropriate (see page 35).

- For the large majority of patients, the use of a **single antipsychotic** (with or without additional mood stabiliser or sedatives) is recommended (see page 40).

- **Polypharmacy** of antipsychotics should only be undertaken where response to a single antipsychotic (including clozapine) has been clearly demonstrated to be inadequate. In such cases, the effect of polypharmacy should be carefully evaluated and documented. Where there is no clear benefit, treatment should revert to single antipsychotic therapy (see page 40).

- In general, **antipsychotics should not be used as 'PRN' sedatives**. Short courses of benzodiazepines or general sedatives (e.g. promethazine) are recommended.

- Responses to antipsychotic drug treatment should be **assessed using recognised rating scales** and be documented in patients' records.

Atypical antipsychotics – summary of NICE guidance[1]

- Choice of antipsychotic should be made jointly by the prescriber and the (properly informed) patient and/or carer.

- When consultation with the patient is not possible and where there is no advance directive, an atypical drug should be used. The patient's carer or advocate should be consulted whenever possible.

- Atypical drugs should be considered in the choice of first-line treatments.

- Atypical drugs should be considered for patients showing or reporting unacceptable adverse effects caused by typical agents (see page 27).

- Patients unresponsive to two different antipsychotics (one an atypical) should be given clozapine.

- Depot medication should be used where there are grounds to suspect that a patient may be unlikely to adhere to prescribed oral therapy.

- Where more than one atypical is appropriate, the drug with the lowest purchase cost should be prescribed.

- 'Advance directives' regarding patients' preference for treatment should be developed and documented.

- Drug treatment should be considered only part of a comprehensive package of care.

- Atypical and typical antipsychotics should not be prescribed together except during changeover of medication.

---

1. National Institute of Clinical Excellence. Health Technology Appraisal No. 43 NICE, London, 2002.

1ˢᵗ episode schizophrenia

Treatment algorithm

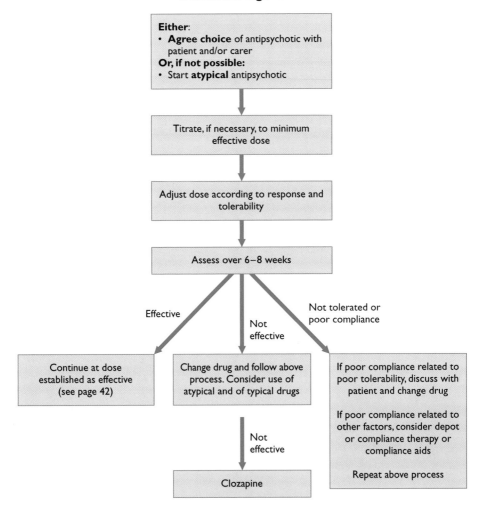

Either:
- **Agree choice** of antipsychotic with patient and/or carer

Or, if not possible:
- Start **atypical** antipsychotic

Titrate, if necessary, to minimum effective dose

Adjust dose according to response and tolerability

Assess over 6–8 weeks

Effective

Not effective

Not tolerated or poor compliance

Continue at dose established as effective (see page 42)

Change drug and follow above process. Consider use of atypical and of typical drugs

If poor compliance related to poor tolerability, discuss with patient and change drug

If poor compliance related to other factors, consider depot or compliance therapy or compliance aids

Not effective

Clozapine

Repeat above process

Relapse or acute exacerbation of schizophrenia

(full adherence to medication confirmed)

Treatment algorithm

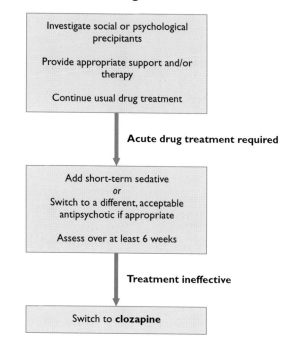

Investigate social or psychological precipitants

Provide appropriate support and/or therapy

Continue usual drug treatment

Acute drug treatment required

Add short-term sedative
or
Switch to a different, acceptable antipsychotic if appropriate

Assess over at least 6 weeks

Treatment ineffective

Switch to **clozapine**

Relapse or acute exacerbation of schizophrenia

(adherence doubtful or known to be poor)

Treatment algorithm

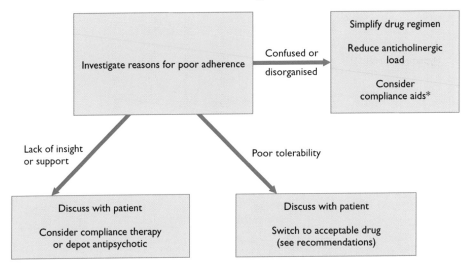

Investigate reasons for poor adherence

Confused or disorganised →

Simplify drug regimen

Reduce anticholinergic load

Consider compliance aids*

Lack of insight or support

Poor tolerability

Discuss with patient

Consider compliance therapy or depot antipsychotic

Discuss with patient

Switch to acceptable drug (see recommendations)

* Compliance aids (e.g. Medidose system) are not a substitute for patient education. The ultimate aim should be to promote independent living, perhaps with the patient filling their own compliance aid, having first been given support and training. Note that such compliance aids are of little use unless the patient is clearly motivated to adhere to prescribed treatment. Note also that some medicines are not suitable for storage in compliance aids.

Switching antipsychotics because of poor tolerability – recommendations

Adverse effect	Suggested drugs	Alternatives	References
Acute EPSEs	Quetiapine Olanzapine Clozapine	Risperidone (<6 mg/day) Sertindole Ziprasidone Aripiprazole	1–5
Hyperprolactinaemia	Quetiapine Olanzapine (small, transient rise in prolactin[6], although symptoms rarely observed[7]) Clozapine	Ziprasidone Aripiprazole Sertindole	8–11
Weight gain	Amisulpride Haloperidol Trifluoperazine	Quetiapine Ziprasidone Aripiprazole	12–15
Tardive dyskinesia	Clozapine	Olanzapine Quetiapine Risperidone (<6 mg/day)	16–19
Impaired glucose tolerance	Amisulpride Risperidone	Ziprasidone Aripiprazole	20–22
QT prolongation	Olanzapine	Amisulpride Aripiprazole	23–24
Sedation	Amisulpride Risperidone Sulpiride Haloperidol	Aripiprazole	–
Postural hypotension	Amisulpride Sulpiride Haloperidol Trifluoperazine	Aripiprazole	–

Note: Experience with ziprasidone and aripiprazole is limited; neither drug licensed in the UK at time of going to press. See page 20.

References

1. Stanniland C, Taylor D. Tolerability of atypical antipsychotics. *Drug Safety* 2000; **22**: 195–214.
2. Daniel T, Baldessarini RJ, Tarazi FI. Effects of newer antipsychotics on extrapyramidal function. *CNS Drugs* 2002; **16**(1): 23–45.
3. Caroff SN, Mann SC, Campbell EC *et al.* Movement disorders associated with atypical antipsychotic drugs. *Journal of Clinical Psychiatry* 2002; **63**(4): 12–19.
4. Lemmens P, Brecher M, Van Baelen B. A combined analysis of double-blind studies with risperidone vs. placebo and other antipsychotic agents: factors associated with extrapyramidal symptoms. *Acta Psychiatrica Scandinavica* 1999; **99**: 160–170.
5. Nyberg S, Olsson H, Nilsson U *et al.* Low striatal and extra-striatal D$_2$ receptor occupancy during treatment with the atypical antipsychotic sertindole. *Psychopharmacology* 2002; **162**: 37–41.

6. Crawford AM, Beasley C, Tollefson GD. The acute and long-term effect of olanzapine compared with placebo and haloperidol on serum prolactin concentrations. *Schizophrenia Research* 1997; **26**: 41–54.
7. Licht R, Arngrim T, Christensen H. Olanzapine-induced galactorrhea. *Psychopharmacology* 2002; **162**: 94–95.
8. Turrone P, Kapur S, Seeman M *et al*. Elevation of prolactin levels by atypical antipsychotics. *American Journal Psychiatry* 2002; **159**: 133–135.
9. David S, Taylor C, Kinon B *et al*. The effects of olanzapine, risperidone and haloperidol on plasma prolactin levels in patients with schizophrenia. *Clinical Therapeutics* 2000; **22**(9): 1085–1095.
10. Hammer MB, Arana GW. Hyperprolactinaemia in antipsychotic-treated patients: guidelines for avoidance and management. *CNS Drugs* 1998; **10**: 209–222.
11. Rapid reduction in hyperprolactinemia upon switching treatment to olanzapine from conventional antipsychotic drugs or risperidone. Poster presented at American Psychiatric Association annual meeting, May 2000, Chicago, Illinois.
12. Taylor DM, McAskill R. Atypical antipsychotics and weight gain – a systemic review. *Acta Psychiatrica Scandinavica* 2000; **101**: 416–432.
13. Allison D, Mentore J, Moonseong H *et al*. Antipsychotic-induced weight gain: A comprehensive research synthesis. *American Journal of Psychiatry* 1999; **156**: 1686–1696.
14. Brecher M, Rak I, Melvin R *et al*. The long-term effect of quetiapine (Seroquel) monotherapy on weight in patients with schizophrenia. *International Journal of Psychiatry in Clinical Practice* 2000; **4**: 287–291.
15. Gibert J, Leal C, Bovio H *et al*. Switching to quetiapine in schizophrenic patients with antipsychotic-induced weight gain. Presented at the 15th European College of Neuropsychopharmacology Congress. October 5–9, 2002, Barcelona, Spain.
16. Lieberman J, Johns C, Cooper T *et al*. Clozapine pharmacology and tardive dyskinesia. *Psychopharmacology* 1989; **99**: S54–S59.
17. O'Brien J, Barber R. Marked improvement in tardive dyskinesia following treatment with olanzapine in an elderly subject. *British Journal Psychiatry* 1998; **172**: 186.
18. Kinon BJ, Milton DR, Stauffer VL *et al*. Effect of chronic olanzapine treatment on the course of presumptive tardive dyskinesia. Poster presented at American Psychiatric Association 152nd Annual Meeting, May 1999, Washington, DC.
19. Llorca P-M, Chereau I, Bayle F-J *et al*. Tardive dyskinesias and antipsychotics: a review. *European Psychiatry* 2002; **17**: 129–38.
20. Berry S, Mahmoud R. Normalization of olanzapine-associated abnormalities of insulin resistance and insulin release after switch to risperidone: the risperidone rescue study. Poster presented at the European College of Neuropsychopharmacology 15th Annual Meeting October 5–9, 2002, Barcelona, Spain.
21. Gianfrancesco F, Grogg A, Mahmoud R *et al*. Differential effects of risperidone, olanzapine, clozapine, and conventional antipsychotics on type 2 diabetes: findings from a large health plan database. *Journal of Clinical Psychiatry* 2002; **63**: 920–930.
22. Mir S, Taylor D. Atypical antipsychotics and hyperglycaemia. *International Clinical Psychopharmacology* 2001; **16**: 63–73.
23. Glassman A, Bigger J. Antipsychotic drugs: prolonged QTc interval, torsade de pointes, and sudden death. *American Journal of Psychiatry* **158**:1774–1782.
24. Taylor D. Antipsychotics and QT prolongation. *Acta Psychiatrica Scandinavica* 2003; **107**(2): 85–95.

Further reading

Van Harten PN, Hoek HW, Kahn RS. Acute dystonia induced by drug treatment. *BMJ* 1999; **319**: 623–626.

Slovenko R (2000). Update on legal issues associated with tardive dyskinesia. *Journal of Clinical Psychiatry* 1999; **61**(Suppl. 4): 45–57.

Devlin MJ, Yanovski SZ, Wilson GT. Obesity: what mental health professionals need to know. *American Journal of Psychiatry* 2000; **157**: 854–866.

National Institute of Clinical Effectiveness. Guidance on the use of newer (atypical) antipsychotic drugs for the treatment of schizophrenia. Health Technology Appraisal No. 43, NICE, London, 2002.

Typical antipsychotics – clinical utility

Typical and atypical antipsychotics are not categorically delineated. Typical drugs are those which can be expected to give rise to acute EPSEs, hyperprolactinaemia and, in the longer term, to tardive dyskinesia. Atypicals, by any sensible definition, might be expected not to be associated with these adverse effects. However, some atypicals show dose-related EPSEs, some induce hyperprolactinaemia and some may eventually give rise to tardive dyskinesia. To complicate matters further, it has been suggested that the therapeutic and adverse effects of typical drugs can be separated by careful dosing[1] – thus making typical drugs atypical (there is much evidence to the contrary, incidentally[2-4]).

Given these observations, it seems unwise to consider so-called typical and atypical drugs as distinct groups of drugs. The essential difference between the two is the therapeutic index in relation to acute EPSEs; for instance, haloperidol has an extremely narrow index (probably substantially less than 0.5 mg/day); olanzapine a wide index (20–40 mg/day).

Typical drugs still play an important role in schizophrenia and offer a valid alternative to atypicals where atypicals are poorly tolerated. Their main drawbacks are, of course, acute EPSEs (see page 62), hyperprolactinaemia and tardive dyskinesia. Hyperprolactinaemia is probably unavoidable in practice and, even when not symptomatic, may grossly affect hypothalamic function[5]. It is firmly associated with sexual dysfunction[6] but be aware that the autonomic effects of some atypicals may also cause sexual dysfunction[7].

Tardive dyskinesia probably occurs more frequently with typicals than atypicals[8,9] (not withstanding difficulties in defining what is atypical), although this is far from certain[10]. Careful observation of patients and the prescribing of the lowest effective dose are essential to help reduce risk of this serious adverse event[11,12].

References

1. Oosthuizen P, Emsley R, Turner J et al. Determining the optimal dose of haloperidol in first-episode psychosis. Journal of Psychopharmacology 2001; 154: 251–255.
2. Zimbroff DL, Kane JM, Tamminga CA et al. Controlled, dose-response study of sertindole and haloperidol in the treatment of schizophrenia. American Journal of Psychiatry 1997; 154: 783–791.
3. Jeste DV, Lacro JP, Palmer B et al. Incidence of tardive dyskinesia in early stages of low-dose treatment with typical neuroleptics in older patients. American Journal of Psychiatry 1999; 156: 309–311.
4. Meltzer HY, Fang VS. The effect of neuroleptics on serum prolactin in schizophrenia patients. Archives of General Psychiatry 1976; 33: 279–286.
5. Smith S, Wheeler M, Murray R et al. The effects of antipsychotic-induced hyperprolactinaemia on the hypothalamic-pituitary-gonadal axis. Journal of Clinical Psychopharmacology 2001; 22: 109–114.
6. Smith S, O'Keane V, Murray R. Sexual dysfunction in patients taking conventional antipsychotic medication. British Journal of Psychiatry 2002; 181: 49–55.
7. Aizenberg D, Modai I, Landa A et al. Comparison of sexual dysfunction in male schizophrenia patients maintained on treatment with classical antipsychotics versus clozapine. Journal of Clinical Psychiatry 2001; 62: 541–544.
8. Tollefson G, Beasley C, Tamura R et al. Double-blind, controlled, long-term study of the comparative incidence of treatment-emergent tardive dyskinesia with olanzapine or haloperidol. American Journal of Psychiatry 1997; 154: 1248–1254.
9. Beasley C, Dellva M, Tamura R et al. Randomised double-blind comparison of the incidence of tardive dyskinesia in patients with schizophrenia during long-term treatment with olanzapine or haloperidol. British Journal of Psychiatry 1999; 174: 23–30.
10. Halliday J, Farrington S, Macdonald S et al. Nithsdale schizophrenia surveys 23: movement disorders. British Journal of Psychiatry 2002; 181: 422–427.
11. Jeste D, Caligiuri M. Tardive dyskinesia. Schizophrenia Bulletin 1993; 19: 303–315.
12. Cavallaro R, Smeraldi E. Antipsychotic-induced tardive dyskinesia: recognition, prevention and management. CNS Drugs 1995; 4: 278–293.

New antipsychotics – recommended monitoring

Table			
Drug	**Obligatory monitoring**		**Suggested**
	Baseline	**Continuation**	**Baseline**
Amisulpride	None	None	Prolactin U&Es Weight
Clozapine	FBC Prescriber and pharmacist must register	FBC – weekly for 18 wks – at least every 2 wks for 1 year – monthly thereafter	HbA$_{1C}$ BP ECG (optional) LFTs U&Es Weight
Olanzapine	None	None	HbA$_{1C}$ BP FBC LFTs U&Es Prolactin Weight
Quetiapine	None	None	HbA$_{1C}$ BP LFTs TFTs U&Es Weight
Risperidone	None	None	HbA$_{1C}$ BP LFTs Prolactin U&Es Weight

additional monitoring		Actions
	Continuation	
Prolactin	– if symptoms occur	Stop if prolactin-related effects intolerable
U&Es	– 6 monthly	
Weight	– as needed	
CPK	– if NMS suspected	Stop if NMS suspected
HbA$_{1C}$ [1,2]	– 3 monthly	Perform OGTT if HbA$_{1C}$ raised
BP	– 4 hourly during titration	Stop if neutrophils below 1.5×10^9/L
CPK	– if NMS suspected	Refer to specialist care if neutrophils below 0.5×10^9/L
ECG[3,4] (optional)	– when maintenance dose is reached	Stop if ECG shows important changes or if signs of heart failure noted
EEG[5,6]	– if myoclonus or seizures occur	Use valproate if EEG show epileptiform changes
LFTs[7]	– every 6 months for first year	Stop if LFTs indicate hepatitis or reduced hepatic function (PT or albumin)
U&Es[8]	– every 6 months	
Weight	– as needed	
HbA$_{1C}$ [1,9,10]	– 3 monthly	Perform OGTT if HbA$_{1C}$ raised
BP	– frequently during initiation	
CPK	– if NMS suspected	Stop if NMS suspected
FBC	– 6 monthly	Stop if neutrophils below 1.5×10^9/L
LFTs	– at 3 and 6 months	Stop if PT or albumin change
U&Es	– 6 monthly	
Prolactin	– if symptoms occur (rare)	
Weight	– as needed	
HbA$_{1C}$ [12]	– 6 monthly	Perform OGTT if HbA$_{1C}$ raised
BP	– frequently during titration	
CPK	– if NMS suspected	Stop if NMS suspected
LFTs	– at 3 and 6 months	Stop if PT or bilirubin change
TFTs	– 6 monthly	
U&Es	– 6 monthly	
Weight	– as needed	
HbA$_{1C}$	- 6 monthly	Perform OGTT if HbA$_{1C}$ raised
BP	- frequently during titration	
CPK	- if NMS suspected	Stop if NMS suspected
LFTs	- 6 monthly	Use with caution in hepatic/renal failure
Prolactin	- if symptoms occur	Stop if prolactin-related effects intolerable
U&Es	- 6 monthly	
Weight	- as needed	

New antipsychotics – recommended monitoring

Drug	Obligatory monitoring		Suggested
	Baseline	Continuation	Baseline
Zotepine	None (ECG in some circumstances)	None (ECG in some circumstances)	HbA$_{1C}$ BP ECG LFTs Prolactin U&Es Weight
Ziprasidone	None (ECG in some circumstances)	None (ECG in some circumstances)	HbA$_{1C}$ BP FBC LFTs U&Es Weight
Aripiprazole	None	None	HbA$_{1C}$ BP FBC LFTs U&Es Weight

KEY: BP = blood pressure
CPK = creatinine phosphokinase
ECG = electrocardiograph
EEG = electro-encephalograph
FBC = full blood count
HbA$_{1C}$= glycosylated haemoglobin
LFTs = liver function tests
OGTT = oral glucose tolerance test
PT = prothrombin time
TFTs = thyroid function tests
U&Es = urea & electrolytes

additional monitoring		Actions
	Continuation	
HbA$_{1C}$	– 6 monthly	Perform OGTT if HbA$_{1C}$ raised
BP	– frequently during titration	
CPK	– if NMS suspected	Stop if NMS suspected
EEG[13]	– if seizures occur	Use valproate if EEG shows epileptiform
ECG	– if necessary when maintenance dose is reached	changes
LFTs	– 6 monthly	Stop if ECG shows important changes
Prolactin	– if symptoms occur	
U&Es	– 6 monthly	Stop if renal function deteriorates
Weight	– as needed	
HbA$_{1C}$	– 6 monthly	Perform OGTT if HbA$_{1C}$ raised
BP	– frequently during initiation	
FBC	– 6–12 monthly	Stop if FBC shows pathological changes
LFTs	– 6 monthly	Stop PT or bilirubin change
U&Es	– 6 monthly	
Weight	– as required	
HbA$_{1C}$	– 6 monthly	Perform OGTT if HbA$_{1C}$ raised
BP	– frequently during initiation	
FBC	– 6–12 monthly	Stop if FBC shows pathological changes
LFTs	– 6 monthly	Stop PT or bilirubin change
U&Es	– 6 monthly	
Weight	– as required	

Sources of information

Monitoring recommendations for new antipsychotics are derived from:
– normal clinical practice with new medicines (e.g. FBC, LFTs, U&Es);
– relevant Summaries of Product Characteristics;
– specific references (see below).

References

1. Wirshing DA, Spellberg BJ, Erhart SM *et al.* Novel antipsychotics and new onset diabetes. *Biological Psychiatry* 1998; **44**: 778–783.
2. Hägg S, Joelsson L, Mjörndal T *et al.* Prevalence of diabetes and impaired glucose tolerance in patients treated with clozapine compared with patients treated with conventional depot neuroleptic medications. *Journal of Clinical Psychiatry* 1998; **59**: 294–299.
3. Leo RJ, Kreeger JL, Kim KY. Cardiomyopathy associated with clozapine. *Annals of Pharmacotherapy* 1996; **30**: 603–605.
4. Low RA, Fuller MA, Popli A.. Clozapine induced atrial fibrillation (Letter). *Clin Psychopharmacology* 1998; **18**: 170.
5. Silvestri RC, Bromfield EB, Khoshbin S. Clozapine-induced seizures and EEG abnormalities in ambulatory psychiatric patients. *Annals of Pharmacotherapy* 1998; **32**: 1147–1151.
6. Taner E, Cosar B, Isik E. Clozapine-induced myoclonic seizures and valproic acid. *International Journal of Psychiatry in Clinical Practice* 1998; **2**: 53–55.
7. Hummer M, Kurz M, Kurzthaler I *et al.* Hepatotoxicity of clozapine. *Journal of Clinical Psychopharmacology* 1997; **17**: 314–317.
8. Elias TJ, Bannister KM, Clarkson AR *et al.* Clozapine: First report of acute interstitial nephritis: case report. *Lancet* 1999; **354**: 1180–1181.
9. Ober SK, Hudak R, Rusterholtz A. Hyperglycemia and olanzapine. *American Journal of Psychiatry* 1999; **156**: 970.
10. Lindenmayer JP, Patel R. Olanzapine-induced ketoacidosis with diabetes mellitus. *American Journal of Psychiatry* 1999; **156**: 1471.
11. Naumann R, Felber W, Heilemann H *et al.* Olanzapine-induced agranulocytosis. *Lancet* 1999; **354**: 566–567.
12. Sobel M, Jaggers ED, Franz MA. New-onset diabetes mellitus associated with the initiation of quetiapine treatment. *Journal of Clinical Psychiatry* 1999; **60**: 556–557.
13. Prakash A, Lamb HM. Zotepine: a review of its pharmacodynamic and pharmacokinetic properties and therapeutic efficacy in the management of schizophrenia. *CNS Drugs* 1998; **9**: 153–175.

Further reading

Taylor D. Monitoring the new antipsychotic drugs. *Progress in Neurology and Psychiatry* 1997; **1**: 13–15.

See also sections on ECG monitoring (page 75), weight gain (page 72) and impaired glucose tolerance (page 80).

Depot antipsychotics

Advice on prescribing depot medication

- **Give a test dose**
  Depots are long-acting. Any adverse effects that result from injection are likely to be long-lived. Thus a small test dose is essential to help avoid severe, prolonged adverse effects. See table below and manufacturer's information.

- **Begin with the lowest therapeutic dose**
  There are few data showing clear dose-response effects for depot preparations. There is some information indicating that low doses are at least as effective as higher ones. Low doses are likely to be better tolerated and are certainly less expensive.

- **Administer at the longest possible licensed interval**
  All depots can be safely administered at their licensed dosing intervals. There is no evidence to suggest that shortening the dose interval improves efficacy. Moreover, injections are painful, so less frequent administration is desirable. The 'observation' that some patients deteriorate in the days before the next depot is due is probably fallacious. For some hours (or even days with some preparations) plasma levels of antipsychotics continue to fall, albeit slowly, after the next injection. Thus patients are most at risk of deterioration immediately after a depot injection and not before it. Moreover, in trials, relapse seems only to occur 3–6 months after withdrawing depot therapy; roughly, the time required to clear steady-state depot drug levels from the blood.

- **Adjust doses only after an adequate period of assessment**
  Attainment of peak plasma levels, therapeutic effect and steady-state plasma levels are all delayed with depot injections. Doses may be *reduced* if adverse effects occur, but should only be *increased* after careful assessment over at least one month, preferably longer. The use of adjunctive oral medication to assess depot requirements may be helpful, but it too is complicated by the slow emergence of antipsychotic effects. Note that at the start of therapy, plasma levels of antipsychotic released from a depot increase over several weeks without increasing the given dose. Dose increases during this time to steady-state plasma levels are thus illogical and impossible to evaluate properly.

Differences between depots

Zuclopenthixol is claimed to be more effective in aggressive patients, flupentixol decanoate in those who are depressed, haloperidol decanoate in the prophylaxis of manic illness and pipothiazine palmitate when EPSEs are problematic. Fluphenazine decanoate is said to be associated with depressed mood (which is common anyway in this patient group). The bulk of the literature in this area originates from the 1970s and 1980s, and the objective data contained therein do little to support the above 'folklore'. Many of these claimed differences are more the result of marketing strategies than of objective scientific evidence. The following *BNF* statement concerning 'choice of antipsychotic' should be borne in mind when considering depot as well as oral antipsychotics:

> *The various drugs differ somewhat in predominant actions and side-effects. Selection is influenced by the degree of sedation required and the patient's susceptibility to extrapyramidal side-effects. However, the differences between antipsychotic drugs are less important than the great variability in patient response; moreover, tolerance to these secondary effects usually develops'.*

One very real difference that does exist is that flupentixol decanoate can be given in very much higher 'neuroleptic equivalent' doses than the other depot preparations and still remain 'within *BNF* limits'. It is doubtful that this confers any real therapeutic advantage.

Table Antipsychotic depot injections – Suggested doses and frequencies[1]

Drug	Trade name	Test dose (mg)	Dose range (mg/week)	Dosing interval (weeks)	Comments
Flupentixol decanoate	Depixol	20	12.5–400	2–4	? Mood elevating; may worsen agitation
Fluphenazine decanoate	Modecate	12.5	6.25–50	2–5	Avoid in depression High EPS
Haloperidol decanoate	Haldol	25*	12.5–75	4	High EPS, low incidence of sedation
Pipothiazine palmitate	Piportil	25	12.5–50	4	? Lower incidence of EPS (unproven)
Zuclopenthixol decanoate	Clopixol	100	100–600	2–4	? Useful in agitation and aggression

Notes:
- Give a quarter or half stated doses in elderly.
- After test dose, wait 4–10 days before starting titration to maintenance therapy (see product information for individual drugs).
- Dose range is given in mg/week for convenience only – avoid using shorter dose intervals than those recommended except in exceptional circumstances (e.g.: long interval necessitates high volume (>3–4 ml) injection).

*Test dose not stated by manufacturer

Intramuscular anticholinergics and depots

Depot antipsychotics do not produce acute EPSEs at the time of administration[2]: this may take hours to days. The administration of intramuscular procyclidine routinely with each depot is illogical, as the effects of the anticholinergic drug will have worn off before plasma antipsychotic levels peak.

References

1. Taylor D, Duncan D. Antipsychotic depot injections – suggested doses and frequencies. *Psychiatric Bulletin* 1995; **19**: 357.
2. Kane JM, Aguglia E, Altamura C *et al*. Guidelines for depot antipsychotic treatment in schizophrenia. *European Neuropsychopharmacology* 1998; **8**: 55–66.

Further reading

Taylor D. Depot antipsychotics revisited. *Psychiatry Bulletin* 1999; **23**: 551–553.

Risperidone long-acting injection

Risperidone is the only atypical drug available as a depot formulation. Doses of 25–50 mg every two weeks appear to be as effective as oral doses of 2–6 mg/day[1]. The long acting injection also seems to be well tolerated – less than 10% experience EPSEs and less than 6% withdrew from a long-term trial because of adverse effects[2]. Few data are available relating to effects on prolactin but problems might be predicted[3].

Risperidone long-acting injection differs importantly from other depots and the following should be noted:

- Risperidone depot is not an esterified form of the parent drug. It contains risperidone coated in polymer to form microspheres. These microspheres have to be suspended in an aqueous base immediately before use.

- The injection must be stored in a fridge (consider the practicalities for CPNs).

- It is available as 25 mg, 37.5 mg and 50 mg. The whole vial must be used (because of the nature of the suspension). This means that there is limited flexibility in dosing. In clinical studies 25 mg was as effective as 50 mg/2 weeks.

- A test dose is not required or sensible. (Testing tolerability with oral risperidone is desirable but not always practical.)

- It takes 3–4 weeks for the first injection to produce therapeutic plasma levels. Patients must be maintained on a full dose of their previous antipsychotic for at least 3 weeks after the administration of the first risperidone injection. If the patient is not already receiving an oral antipsychotic, oral risperidone should be prescribed. (See table for advice on switching from depots.)

- Risperidone depot must be administered every 2 weeks. The pharmacokinetic profile does not allow longer intervals between doses. There is no flexibility to negotiate with patients about the frequency of administration.

For guidance on switching to risperidone long-acting injection see the table on page 38.

References

1. Chue P, Eerdekens M, Augustyns I et al. Efficacy and safety of long-acting risperidone microspheres and risperidone oral tablets. Poster presented at the 11th Biennial Winter Workshop on Schizophrenia, February 24–March 1, Davos, Switzerland, 2002.
2. Eerdekens, M., Fleischhacker, WW, Xie Y et al. Long term safety of long-acting risperidone microspheres. Poster presented at the 11th Biennial Winter Workshop on Schizophrenia, February 24–March 1, 2002, Davos, Switzerland, 2002.
3. Kleinber DL, Davies JM de Costa R et al. Prolactin levels and adverse events in patients treated with risperidone. *Journal of Clinical Psychopharmacology* 1999; 19: 57–61.

Switching to risperidone long-acting injection (RLAI)

Table		
Switching from	*Recommended method of switching*	*Comments*
No treatment (new patient or recently non-compliant)	Start risperidone oral at 2 mg day and increase to 3 or 4 mg/day on day two. If tolerated, give RLAI 25 mg on day three. Continue with oral risperidone for at least three weeks then taper over 1–2 weeks	Use oral risperidone before giving injection to assure good tolerability
Oral risperidone	Give RLAI 25 mg. Continue with oral risperidone for at least 3 weeks, then taper over 1–2 weeks	RLAI 25 mg and 50 mg appear to have the same efficacy. However, for patients maintained on more than 4 mg/day oral risperidone, higher doses of RLAI may, in theory, be required
Oral antipsychotics (not risperidone)	*Either:* (a) Switch to oral risperidone and then, if tolerated give injection (25 mg) *or:* (b) Give RLAI 25 mg and then slowly discontinue oral antipsychotics after 3–4 weeks	Suggest switching all patients to 25 mg every 2 weeks. Higher doses appear to be no more effective. Note that steady-state levels are not achieved for at least 6 weeks after first injection. Higher doses of RLAI may eventually be required but all patients should start on 25 mg
Depot antipsychotic	Give RLAI 25 mg one week *before* the last depot injection is given, or give RLAI in place of the last depot injection	As above, 25 mg every 2 weeks is recommended for all patients, at least initially. Increase dose only after response at steady state has been evaluated
Antipsychotic polypharmacy with depot	Give RLAI 25 mg one week before the last depot injection is given, or in place of the last depot injection. Slowly taper oral antipsychotics 3–4 weeks later	Aim to treat patient with RLAI as the sole antipsychotic. As before, 25 mg every 2 weeks is recommended initially for all patients, regardless of previous therapy
Note: These recommendations differ somewhat from those of the manufacturer. The main difference is that 25 mg every 2 weeks is recommended as initial therapy for all patients, regardless of previous treatment. The reasoning behind this is that 25 mg and 50 mg were equivalent in all clinical trials. There is a possibility that higher doses are more effective in certain individuals but, given that higher doses are more expensive and possibly less well tolerated, it seems prudent to suggest that all patients receive a trial of 25 mg every 2 weeks before any dose increase is contemplated.		

Management of patients on long-term depots

Such patients should be seen by their consultant at least once a year (ideally more frequently) in order to review their progress and treatment. There is no simple formula for deciding when to reduce the dose, therefore a risk/benefit analysis must be done for every patient, taking the following factors into consideration:

- Is the patient symptom-free and if so for how long? Long-standing, non-distressing symptoms which have not previously been responsive to medication may be excluded.

- What is the severity of the side-effects (EPSEs, TD, obesity, etc.)?

- What is the previous pattern of illness? Consider the speed of onset, duration and severity of episodes and any danger posed to self or others.

- Has dosage reduction been attempted before and if so, what was the outcome?

- What are the patient's current social circumstances? Is it a period of relative stability, or are stressful life events anticipated?

- What is the social cost of relapse (e.g. is the patient the sole breadwinner for a family)?

- Is the patient able to monitor his/her own symptoms, and if so, will he/she seek help?

If after consideration of the above, the decision is taken to reduce medication, the patient's family should be involved and a clear explanation given of what should be done if symptoms return/worsen. It would then be reasonable to proceed in the following manner:

- If it has not already been done, oral antipsychotic medication should be discontinued first.

- The interval between injections should be increased to up to 4 weeks before decreasing the dose given each time. Note: *not* with risperidone.

- The dose should be reduced by no more than a third at any one time. Note: special considerations apply to risperidone.

- Decrements should, if possible, be made no more frequently than every 3 months.

- Discontinuation should be seen as the end point of the above process.

If the patient becomes symptomatic, this should be seen not as a failure, but rather as an important step in determining the minimum effective dose that the patient requires.

Antipsychotic polypharmacy

There is no good objective evidence that antipsychotic polypharmacy offers any efficacy advantage over the use of a single antipsychotic, but such prescriptions are commonly seen[1]. National surveys have repeatedly shown that up to 50% of patients prescribed atypical antipsychotics receive a typical drug as well[2,3]. Anticholinergic medication is then often required[3].

A UK audit of antipsychotic prescribing in hospitalised patients found that 20% of all patients prescribed antipsychotics were prescribed doses above the *BNF* maximum. Very few of these prescriptions were for single antipsychotics[1] (high doses were the result of antipsychotic polypharmacy). Monitoring of patients receiving high doses or combinations was very poor. Prescribers would seem not to be aware of the additive side-effects resulting from antipsychotic polypharmacy. Clinical factors such as age (young), gender (male) and diagnosis (schizophrenia) were associated with antipsychotic polypharmacy, albeit only a small proportion of the total[4]. One study has shown a past history of violence to be an important factor[5]. The majority of such prescribing, however, remains unexplained.

Another study which followed a cohort of patients with schizophrenia prospectively over a 10-year period found that receiving more than one antipsychotic concurrently was associated with increased mortality[6]. There was no association with the total number of antipsychotics given sequentially as monotherapy, the maximum daily antipsychotic dose, duration of exposure, lifetime intake, or any other measure of illness severity. Interestingly, the prescription of anticholinergics was associated with increased survival. Although these data should be interpreted with some important caveats in mind, they should serve to remind us that antipsychotic monotherapy is desirable and should be the norm. It follows that it should be standard practice to document the rationale for using antipsychotic polypharmacy in individual cases in clinical notes along with a clear account of any benefits and side-effects. Medicolegally, that would seem to be wise.

Note that NICE explicitly demand that atypicals and typicals be not prescribed together except when switching[7].

References

1. Harrington M, Lelliott P, Paton C *et al.* The results of a multi-centre audit of the prescribing of antipsychotic drugs for in-patients in the UK. *Psychiatric Bulletin* 2002; **26**: 414–418.
2. Taylor D, Mace S, Mir S *et al.* A prescription survey of the use of atypical antipsychotics for hospital patients in the UK. *International Journal of Psychiatry in Clinical Practice* 2000; **4**: 41–46.
3. Paton C, Lelliott P, Harrington M *et al.* Patterns of antipsychotic and anticholinergic prescribing for hospital inpatients. *Journal of Clinical Psychopharmacology* 2003; **26**: 419–423.
4. Lelliott P, Paton C, Harrington M. The influence of patient variables on polypharmacy and combined high dose of antipsychotic drugs prescribed for in-patients. *Psychiatric Bulletin* 2002; **26**: 411–414.
5. Wilkie A, Preston N, Wesby R. High dose neuroleptics – who gives them and why? *Psychiatric Bulletin* 2001; **25**: 179–183.
6. Waddington JL, Youssef HA, Kinsella A. Mortality in schizophrenia: antipsychotic polypharmacy and absence of adjunctive anticholinergics over the course of a 10 year prospective study. *British Journal of Psychiatry* 1998; **173**: 325–329.
7. National Institute for Clinical Excellence. *Guidance on the use of newer (atypical) antipsychotic drugs for the treatment of schizophrenia.* London: NICE, June 2002.

Negative symptoms

A good deal of advertising material for new antipsychotics emphasises improved efficacy against negative symptoms when compared to older alternatives. Some points are worthy of consideration.

The aetiology of negative symptoms is complex and it is important to determine the most likely cause in any individual case before embarking on a treatment regimen. Negative symptoms can be either primary (transient or enduring), or secondary to positive symptoms (e.g. asociality secondary to paranoia), EPSEs (e.g. bradykinesia, lack of facial expression), depression (e.g. social withdrawal) or institutionalisation[1]. Secondary negative symptoms are obviously best dealt with by treating the relevant cause (EPSEs, depression etc.). In general:

- The earlier a psychotic illness is effectively treated, the less likely is the development of negative symptoms over time[2].

- Older antipsychotics have only a small effect against primary negative symptoms and can cause secondary negative symptoms (EPSEs).

- Atypical antipsychotics cause few EPSEs but are not strikingly effective against primary negative symptoms. Many trials report statistically significant differences in favour of the atypical, but the clinical significance of the small mean changes observed is questionable. More robust data support the effectiveness of amisulpride in primary negative symptoms.

References

1. Carpenter WT. The treatment of negative symptoms: pharmacological and methodological issues. *British Journal of Psychiatry* 1996; **168**(Suppl. 29): 17–22.
2. Waddington JL, Youssef HA, Kinsella A. Sequential cross sectional and 10 year prospective study of severe negative symptoms in relation to duration of initially untreated psychosis in chronic schizophrenia. *Psychological Medicine* 1995; **25**: 849–857.

Antipsychotic prophylaxis

First episode of psychosis

A placebo-controlled study has shown that when no prophylactic treatment is given, 57% of first-episode patients have relapsed at 1 year[1]. After 1–2 years of being well on antipsychotic medication, the risk of relapse remains high (figures of 10–15% per month have been quoted), but this area is less well researched[2,3]. Although current consensus is that antipsychotics should be prescribed for 1–2 years after a first episode of schizophrenia[4,5], Gitlan et al.[6] found that withdrawing antipsychotic treatment in line with this consensus led to a relapse rate of almost 80% after 1 year medication-free and 98% after 2 years. In practice, a firm diagnosis of schizophrenia is rarely made after a first episode and the majority of prescribers and/or patients will have at least attempted to stop antipsychotic treatment within 1 year[7]. It is vital that patients, carers and keyworkers are aware of the early signs of relapse and how to access help. Antipsychotics should not be considered the only intervention. Psychosocial and psychological interventions are clearly also important.

Multi-episode schizophrenia

The majority of those who have one episode of schizophrenia will go on to have further episodes. With each subsequent episode, the baseline level of functioning deteriorates[8] and the majority of this decline is seen in the first decade of illness. Suicide risk (10%) is also concentrated in the first decade of illness. Those who receive targeted antipsychotics (i.e. only when symptoms re-emerge) have a worse outcome than those who receive prophylactic antipsychotics[9,10] and the risk of TD may also be higher. The figure below depicts the relapse rate in a large cohort of patients with psychotic illness, the majority of whom had already experienced multiple episodes[11]. All had originally received, or were still receiving treatment with typical antipsychotics. Note that many of the studies included in this data set were old and unstandardised diagnostic criteria were used. Variable definitions of relapse and short follow-up periods were the norm and other psychotropic drugs were not controlled for.

Figure   Effect of prophylactic antipsychotics

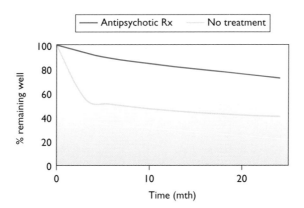

There is some evidence to support improved long-term outcomes with atypical antipsychotics. Csernansky *et al.*[12] found that relapse rates over 2 years were 34% for risperidone and 60% for haloperidol. A naturalistic study found that almost 70% of those discharged from hospital on risperidone or olanzapine were not re-admitted over the next 2 years, compared with 52% of those who were treated with conventional antipsychotics[13]. Another naturalistic study found relapse rates and service costs to be significantly lower with risperidone than with conventional drugs[14].

Dose for prophylaxis

Many patients probably receive higher doses than necessary (particularly of the older drugs) when acutely psychotic[15,16]. In the longer term a balance needs to be made between effectiveness and side-effects. Lower doses of the older drugs (8 mg haloperidol/day or equivalent) are, when compared with higher doses, associated with less severe side-effects[17], better subjective state and better community adjustment[18]. Very low doses increase the risk of psychotic relapse[15,19]. There are no data to support the use of lower than standard doses of the newer drugs as prophylaxis.

How and when to stop[20]

The decision to stop antipsychotic drugs requires a risk–benefit analysis for each patient. Withdrawal of antipsychotic drugs after long-term treatment should be gradual and closely monitored. The relapse rate in the first 6 months after abrupt withdrawal is double that seen after gradual withdrawal (defined as slow taper down over at least 3 weeks for oral antipsychotics or abrupt withdrawal of depot preparations)[21]. Abrupt withdrawal may also lead to discontinuation symptoms (e.g. headache, nausea, insomnia) in some patients[22].

The following factors should be considered[20]:

- Is the patient symptom-free, and if so, for how long? Long-standing, non-distressing symptoms which have not previously been responsive to medication may be excluded.

- What is the severity of side-effects (e.g. EPSEs, TD, obesity, etc.)?

- What was the previous pattern of illness? Consider the speed of onset, duration and severity of episodes and any danger posed to self and others.

- Has dosage reduction been attempted before, and if so, what was the outcome?

- What are the patient's current social circumstances? Is it a period of relative stability, or are stressful life events anticipated?

- What is the social cost of relapse (e.g. is the patient the sole breadwinner for a family)?

- Is the patient/carer able to monitor symptoms, and if so, will they seek help?

As with first-episode patients, patients, carers and keyworkers should be aware of the early signs of relapse and how to access help. Those with a history of aggressive behaviour or serious suicide attempts and those with residual psychotic symptoms should be considered for life-long treatment.

Key points that patients should know

- Antipsychotics do not 'cure' schizophrenia. They treat symptoms in the same way that insulin treats diabetes.

- Long-term treatment is required to prevent relapses.

- Many antipsychotic drugs are available. Different drugs suit different patients. Perceived side-effects should always be discussed, so that the best tolerated drug can be found.

- Antipsychotics should not be stopped suddenly.

References

1. Crow TJ, McMillan JP, Johnson AL *et al*. The Northwick Park study of first episodes of schizophrenia 11. A randomised controlled trial of prophylactic neuroleptic treatment. *British Journal of Psychiatry* 1986; **148**: 120–127.
2. Neuchterlein KH, Gitlin M, Subotnik KL. The early course of schizophrenia and long–term maintenance neuroleptic therapy. *Archives of General Psychiatry* 1995; **52**: 193–195.
3. Davis JM, Metalon L, Watanabe MD *et al*. Depot antipsychotic drugs: place in therapy. *Drugs* 1994; **47**: 741–773.
4. Sheitman BB, Lee H, Strausi R *et al*. The evaluation and treatment of first-episode psychosis. *Schizophrenia Bulletin* 1997; **23**: 653–661.
5. American Psychiatric Association. Practice guideline for the treatment of patients with schizophrenia. *American Journal of Psychiatry* 1997; **154**(4 Suppl. 1): 1–63.
6. Gitlin M, Neuchterlein K, Subotnik KL. Clinical outcome following neuroleptic discontinuation in patients with remitted recent-onset psychosis. *American Journal of Psychiatry* 2001; **158**: 1835–1842.
7. Johnson DAW, Rasmussen JGC. Professional attitudes in the UK towards neuroleptic maintenance therapy in schizophrenia: the problem of inadequate prophylaxis. *Psychiatric Bulletin* 1997; **21**: 394–397.
8. Wyatt RJ. Neuroleptics and the natural course of schizophrenia. *Schizophrenia Bulletin* 1991; **17**: 325–351.
9. Jolly AG, Hirsch SR, McRink A *et al*. Trial of brief intermittent neuroleptic prophylaxis for selected schizophrenic outpatients: clinical outcomes at one year. *BMJ* 1989; **298**: 985–990.
10. Herz MI, Glazer WM, Mostert MA *et al*. Intermittent vs maintenance medication in schizophrenia: 2 year results. *Archives of General Psychiatry* 1991; **48**: 333–339.
11. Gilbert PL, Harris MJ, McAdams LA *et al*. Neuroleptic withdrawal in schizophrenic patients. *Archives of General Psychiatry* 1995; **52**: 173–188.
12. Csernansky JG, Mahmoud R, Brenner R. A comparison of risperidone and haloperidol for the prevention of relapse in patients with schizophrenia. *New England Journal of Medicine* 2002; **346**: 16–22.
13. Rabinowitz J, Lichtenberg P, Kaplan Z *et al*. Rehospitalisation rates of chronically ill schizophrenic patients discharged on a regimen of risperidone, olanzapine or conventional antipsychotics. *American Journal of Psychiatry* 2001; **158**: 266–269.
14. Malla AK, Norman RM, Scholten DJ *et al*. A comparison of long-term outcome in first-episode schizophrenia following treatment with risperidone or a typical antipsychotic. *Journal of Clinical Psychiatry* 2001; **62**(3): 179–184.
15. Baldessarini RJ, Cohen BM, Teicher MH. Significance of neuroleptic dose and plasma level in the pharmacological treatment of psychoses. *Archives of General Psychiatry* 1988; **45**: 79–90.
16. Harrington M, Lelliott P, Paton C *et al*. The results of a multi-centre audit of the prescribing of antipsychotic drugs for in-patients in the UK. *Psychiatric Bulletin* 2002; **26**: 414–418.
17. Geddes J, Freemantle N, Harrison P *et al*. Atypical antipsychotics in the treatment of schizophrenia: systematic overview and meta-regression analysis. *BMJ* 2000; **321**: 1371–1376.
18. Hogarty GE, McEvoy JP, Munetz M *et al*. Dose of fluphenazine, familial expressed emotion, and outcome in schizophrenia: results of a two-year controlled study. *Archives of General Psychiatry* 1988; **45**: 797–805.
19. Marder SR, van Putten T, Mintz J. Low and conventional dose maintenance therapy with fluphenazine decanoate: two-year outcome. *Archives of General Psychiatry* 1987; **44**: 518–521.
20. Wyatt J. Risks of withdrawing antipsychotic medications. *Archives of General Psychiatry* 1995; **52**: 196–199.
21. Viguera AC, Baldessarini RJ, Hegarty JD. Clinical risk following abrupt and gradual withdrawal of maintenance neuroleptic treatment. *Archives of General Psychiatry* 1997; **54**: 49–55.
22. Chouinard G, Bradvejn J, Annable L *et al*. Withdrawal symptoms after long-term treatment with low-potency neuroleptics. *Journal of Clinical Psychiatry* 1984; **45**: 500–502.

Further reading

Bosveld-van Haandel LJM, Slooff CJ, van den Bosch RJ. Reasoning about the optimal duration of prophylactic antipsychotic medication in schizophrenia: evidence arguments. *Acta Psychiatrica Scandinavica* 2001; **103**: 335–346.

Csernansky JG, Schuchart EK. Relapse and rehospitalisation rates in patients with schizophrenia: effects of second generation antipsychotics. *CNS Drugs* 2002; **16**: 473–484.

Refractory schizophrenia

Clozapine – dosing regimen

Many of the adverse effects of clozapine are dose-dependent and associated with speed of titration. Adverse effects also tend to be more common at the beginning of therapy. To minimise these problems it is important to start therapy at a low dose and to increase dosage slowly.

Clozapine should be started at a dose of 12.5 mg once a day. Blood pressure should be monitored hourly for six hours because of the hypotensive effect of clozapine. This monitoring is not usually necessary if the first dose is given at night. On day 2, the dose can be increased to 12.5 mg twice daily. If the patient is tolerating clozapine, the dose can then be increased by 25–50 mg a day, until a dose of 300 mg a day is reached. This can usually be achieved in 2–3 weeks. Further dosage increases should be made slowly in increments of 50–100 mg each week. A dose of 450 mg/day or a plasma level of 350 μg/l should be aimed for. The total clozapine dose should be divided and, if sedation is a problem, the larger portion of the dose can be given at night.

The following table is a suggested starting regime for clozapine. This is a cautious regimen – more rapid increases have been used in exceptional circumstances. Slower titration may be necessary where sedation is severe. If the patient is not tolerating a particular dose, decrease to one that was tolerated. If the adverse effect resolves, increase the dose again but at a slower rate. If for any reason a patient misses *less than* 2 days' clozapine, restart at the dose prescribed before the event. Do not administer extra tablets to catch up. If more than 2 days are missed, restart at 12.5 mg once daily and increase slowly (but at a faster rate than in drug-naïve patients).

Table	Suggested starting regime for clozapine (in-patients)	
Day	Morning dose (mg)	Evening dose (mg)
1	–	12.5
2	12.5	12.5
3	25	25
4	25	25
5	25	50
6	25	50
7	50	50
8	50	75
9	75	75
10	75	100
11	100	100
12	100	125
13	125	125
14	125	150
15	150	150
18	150	200
21	200	200
28	200	250

Optimising clozapine treatment

Optimising clozapine treatment	
Target dose *(Note that dose is best adjusted according to) patient tolerability*	• Average dose in UK is around 450 mg/day[1] • Response usually seen in the range 150–900 mg/day[2] • Lower doses required in the elderly, females and non-smokers, and in those prescribed certain enzyme inhibitors[3,4]
Plasma levels	• Most studies indicate that threshold for response is in the range 350–420 µg/l[5,6] Threshold may be as high as 500 µg//l[7] (see page 4) • Importance of norclozapine levels not established

References

1. Taylor D, Mace S, Mir S, Kerwin R. A prescription survey of the use of atypical antipsychotics for hospital inpatients in the United Kingdom. *International Journal of Psychiatry in Clinical Practice* 2000; 4: 41–46.
2. Murphy B, Long C, Paton C. Maintenance doses for clozapine. *Psychiatric Bulletin* 1998; 22: 12–14.
3. Taylor D. Pharmacokinetic interactions involving clozapine. *British Journal of Psychiatry* 1997; 171: 109–112.
4. Lane HY, Chang YC, Chang WH *et al.* Effects of gender and age on plasma levels of clozapine and its metabolites: analysed by critical statistics. *Journal of Clinical Psychiatry* 1999; 60: 36–40.
5. Taylor D, Duncan D. The use of clozapine plasma levels in optimising therapy. *Psychiatric Bulletin*1995; 19: 753–755.
6. Spina E, Avenoso A, Facciolà G *et al.* Relationship between plasma concentrations of clozapine and norclozapine and therapeutic response in patients with schizophrenia resistant to conventional neuroleptics. *Psychopharmacology* 2000; 148: 83–89.
7. Perry PJ. Therapeutic drug monitoring of atypical antipsychotics: is it of potential clinical value? *CNS Drugs* 2000; 13: 167–171.

The table below shows other suggested options where 3–6 months of clozapine alone has provided unsatisfactory benefit.

Table	Suggested options for augmenting clozapine
Option	**Comment**
Add sulpiride[1] (400 mg/day)	● May be useful in partial or non-responders. The only augmentation strategy supported by a randomised trial
Add lamotrigine[2–4] (25–300 mg/day)	● May be useful in partial or non-responders
Add risperidone[5,6] (2 mg/day)	● Increases clozapine plasma levels. May have additive antipsychotic effects
Add omega-3 triglycerides [7,8] (2–3 g EPA daily)	● Modest, if contested, evidence to support efficacy in non- or partial responders to antipsychotics, including clozapine (see page 60)
Try amisulpride[9] (400–800 mg/day)	● Developing evidence and experience suggests amisulpride augmentation is worthwhile
Try haloperidol (2 mg/day)	● Anecdotal reports of clinical improvement. No published evidence

Notes:
- For discussion of augmentation strategies see Chong S-A, Remington G. Clozapine augmentation: safety and efficacy. *Schizophrenia Bulletin* 2000; **26**: 421–440
- Always consider the use of mood stabilisers and/or antidepressants where mood disturbance is thought to contribute to symptoms
- Topiramate has also been suggested, either to augment clozapine or to induce weight loss. It is probably not effective as augmentation and may even worsen psychosis[3,10]
- Other options include adding pimozide[11] and olanzapine[12]. Neither is recommended: pimozide has important cardiac toxicity and the addition of olanzapine is expensive and poorly supported

References

1. Shiloh R, Zemishlany Z, Aizenberg D *et al.* Sulpiride augmentation in people with schizophrenia partially responsive to clozapine. *British Journal of Psychiatry* 1997; **171**: 569–573.
2. Dursun SM, McIntosh D. Clozapine plus lamotrigine in treatment-resistant schizophrenia. *Archives of General Psychiatry* 1999; **56**: 950.
3. Dursun SM, Deakin J. Augmenting antipsychotic treatment with lamotrigine or topiramate in patients with treatment-resistant schizophrenia: a naturalistic case-series outcome study. *Journal of Psychopharmacology* 2001; **15**: 297–301
4. Dumortier S, Kalalou K, Benadhira R *et al.* Lamotrigine clozapine combination in refractory schizophrenia: three cases. *Journal of Neuropsychiatry & Clinical Neurosciences* 2002; **14**: 86
5. Morera AL, Barreiro P, Cano-Muñoz JL. Case report: risperidone and clozapine combination for the treatment of refractory schizophrenia. *Acta Psychiatrica Scandinavica* 1999; **99**: 305–307.
6. Raskin S, Katz G, Zislin Z *et al.* Clozapine and risperidone: combination/augmentation treatment of refractory schizophrenia: a preliminary observation. *Acta Psychiatrica Scandinavica* 2000; **101**: 334–336.
7. McGorry PD, Yung AR, Phillips L *et al.* Double-blind placebo controlled trial of N-3 polyunsaturated fatty acids as an adjunct to neuroleptics. *Schizophrenia Research* 1998; **29**: 160–161.
8. Puri BK, Richardson AJ. Sustained remission of positive and negative symptoms of schizophrenia following treatment with eicosapentaenoic acid. *Archives of General Psychiatry* 1998; **55**: 188–189.
9. Mathiasson P, Costa D, Erlandsson K *et al.* The relationship between dopamine D2 receptor occupancy and clinical response in amisulpride augmentation of clozapine non-response. *Journal of Psychopharmacology* 2001; **15**(Suppl.): S41.
10. Millson R, Owen J, Lorberg G *et al.* Topiramate for refractory schizophrenia. *American Journal of Psychiatry* 2002; **159**: 675.
11. Friedman J, Ault K, Powchik P. Pimozide augmentation for the treatment of schizophrenic patients who are partial responders to clozapine. *Biological Psychiatry* 1997; **42**: 522–523.
12. Sonnerberg G, Frank S. Olanzapine augmentation of clozapine. *Annals of Clinical Psychiatry* 1998; **10**: 113–115.

Refractory schizophrenia – alternatives to clozapine

The table below lists alternatives to clozapine (where clozapine has proved toxic or is contra-indicated).

Table Alternatives to clozapine

Treatment	Comments
Risperidone[1,2] 4–8 mg/day	Doubtful efficacy in true treatment-refractory schizophrenia, but some supporting evidence.
Olanzapine[3–6] 5–25 mg/day	Probably not effective, but some studies suggest it may be worth a carefully-monitored trial
Olanzapine high dose[7–9] 30–60 mg/day	Possibly effective, but expensive and unlicensed. No controlled trial as yet
	Note that olanzapine may lose atypicality at higher doses[10]
Omega-3-triglycerides[11,12]	Suggested efficacy but scant data (see page 60)
Antipsychotic + *Ginkgo biloba*[13,14] (360 mg/day)	Very limited evidence of benefit; very little clinical experience in UK
Quetiapine[15–17]	Very limited evidence of benefit; clinical experience is not encouraging
ECT[18]	Well-used option; effect may be short-lived

Notes:

- Judged by evidence-based criteria, only clozapine is effective in refractory schizophrenia.

- Above treatments should only be used instead of clozapine where clozapine cannot be used because of toxicity or very poor tolerability.

- Switching from clozapine to other atypicals is usually unsuccessful or disastrous and should not be attempted unless a severe clozapine-related adverse effect has occurred.

References

1. Breier AF, Malhotra AK, Su TP *et al*. Clozapine and risperidone in chronic schizophrenia: effects on symptoms, Parkinsonian side effects, and neuroendocrine response. *American Journal of Psychiatry* 1999; **156**: 294–298.
2. Bondolfi G, Dufour H, Patris M *et al*. Risperidone versus clozapine in treatment-resistant chronic schizophrenia: a randomized double-blind study. *American Journal of Psychiatry* 1998; **155**: 499–504.
3. Breier A, Hamilton SH. Comparative efficacy of olanzapine and haloperidol for patients with treatment-resistant schizophrenia. *Biological Psychiatry* 1999; **45**: 403–411.
4. Conley RR, Tamminga CA, Bartko JJ *et al*. Olanzapine compared with chlorpromazine in treatment-resistant schizophrenia. *American Journal of Psychiatry* 1998; **155**: 914–920.
5. Sanders RD, Mossman D. An open trial of olanzapine in patients with treatment-refractory psychoses. *Journal of Clinical Psychopharmacology* 1999; **19**: 62–66.
6. Taylor D, Mir S, Mace S. Olanzapine in practice: a prospective naturalistic study. *Psychiatric Bulletin* 1999; **23**: 178–180.
7. Sheitman BB, Lindgren JC, Early J *et al*. High-dose olanzapine for treatment-refractory schizophrenia. *American Journal of Psychiatry* 1997; **154**: 1626.
8. Fanous A, Lindenmayer JP. Schizophrenia and schizoaffective disorder treated with high doses of olanzapine. *Journal of Clinical Psychopharmacology* 1999; **19**: 275–276.
9. Dursun SM, Gardner DM, Bird DC *et al*. Olanzapine for patients with treatment-resistant schizophrenia: a naturalistic case-series outcome study. *Canadian Journal of Psychiatry* 1999; **44**: 701–704.
10. Bronson BD, Lindenmayer J-P. Adverse effects of high dose olanzapine in treatment-refractory schizophrenia (letter). *Journal of Clinical Psychopharmacology* 2000; **20**: 382–384.
11. Mellor JE, Laugharne JDE, Peet M. Omega-3 fatty acid supplementation in schizophrenic patients. *Human Psychopharmacology* 1996; **11**: 39–46.
12. Puri BK, Steiner R, Richardson AJ. Sustained remission of positive and negative symptoms of schizophrenia following treatment with eicosapentaenoic acid. *Archives of General Psychiatry* 1998; **55**: 188–189.
13. Zhou D, Zhang X, Su J *et al*. The effects of classic antipsychotic haloperidol plus the extract of ginkgo biloba on superoxide dismutase in patients with chronic refractory schizophrenia. *Chinese Medical Journal* 1999; **112**(12): 1093–1096.
14. Zhang X, Zhou D, Zhang P *et al*. A double-blind, placebo-controlled trial of extract of *Ginkgo biloba* added to haloperidol in treatment-resistant patients with schizophrenia. *Journal of Clinical Psychiatry* 2001; **62**(11): 878–883.
15. Reznik I, Benatov R, Sirota P *et al*. Long-term efficacy and safety of quetiapine in treatment-refractory schizophrenia: A case report. *International Journal of Psychiatry in Clinical Practice* 2000; **4**: 77–80.
16. Windhager E, Whiteford J, Jones A *et al*. Patients switched to quetiapine demonstrated improved efficacy and tolerability irrespective of previous medication. Poster presented at the 15ᵗʰ European College of Neuropsychopharmacology Congress, Barcelona, Spain, 5–9 October 2002.
17. Nayer A, Jones A, Whiteford J *et al*. Improved efficacy gained from switching to quetiapine in patients with schizophrenia. Poster presented at the 15ᵗʰ European College of Neuropsychopharmacology Congress, Barcelona, Spain, 5–9 October 2002.
18. Chanpattana W, Chakrabhand M. Combined ECT and neuroleptic therapy in treatment-refractory schizophrenia: prediction of outcome. *Psychiatry Research* 2001; **105**: 107–115.

Further reading

Still DJ, Dorson PG, Crismon MH *et al*. Effects of switching inpatients with treatment-resistant schizophrenia from clozapine to risperidone. *Psychiatric Services* 1996; **47**: 1382–1384.

Henderson DC, Nasrallah RA, Goff DC. Switching from clozapine to olanzapine in treatment-refractory schizophrenia: safety, clinical efficacy, and predictors of response. *Journal of Clinical Psychiatry* 1998; **59**: 585–588.

Lindenmayer J-P, Czobar P, Volavka J *et al*. Olanzapine in refractory schizophrenia after failure of typical or atypical antipsychotic treatment: an open-label switch study. *Journal of Clinical Psychiatry* 2002; **63**: 931–935.

Clozapine – management of adverse effects

Table

Adverse effect	Timecourse	Action
Sedation	First 4 weeks. May persist, but usually wears off	Give smaller dose in the morning. Some patients can only cope with single night-time dosing. Reduce dose if necessary
Hypersalivation	First 4 weeks. May persist, but usually wears off. Often very troublesome at night	Give hyoscine 300 µg (Kwells) sucked and swallowed at night. Pirenzepine[1] (not licensed in the UK) up to 50 mg tds may be tried (see page 54)
Constipation	Usually persists	Recommend high fibre diet. Bulk forming laxatives +/- stimulants may be used
Hypotension	First 4 weeks	Advise patient to take time when standing up. Reduce dose or slow down rate of increase. If severe, consider moclobemide and Bovril[2], or fludrocortisone
Hypertension	First 4 weeks, sometimes longer	Monitor closely and increase dose as slowly as is necessary. Hypotensive therapy (e.g. atenolol 25 mg/day) is sometimes necessary
Tachycardia	First 4 weeks, but sometimes persists	Very common in early stages of treatment but usually benign. Tachycardia, if persistent at rest and associated with fever, hypotension or chest pain, may indicate myocarditis[3,4]. Referral to a cardiologist is advised. Clozapine should be stopped if tachycardia occurs in the context of chest pain or heart failure
Weight gain	Usually during the first year of treatment	Dietary counselling is essential. Advice may be more effective if given before weight gain occurs. Weight gain is common and often profound (>10 lb) (see page 72)
Fever	First 3 weeks	Give antipyretic but check FBC. This fever is not usually related to blood dyscrasias[5] but beware myocarditis
Seizures	May occur at any time[6]	Dose-/dose increase-related. Consider prophylactic valproate* if on high dose. After a seizure: withhold clozapine for one day; restart at reduced dose; give sodium valproate. Note that EEG abnormalities are common in those on clozapine[7]
Nausea	First 6 weeks	May give anti-emetic. Avoid prochlorperazine and metoclopramide if previous EPSEs
Nocturnal enuresis	May occur at any time	Try manipulating dose schedule. Avoid fluids before bedtime. May resolve spontaneously[8]. In severe cases, desmopressin is usually effective[9]
Neutropenia/ agranulocytosis	First 18 weeks (but may occur at any time)	Stop clozapine; admit to hospital

* Usual dose is 1000–2000 mg/day. Plasma levels may be useful as a rough guide to dosing – aim for 50–100 mg/l. Use of modified-release preparation (Epilim Chrono) may aid compliance: can be given once-daily and may be better tolerated.

References

1. Fritze J, Tilmann E. Pirenzepine for clozapine-induced hypersalivation. *Lancet* 1995; **346**: 1034.
2. Taylor D, Reveley A, Faivre F. Clozapine-induced hypotension treated with moclobemide and Bovril. *British Journal of Psychiatry* 1995; **167**: 409–410.
3. Committee on Safety of Medicines. Clozapine and cardiac safety: updated advice for prescribers. *Current Problems in Pharmaco-vigilance* 2002; **28**: 8–9.
4. Hägg S, Spigset O, Bate A *et al*. Myocarditis related to clozapine treatment. *Journal of Clinical Psychopharmacology* 2001; **21**: 382–388.
5. Tham JC, Dickson RA. Clozapine-induced fevers and 1-year clozapine discontinuation rate. *Journal of Clinical Psychiatry* 2002; **63**: 880–884.
6. Pacia SV, Devinsky O. Clozapine-related seizures: experience with 5,629 patients. *Neurology* 1994; **44**: 2247–2249.
7. Centorrino F, Price BH, Tuttle M *et al*. EEG abnormalities during treatment with typical and atypical antipsychotics. *American Journal of Psychiatry* 2002; **159**: 109–115.
8. Warner MP, Harvey CA, Barnes TRE. Clozapine and urinary incontinence. *International Clinical Psychopharmacology* 1994; **9**: 207–209.
9. Use of desmopressin to treat clozapine-induced nocturnal enuresis (Letter). *Journal of Clinical Psychiatry* 1994; **55**: 315–316.

Further reading

Lieberman JA. Maximizing clozapine therapy: managing side effects. *Journal of Clinical Psychiatry* 1998; **59**(Suppl. 3): 38–43.

Clozapine – serious adverse effects

Agranulocytosis, thromboembolism, cardiomyopathy and myocarditis

Clozapine clearly and substantially *reduces* overall mortality in schizophrenia, largely because of a considerable reduction in the rate of suicide[1,2].

Nevertheless, clozapine can cause serious, life-threatening adverse effects, of which **agranulocytosis** is the best known. In the UK, there have been three deaths due to clozapine-associated agranulocytosis – a risk of less than 1 in 5000 patients treated. Risk is well managed by the Clozaril Patient Monitoring Scheme (CPMS).

A possible association between clozapine and **pulmonary embolism** has been suggested. Initially, Walker *et al.*[1] uncovered a risk of fatal pulmonary embolism of 1 in 4500 – about 20 times the risk in the population as a whole. Following a case report of non-fatal pulmonary embolism possibly related to clozapine,[3] data from the Swedish authorities were published[4]. Twelve cases of venous thromboembolism were described, of which 5 were fatal. The risk of thromboembolism was estimated to be 1 in 2000–6000 patients treated. Thromboembolism may be related to clozapine's observed effect on antiphospholipid antibodies.[5] It seems most likely to occur in the first 3 months of treatment.

It has also been suggested that clozapine is associated with **myocarditis** and **cardiomyopathy**. Australian data identified 23 cases (15 myocarditis, 8 cardiomyopathy), of which 6 were fatal[6]. Risk of death from either cause is estimated from these data to be 1 in 1300. Myocarditis seems to occur within 6–8 weeks of starting clozapine; cardiomyopathy may occur later in treatment. It is notable that other data sources give rather different risk estimates: in Canada the risk of fatal myocarditis was estimated to be 1 in 12,500, and in the USA, 1 in 67,000[7].

Note also that, despite an overall reduction in mortality, younger patients may have an increased risk of sudden death[8], perhaps because of clozapine-induced ECG changes[9]. The overall picture remains very unclear but caution is required. There may, of course, be similar problems with other antipsychotics[10,11].

Summary

- Overall mortality appears to be lower for those on clozapine than in schizophrenia as a whole.
- Risk of fatal agranulocytosis is less than 1 in 5000 patients treated under the UK Clozaril Patient Monitoring Scheme.
- Risk of fatal pulmonary embolism is estimated to be around 1 in 4500 patients treated.
- Risk of fatal myocarditis or cardiomyopathy may be as high as 1 in 1300 patients.
- Careful monitoring is essential especially during the first 3 months of treatment.

References

1. Walker AM. Mortality in current and former users of clozapine. *Epidemiology* 1997; **8**: 671–677.
2. Munro J, O'Sullivan D, Andrews C *et al.* Active monitoring of 12,760 clozapine recipients in the UK and Ireland: Beyond pharmacovigilance. *British Journal of Psychiatry* 1999; **175**: 576–580.
3. Lacika S, Cooper JP. Pulmonary embolus possibly associated with clozapine treatment (Letter). *Canadian Journal of Psychiatry* 1999; **44**: 396–397.
4. Hägg S, Spigset O, Söderström TG. Association of venous thromboembolism and clozapine. *Lancet* 2000; **355**: 1155–1156.
5. Davis S. Antiphospholipid antibodies associated with clozapine treatment. *American Journal of Hematology* 1994; **46**: 166–167.
6. Kilian JG, Kerr K, Lawrence C *et al.* Myocarditis and cardiomyopathy associated with clozapine. *Lancet* 1999; **354**: 1841–1845.
7. Warner B, Alphs L, Schaedelin J *et al.* Myocarditis and cardiomyopathy associated with clozapine (Letter). *Lancet* 2000; **355**: 842–843.
8. Modal I, Hirschman S, Rava A *et al.* Sudden death in patients receiving clozapine treatment: a preliminary investigation. *Journal of Clinical Psychopharmacology* 2000; **20**: 325–327.
9. Kang UG, Kwon JS, Ahn YM *et al.* Electrocardiographic abnormalities in patients treated with clozapine. *Journal of Clinical Psychiatry* 2000; **61**: 441–446.
10. Thomassen R, Vandenbroucke JP, Rosendaal FR. Antipsychotic drugs and thromboembolism (Letter). *Lancet* 2000; **356**: 252.
11. Hägg S, Spigset O. Antipsychotic-induced venous thromboembolism: a review of the evidence. *CNS Drugs* 2002; **16**: 765–776.

Clozapine-related hypersalivation

Clozapine is well known to be causally associated with apparent hypersalivation (drooling, particularly at night). This seems to be chiefly problematic in the early stages of treatment and is probably dose-related. Clinical observation suggests that hypersalivation reduces in severity over time (usually several months) but may persist. Clozapine-induced hypersalivation is socially embarrassing and potentially life-threatening[1], so treatment is a matter of some urgency.

The pharmacological basis of clozapine-related hypersalivation remains unclear. Suggested mechanisms include muscarinic M_4 agonism, adrenergic α_2 antagonism and inhibition of the swallowing reflex[2,3]. The last of these is supported by trials which suggest that saliva production is *not* increased in clozapine-treated patients[4,5].

Whatever the mechanism, drugs which reduce saliva production are likely to diminish the severity of this adverse effect. The table below describes drug treatments so far examined.

References

1. Hinkes R, Quesada TV, Currier MB *et al.* Aspiration pneumonia possibly secondary to clozapine-induced sialorrhea. *Journal of Clinical Psychopharmacology* 1997; 16: 462–463.
2. Davydov L, Botts SR. Clozapine-induced hypersalivation. *Annals of Pharmacotherapy* 2001; 34: 662–665.
3. Rogers DP, Shramko JK. Therapeutic options in the treatment of clozapine-induced sialorrhea. *Pharmacotherapy* 2000; 20: 1092–1095.
4. Rabinowitz T, Frankenburg FR, Centorrino F *et al.* The effect of clozapine on saliva flow rate: a pilot study. *Biological Psychiatry* 1996; 40: 1132–1134.
5. Ben-Aryeh H, Jungerman T, Szargel R *et al.* Salivary flow-rate and composition in schizophrenic patients on clozapine: subjective reports and laboratory data. *Biological Psychiatry* 1996; 39: 946–949.
6. Fritze J, Elliger T. Pirenzepine for clozapine-induced hypersalivation. *Lancet* 1995; 346: 1034.
7. Bai Y-M, Lin C-C, Chen J-Y *et al.* Therapeutic effect of pirenzepine for clozapine-induced hypersalivation: a randomized, double-blind, placebo-controlled, cross-over study. *Journal of Clinical Psychopharmacology* 2001; 21: 608–611.
8. Spivak B, Adlersberg S, Rosen L *et al.* Trihexyphenidyl treatment of clozapine-induced hypersalivation. *International Clinical Psychopharmacology* 1997; 12: 213–215.
9. Reinstein MJ, Sirotovskaya LA, Chasanov MA *et al.* Comparative efficacy and tolerability of benzatropine and terazosin in the treatment of hypersalivation secondary to clozapine. *Clinical Drug Investigations* 1999; 17: 97–102.
10. Copp P, Lament R, Tennent TG. Amitriptyline in clozapine-induced sialorrhoea. *British Journal of Psychiatry* 1991; 159: 166.
11. Calderon J, Rubin E, Sobota WL. Potential use of ipratropium bromide for the treatment of clozapine-induced hypersalivation: a preliminary report. *International Clinical Psychopharmacology* 2000; 15: 49–52.
12. Antonello C, Tessier P. Clozapine and sialorrhea: a new intervention for this bothersome and potentially dangerous side effect. *Revue de Psychiatrie et de Neuroscience* 1999; 24: 250.
13. Grabowski J. Clonidine treatment of clozapine-induced hypersalivation. *Journal of Clinical Psychopharmacology* 1992; 12: 69.
14. Corrigan FM, Macdonald S. Clozapine-induced hypersalivation and the alpha 2 adrenoceptor. *British Journal Psychiatry* 1995; 167: 412.

Further reading

Cree A, Mir S, Fahy T. A review of the treatment options for clozapine-induced hypersalivation. *Psychiatric Bulletin* 2001; 25: 114–116.

Table Summary

Treatment	Comments	References*
Pirenzepine 25–100 mg/day	Selective M_1, M_4 antagonist	6,7
	Extensive clinical experience suggests efficacy in some but randomised trial suggests no effect. Still widely used	
Benzhexol (trihexyphenidyl) 5–15 mg/day	Small, open study suggests useful activity	8
	Widely used in some centres but may impair cognitive function	
Benztropine 2 mg/day + terazosin 2 mg/day	Combination shown to be better than either drug alone	9
	Not widely used	
Amitriptyline 75–100 mg/day	Limited literature support. Adverse effects may be troublesome	10
Ipratropium Nasal spray (0.03%) – given sublingually	Limited literature support. Rarely used	11
Atropine eye drops (1%) – given sublingually	Limited literature support. Rarely used	12
Clonidine (0.1 mg patch weekly or 0.1 mg orally at night)	α_2 partial agonist. Limited literature support. May exacerbate psychosis and depression	13
Lofexidine 0.2 mg twice daily	α_2 agonist. Very few data. May exacerbate psychosis and depression	14
Propantheline 7.5 mg at night	Peripheral anticholinergic. No central effects No published data	–
Hyoscine 0.3 mg sucked and swallowed up to 3 times daily	Peripheral and central anticholinergic	–
	Very widely used but no published data available	
	May cause cognitive impairment, drowsiness and constipation	

* References listed on page 54

Guidelines for the initiation of clozapine for patients based in the community

Note: this section provides general guidance – refer to manufacturer's and local policies (where available) for detailed guidance.

Some points to check before starting

- Is the patient likely to be compliant with oral medication?

- Has the patient understood the need for regular blood tests?

- Is it possible for the patient to be seen every day during the early titration phase?

- Is the patient able to attend the team base or pharmacy to collect medication every week?

- Does the patient need medication delivered to their home?

    Mandatory blood monitoring and registration with the Clozaril® Patient Monitoring Service (CPMS) or equivalent

- Register with the relevant monitoring service.

- Perform baseline blood tests (WCC and differential count) before starting clozapine.

- Further blood testing continues weekly for the first 18 weeks and then every 2 weeks for the remainder of the year. After that, the blood monitoring is done monthly.

Dosing (see table opposite)

Note: other schedules than that described below are possible (e.g. 12-week titration with twice-weekly monitoring).

- Day 1: start at 12.5 mg at night.

- Day 2: increase to 12.5 mg twice a day (unless the dose on day 1 is not tolerated).

- Day 3 and onwards: the dose may be increased by 25–50 mg a day, until a dose of 300 mg is reached. Estimate plasma level of clozapine at this point.

- Further dose increases should be made in increments of 50 mg a week until a dose of 450 mg or level of between 350 and 500 µg/l is achieved (see page 4).

- Doses up to 200 mg maybe given as a single dose at night.

- See table for a suggested titration regime.

- Clozapine levels are lower in males, smokers and younger adults (see page 4).

Switching from other antipsychotics

- The switching regime will be largely dependent on the patient's mental state.

- Consider additive side-effects of the antipsychotics (e.g. effect on QTc interval) (see page 75)

- Consider drug interactions (e.g. risperidone may increase clozapine levels).

- All depots, sertindole, pimozide, ziprasidone and thioridazine should be stopped before clozapine is started.

- Other antipsychotics and clozapine may be cross-tapered with varying degrees of caution.

Table Suggested titration regime – clozapine in the community

Day	Day of the week	Morning dose (mg)	Evening dose (mg)	Percentage dose of previous antipsychotic
1	Monday	–	12.5	100
2	Tuesday	12.5	12.5	
3	Wednesday	12.5	25	
4	Thursday	25	25	
5	Friday	25	50	
6	Saturday	25	50	
7	Sunday	25	50	
8	Monday	50	50	75
9	Tuesday	50	75	
10	Wednesday	50	75	
11	Thursday	50	100	
12	Friday	50	100	
13	Saturday	50	100	
14	Sunday	50	100	
15	Monday	75	100	50
16	Tuesday	75	100	
17	Wednesday	75	100	
18	Thursday	100	100	
19	Friday	100	100	
20	Saturday	100	100	
21	Sunday	100	100	
22	Monday	100	125	25
23	Tuesday	100	150	
24	Wednesday	100	175	
25	Thursday	100	200	
26	Friday	100	200	
27	Saturday	100	200	
28	Sunday	100	200	0

Clozapine in the community – acute monitoring requirements

- *Blood pressure (BP), temperature and pulse.* After the first dose, monitor BP, temperature and pulse 1–3 hours afterwards. (This may not be necessary if the first dose is given at bedtime.) Thereafter, the patient should be seen at least once a day and all 3 parameters should be monitored before and after the morning dose.

- Continue daily monitoring for at least 2 weeks or until there are no unacceptable adverse effects. Alternate day monitoring may then be undertaken until a stable dose is reached. Thereafter monitor at time of blood testing.

- The formal carer (usually the CPN) should inform the prescriber if:

  - **Temperature** rises above **38°C** (this is very common and is not a good reason, on its own, for stopping clozapine)

  - **Pulse** is **>100 bpm** (also common but may rarely be linked to myocarditis)

  - **Postural drop** of **>30 mmHg**

  - Patient is clearly over-sedated

  - Any other **adverse effect is intolerable**

Additional monitoring requirements (see page 30)

Baseline	I month	3 months	6 months	12 months
Weight	Weight	Weight	Weight	Weight
HbA$_{1C}$*	Plasma glucose*	HbA$_{1c}$*	HbA$_{1c}$*	HbA$_{1c}$*
LFTs			LFTs	
*Perform OGTT if HbA$_{1C}$ or plasma glucose raised				

Where available, consider also use of ECG (benefit not established). Consider monitoring plasma lipids.

Adverse effects

- Sedation and hypotension are common at the start of treatment. These effects can usually be managed by reducing the dose or slowing down the rate of titration.

- Many other adverse effects associated with clozapine can also be managed by dose reduction.

Management of adverse effects

See page 50.

Serious cardiac adverse effects (see page 52)

Patients who have a *persistent* tachycardia at rest, especially during the first 2 months of treatment, should be closely observed for other signs or symptoms of myocarditis or cardiomyopathy. These include palpitations, arrhythmias, symptoms mimicking myocardial infarction, chest pain and other unexplained symptoms of heart failure.

In patients with suspected clozapine-induced myocarditis or cardiomyopathy, the drug must be stopped and the patient be referred to a cardiologist. If clozapine-induced myocarditis or cardiomyopathy is confirmed the patient must not be re-exposed to clozapine.

Fish oils in schizophrenia

Fish oils contain the omega-3 fatty acids, eicosapentanoic acid (EPA) and docosahexanoic acid (DHA). These compounds are thought to be involved in maintaining neuronal membrane structure, in the modulation of membrane proteins and in the production of prostaglandins and leukotrienes[1]. They have been suggested as treatments for a variety of psychiatric illnesses[2] but most research relates to their use in schizophrenia, where case reports[3–5] and prospective trials suggest useful efficacy (see table).

Table A summary of the evidence – fish oils in schizophrenia

References	n	Design	Outcome
Mellor et al. 1995[6]	20	Open label evaluation of fish oil (EPA+DHA) added to usual medication	Significant improvement in symptoms
Peet et al. 2001[7]	45	Double-blind, randomised comparison of EPA (2 g daily), DHA and placebo (12 weeks)	EPA significantly more effective than DHA or placebo
Peet et al. 2001[7]	26	Double-blind, randomised comparison of EPA (2 g daily) or placebo as sole drug treatment (12 weeks)	All 12 patients given placebo required conventional antipsychotic treatment; 8 of 14 given EPA required antipsychotics. EPA more effective
Peet & Horrobin 2002[8]	115	Double-blind randomised comparison of ethyl-EPA (1, 2 or 4 g/day) and placebo added to antipsychotic treatment conventional, atypical or clozapine) (12 weeks)	Ethyl-EPA significantly improved response in patients receiving clozapine. 2 g/day most effective dose
Fenton et al. 2001[9]	87	Double-blind, randomised comparison of EPA (3 g daily) and placebo added to standard drug treatment (16 weeks)	No differences between EPA and placebo
Emsley et al. 2002[10]	40	Double-blind, randomised comparison of EPA (3 g daily) and placebo added to standard drug treatment (12 weeks)	EPA associated with significantly greater reduction in symptoms and tardive dyskinesia (9 patients in each group received clozapine)

On balance, evidence suggests that EPA (2–3 g daily) is a worthwhile option in schizophrenia when added to standard treatment, particularly clozapine. However, doubt still remains over the true extent of the beneficial effect derived from fish oils. Set against doubts over efficacy are the observations that fish oils are relatively cheap, well tolerated (mild GI symptoms may occur) and may benefit physical health[1].

Fish oils are therefore very tentatively recommended for the treatment of residual symptoms of schizophrenia but particularly in patients responding poorly to clozapine. Careful assessment of response is essential and fish oils should be withdrawn if no effect is observed after 3 months' treatment.

The recommended dose is
Omacor (414 mg EPA) 5 capsules daily *or* **Maxepa (170 mg EPA) 10 capsules daily**

References

1. Fenton WS, Hibbeln J, Knable M. Fatty acids in schizophrenia. *Biological Psychiatry* 2000; **47**: 821.
2. Freeman MP. Omega-3 fatty acids in psychiatry: a review. *Annals of Clinical Psychiatry* 2000; **12**: 159–165.
3. Richardson AJ, Easton T, Puri BK. Red cell and plasma fatty acid changes accompanying symptom remission in a patient with schizophrenia treated with eicosapentaenoic acid. *European Neuropsychopharmacology* 2000; **10**: 189–193.
4. Puri BK, Richardson AJ, Horrobin DF *et al*. Eicosapentaenoic acid treatment in schizophrenia associated with symptom remission, normalisation of blood fatty acids, reduced neuronal membrane phospholipid turnover and structural brain changes. *International Journal of Clinical Practice* 2000; **54**: 57–63.
5. Su K-P, Shen W, Huang S-Y. Omega-3 fatty acids as a psychotherapeutic agent for a pregnant schizophrenic patient. *European Neuropsychopharmacology* 2001; **11**: 295–299.
6. Mellor JE, Laugharne JD, Peet M. Schizophrenic symptoms and dietary intake of n3 fatty acids. *Schizophrenia Research* 1995; **18**: 85–86.
7. Peet M, Brind J, Ramchand CN *et al*. Two double-blind placebo-controlled pilot studies of eicosapentaenoic acid in the treatment of schizophrenia. *Schizophrenia Research* 2001; **49**: 243–251.
8. Peet M, Horrobin DF. A dose-ranging exploratory study of the effects of ethyl-eicosapentaenoate in patients with persistent schizophrenic symptoms. *Journal of Psychiatric Research* 2002; **36**: 7–18.
9. Fenton WS, Dickerson F, Boronow J *et al*. A placebo-controlled trial of omega-3 fatty acid (ethyl eicosapentaenoic acid) supplementation for residual symptoms and cognitive impairment in schizophrenia. *American Journal of Psychiatry* 2001; **158**: 2071–2074.
10. Emsley R, Myburgh C, Oosthuizen P *et al*. Randomized, placebo-controlled study of ethyl-eicosapentaenoic acid as supplemental treatment in schizophrenia. *American Journal of Psychiatry* 2002; **159**: 1596–1598.

Further reading

Joy CB, Mumby-Croft R, Joy LA. Polyunsaturated fatty acid (fish or evening primrose oil) for schizophrenia (Cochrane Review). In: The Cochrane Library, Issue 4. Oxford: Update software, 2002.

Extrapyramidal side-effects

Table Most common extrapyramidal side-effects

	Dystonia (uncontrolled muscular spasm)	Pseudo-parkinsonism (tremor, etc.)	Akathisia (restlessness)	Tardive dyskinesia (abnormal movements)
Signs & symptoms[1]	Muscle spasm in any part of the body, e.g. • Eyes rolling upwards (oculogyric crisis) • Head and neck twisted to the side (torticollis) *The patient may be unable to swallow or speak clearly. In extreme cases, the back may arch or the jaw dislocate* Acute dystonia can be both painful and very frightening	• Tremor and/or rigidity • Bradykinesia (decreased facial expression, flat monotone voice, slow body movements, inability to initiate movement) • Bradyphrenia (slowed thinking) • Salivation Pseudoparkinsonism can be mistaken for depression or the negative symptoms of schizophrenia	A subjectively unpleasant state of inner restlessness where there is a strong desire or compulsion to move • Foot stamping when seated • Constantly crossing/uncrossing legs • Rocking from foot to foot • Constantly pacing up and down Akathisia can be mistaken for psychotic agitation and has been linked with suicide and aggression towards others	A wide variety of movements can occur such as: • Lip smacking or chewing • Tongue protrusion (fly catching) • Choreiform hand movements (pill rolling or piano playing) • Pelvic thrusting Severe orofacial movements can lead to difficulty speaking, eating or breathing. Movements are worse when under stress
Rating scales	No specific scale Small component of general EPSE scales	Simpson–Angus EPSE Rating Scale[2]	Barnes Akathisia Scale[3]	Abnormal Involuntary Movement Scale[4] (AIMS)
Prevalence (with older drugs)	Approximately 10%[5], but more common[6]: • In young males • In the neuroleptic-naive • With high potency drugs (e.g. haloperidol) Dystonic reactions are rare in the elderly	Approximately 20%[7], but more common in: • Elderly females • Those with pre-existing neurological damage (head injury, stroke, etc.)	Approximately 25%[8]	5% of patients per year of anti-psychotic exposure[9]. More common in: • Elderly women • Those with affective illness • Those who have had acute EPSEs early on in treatment

	Dystonia (uncontrolled muscular spasm)	Pseudo-parkinsonism (tremor, etc.)	Akathisia (restlessness)	Tardive dyskinesia (abnormal movements)
Time taken to develop	Acute dystonia can occur within hours of starting antipsychotics (minutes if the IM or IV route is used) Tardive dystonia occurs after months to years of antipsychotic treatment	Days to weeks after antipsychotic drugs are started or the dose is increased	Acute akathisia occurs within hours to weeks of starting antipsychotics or increasing the dose. Tardive akathisia takes longer to develop and can persist after antipsychotics have been withdrawn	Months to years Approximately 50% of cases are reversible[9]
Treatment	Anticholinergic drugs given orally, IM or IV depending on the severity of symptoms[6] • Remember the patient may be unable to swallow • Response to IV administration will be seen within 5 minutes • Response to IM administration takes around 20 minutes	Several options are available depending on the clinical circumstances: • Reduce the antipsychotic dose • Change to an atypical drug (as antipsychotic monotherapy!) • Prescribe an anticholinergic. The majority of patients do not require long-term anticholinergics. Use should be reviewed at least every 3 months	• Reduce the antipsychotic dose • Change to an atypical drug • A reduction in symptoms may be seen with[10]: – Propranolol 30–80 mg/day – Cyproheptadine 8–16 mg/day – Clonazepam (low dose) All are unlicenced for this indication Anticholinergics are generally unhelpful	• Stop anticholinergic if prescribed • Reduce dose of antipsychotic • Change to an atypical drug[11] • Clozapine is the most likely antipsychotic to be associated with resolution of symptoms[12] • Other drugs such as valproate, tetrabenazine, clonazepam etc., but the evidence base is poor[13]

63

EPSEs are:

- dose-related

- uncommon with atypicals

- more likely with high-potency typicals.

References

1. Gervin M, Barnes TRE. Assessment of drug-related movement disorders in schizophrenia. *Advances in Psychiatric Treatment* 2000; **6**: 332–334.
2. Simpson GM, Angus JWS. A rating scale for extrapyramidal side-effects. *Acta Psychiatrica Scandinavica* 1970; **212**: 11–19.
3. Barnes TRE. A rating scale for drug-induced akathisia. *British Journal of Psychiatry* 1989; **154**: 672–676.
4. Guy W. *ECDEU assessment manual for psychopharmacology.* Washington DC: US Department of Health, Education and Welfare, 1976, pp. 534–537.
5. American Psychiatric Association. Practice guideline for the treatment of schizophrenia. *American Journal of Psychiatry* 1997; **154**(4 Suppl.): 1–63.
6. van Harten PN, Hoek HW, Kahn RS. Acute dystonia induced by drug treatment. *BMJ* 1999; **319**: 623–626.
7. Bollini P, Pampallona S, Orgam J *et al.* Antipsychotic drugs: is more worse? A meta-analysis of the randomised controlled trials. *Psychological Medicine* 1994; **24**: 307–316.
8. Halstead SM, Barnes TRE, Speller JC. Akathisia: prevalence and associated dysphoria in an in-patient population with chronic schizophrenia. *British Journal of Psychiatry* 1994; **164**: 177–183.
9. American Psychiatric Association. *Tardive dyskinesia: a task force report of the American Psychiatric Association.* Washington DC: American Psychiatric Association, 1992.
10. Miller CH, Fleischaker WW. Managing antipsychotic induced acute and chronic akathisia. *Drug Safety* 2000; **22**: 73–81.
11. Glazer W. Expected incidence of tardive dyskinesia associated with atypical antipsychotics. *Journal of Clinical Psychiatry* 2000; **61**(Suppl. 4): 21–26.
12. Simpson GM. The treatment of tardive dyskinesia and tardive dystonia. *Journal of Clinical Psychiatry* 2000; **61**(Suppl. 4): 39–44.
13. Duncan D, McConnell H, Taylor D. Tardive dyskinesia: how is it prevented and treated? *Psychiatric Bulletin* 1997; **21**: 422–425.

Treatment of symptomatic, antipsychotic-induced hyperprolactinaemia

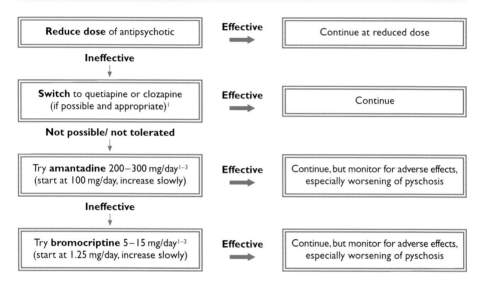

Reduce dose of antipsychotic	**Effective** →	Continue at reduced dose

Ineffective ↓

Switch to quetiapine or clozapine (if possible and appropriate)[1]	**Effective** →	Continue

Not possible/ not tolerated ↓

Try **amantadine** 200–300 mg/day[1–3] (start at 100 mg/day, increase slowly)	**Effective** →	Continue, but monitor for adverse effects, especially worsening of pyschosis

Ineffective ↓

Try **bromocriptine** 5–15 mg/day[1–3] (start at 1.25 mg/day, increase slowly)	**Effective** →	Continue, but monitor for adverse effects, especially worsening of pyschosis

Notes:
- Hyperprolactinaemia is often asymptomatic. Adverse effects, when they do occur, are sometimes mild and do not affect quality of life. However, subtle long-term effects may occur. These include osteoporosis[4] and suppression of the hypothalamic–pituitary gonadal axis[5].
- Before starting treatment, take a full sexual/menstrual history to establish whether or not symptoms are related to antipsychotic use.
- Other causes of hyperprolactinaemia (e.g. prolactin-secreting tumour) must be considered.
- Evaluate efficacy of each treatment option over at least one month: prolactin levels may fall within days, but adverse effects such as gynaecomastia respond more slowly.
- Withdraw previously ineffective treatments before starting the next option in the algorithm.
- Olanzapine causes dose-dependent, transient hyperprolactinaemia[6]. Symptoms are rare, especially at 10 mg/day. Ziprasidone[7] and aripiprazole[8], too, have minimal effects on prolactin but experience is limited.
- Risk of psychosis with amantadine and bromocriptine renders them effectively obsolete, given alternatives available.

References

1. Hammer MB, Arana GW. Hyperprolactinaemia in antipsychotic-treated patients: guidelines for avoidance and management. *CNS Drugs* 1998; Sept 10: 209–222.
2. Duncan D, Taylor D. Treatment of psychotropic-induced hyperprolactinaemia. *Psychiatric Bulletin* 1995; **19**: 755–757.
3. Marken PA, Haykal RF, Fisher JN. Management of psychotropic-induced hyperprolactinemia. *Clinical Pharmacology* 1992; **11**: 851–856.
4. Halbreich U, Palter S. Accelerated osteoporosis in psychiatric patients: possible pathophysiological processes. *Schizophrenia Bulletin* 1996; **22**: 447–454.
5. Smith S, Wheeler MJ, Murrey R *et al.* The effects of antipsychotic-induced hyperprolactinaemia on the hypothalamic-pituitary-gonadal axis. *Journal of Clinical Psychopharmacology* 2002; **22**: 109–114.
6. David SR, Taylor Cc, Kinon BJ *et al.* The effects of olanzapine, risperidone, and haloperidol on plasma prolactin levels in patients with schizophrenia. *Clinical Therapeutics* 2000; **22**: 1085–1095.
7. Taylor D. Ziprasidone – an atypical antipsychotic. *Pharmaceutical Journal* 2001; **266**: 396–401.
8. Taylor D. Aripiprazole: a review of its pharmacology and clinical use. *International Journal of Clinical Practice* 2003; **57**: 49–54.

Algorithm for the treatment of antipsychotic-induced akathisia

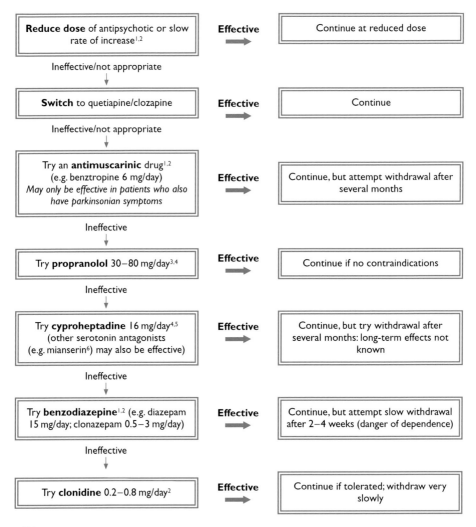

Reduce dose of antipsychotic or slow rate of increase[1,2]	Effective ⟹	Continue at reduced dose

Ineffective/not appropriate ↓

Switch to quetiapine/clozapine	Effective ⟹	Continue

Ineffective/not appropriate ↓

Try an **antimuscarinic** drug[1,2] (e.g. benztropine 6 mg/day) *May only be effective in patients who also have parkinsonian symptoms*	Effective ⟹	Continue, but attempt withdrawal after several months

Ineffective ↓

Try **propranolol** 30–80 mg/day[3,4]	Effective ⟹	Continue if no contraindications

Ineffective ↓

Try **cyproheptadine** 16 mg/day[4,5] (other serotonin antagonists (e.g. mianserin[6]) may also be effective)	Effective ⟹	Continue, but try withdrawal after several months: long-term effects not known

Ineffective ↓

Try **benzodiazepine**[1,2] (e.g. diazepam 15 mg/day; clonazepam 0.5–3 mg/day)	Effective ⟹	Continue, but attempt slow withdrawal after 2–4 weeks (danger of dependence)

Ineffective ↓

Try **clonidine** 0.2–0.8 mg/day[2]	Effective ⟹	Continue if tolerated; withdraw very slowly

Notes:
- Akathisia is sometimes difficult to diagnose with certainty. A careful history of symptoms and drug use is essential. Note that severe akathisia may be linked to violent or suicidal behaviour[7–9].
- Evaluate efficacy of each treatment option over at least one month. Some effect may be seen after a few days but it may take much longer to become apparent in those with chronic akathisia.
- Withdraw previously ineffective treatments before starting the next option in the algorithm.
- Combinations of treatment may be used in refractory cases if carefully monitored.
- Consider tardive akathisia in patients on long-term therapy.

References

1. Fleischhacker WW, Roth SD, Kane JM. The pharmacologic treatment of neuroleptic-induced akathisia. *Journal of Clinical Psychopharmacology* 1990; **10**: 12–21.
2. Sachdev P. The identification and management of drug-induced akathisia. *CNS Drugs* 1995; **4**: 28–46.
3. Adler L, Angrist B, Peselow E, *et al*. A controlled assessment of propranolol in the treatment of neuroleptic-induced akathisia. *British Journal of Psychiatry* 1986; **149**: 42–45.
4. Fischel T, Hermesh H, Aizenberg D *et al*. Cyproheptadine versus propranolol for the treatment of acute neuroleptic-induced akathisia: a comparative double-blind study. *Journal of Clinical Psychopharmacology* 2001; **21**: 612–615.
5. Weiss D, Aizenberg D, Hermesh H *et al*. Cyproheptadine treatment of neuroleptic-induced akathisia. *British Journal of Psychiatry* 1995; **167**: 483–486.
6. Poyurovsky M, Shadorodsky M, Fuchs M *et al*. Treatment of neuroleptic-induced akathisia with the 5HT$_2$ antagonist mianserin. *British Journal of Psychiatry* 1999; **174**: 238–242.
7. Drake RE, Ehrlich J. Suicide attempts associated with akathisia. *American Journal of Psychiatry* 1985; **142**: 499–501.
8. Azhar MZ, Varma SL. Akathisia-induced suicidal behaviour. *European Psychiatry* 1992; 7: 239–241.
9. Hansen L. A critical review of akathisia, and its possible association with suicidal behaviour. *Human Psychopharmacology* 2001; **16**: 495–505.

Further reading

Maidment I. Use of serotonin antagonists in the treatment of neuroleptic-induced akathisia. *Psychiatric Bulletin* 2000; **24**: 348–351.

Treatment of tardive dyskinesia

Despite the introduction and widespread use of atypical antipsychotics, tardive dyskinesia (TD) remains a commonly encountered phenomenon[1]. Treatment of established TD is often unsuccessful, so prevention and early detection are essential. There is some evidence that the use of some atypical drugs is associated with lower rates of TD[2,3] but this is somewhat controversial. Clozapine seems to have an extremely low rate of TD[4].

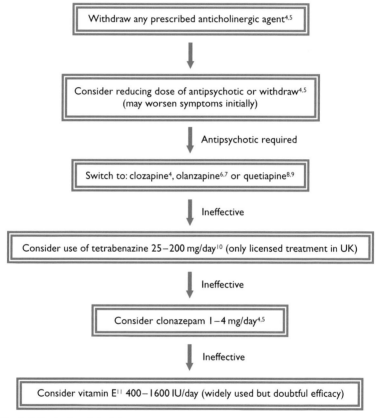

Other putative treatments include:

$5HT_3$ antagonists[12,13]
(e.g. ondansetron 12 mg/day)

Pyridoxine (B_6) up to 400 mg/day[14]

Melatonin 10 mg/day[15]

Donepezil 10 mg/day[16]

References

1. Halliday J, Farrington S, MacDonald S *et al.* Nithsdale schizophrenia surveys 23: movement disorders – 20-year review. *British Journal of Psychiatry* 2002; **181**: 422–427.
2. Beasley CM, Dellva MA, Tamura RN. Randomised double-blind comparison of the incidence of tardive dyskinesia in patients with schizophrenia during long-term treatment with olanzapine or haloperidol. *British Journal of Psychiatry* 1999; **174**: 23–30.
3. Glazer WM. Expected incidence of tardive dyskinesia associated with atypical antipsychotics. *Journal of Clinical Psychiatry* 2000; **61**(Suppl. 4): 21–26.
4. Duncan D, McConnell H, Taylor D. Tardive dyskinesia – how is it prevented and treated? *Psychiatric Bulletin* 1977; **21**: 422–425.
5. Simpson GM. The treatment of tardive dyskinesia and tardive dystonia. *Journal of Clinical Psychiatry* 2000; **61**(Suppl. 4): 39–44.
6. Soutullo CA, Keck PE, McElroy SL. Olanzapine in the treatment of tardive dyskinesia: a report of two cases. *Journal of Clinical Psychopharmacology* 1999; **19**: 100–101 (Letter).
7. Kinon BJ, Milton DR, Stauffer VL, *et al.* Effect of chronic olanzapine treatment on the course of presumptive tardive dyskinesia. Presented at American Psychiatric Association 152nd Annual Meeting, May 1999, Washington DC.
8. Vesely C, Küfferle B, Brücke T, *et al.* Remission of severe tardive dyskinesia in a schizophrenic patient treated with the atypical antipsychotic substance quetiapine. *International Clinical Psychopharmacology* 2000; **15**: 57–60.
9. Alptekin K and Kivircik AK. Quetiapine-induced improvement of tardive dyskinesia in three patients with schizophrenia. *International Clinical Psychopharmacology* 2002; **17**: 263–264.
10. Jankovic J and Beach J. Long-term effects of tetrabenazine in hyperkinetic movement disorders. *Neurology* 1997; **48**: 358–362.
11. Adler LA, Rotrosen J, Edson R *et al.* Vitamin E treatment for tardive dyskinesia. *Archives of General Psychiatry* 1999; **56**: 836–841.
12. Sirota P, Mosheva T, Shabtay H *et al.* Use of the selective serotonin 3 receptor antagonist ondansetron in the treatment of neuroleptic-induced tardive dyskinesia. *American Journal of Psychiatry* 2000; **157**: 287–289.
13. Naidu PS, Kulkarni SK. Reversal of neuroleptic-induced orofacial dyskinesia by 5-HT3 receptor antagonists. *European Journal of Pharmacology* 2001; **420**: 113–117.
14. Lerner V, Miodownik C, Kaptsan A *et al.* Vitamin B6 in the treatment of tardive dyskinesia: a double-blind, placebo-controlled study. *American Journal of Psychiatry* 2001; **158**: 1511–1514.
15. Shamir E, Barak Y, Shalman I *et al.* Melatonin treatment for tardive dyskinesia: a double-blind, placebo-controlled, crossover study. *Archives of General Psychiatry* 2001; **58**: 1049–1052.
16. Caroff SN, Campbell EC, Havey JC *et al.* Treatment of tardive dyskinesia with donepezil. *Journal of Clinical Psychiatry* 2001; **62**: 128–129.

Neuroleptic malignant syndrome

Neuroleptic malignant syndrome (NMS) is a rare but potentially serious even fatal adverse effect of all antipsychotics. NMS is a syndrome largely of sympathetic hyperactivity occurring as a result of dopaminergic antagonism in the context of psychological stressors and genetic predisposition[1]. Although widely seen as an acute, severe syndrome, NMS may, in many cases, have few signs and symptoms; 'full blown' NMS may thus represent the extreme of a range of non-malignant related symptoms[2].

The incidence and mortality of NMS are difficult to establish and probably vary as drug use changes and recognition increases. It has been estimated that less than 1% of all patients treated with conventional antipsychotics will experience NMS[3]. Incidence figures for atypical drugs are not available, but all have been reported to be associated with the syndrome[4-7]. NMS is also very rarely seen with other drugs such as antidepressants[8,9].

Table Neuroleptic malignant syndrome	
Signs and symptoms[1,3,10,11]	Fever, diaphoresis, rigidity, confusion, fluctuating consciousness
	Fluctuating blood pressure, tachycardia
	Elevated creatinine kinase, leukocytosis, altered liver function tests
Risk factors[10-13]	High potency typical drugs, recent or rapid dose increase, rapid dose reduction, abrupt withdrawal of anticholinergics
	Psychosis, organic brain disease, alcoholism, Parkinson's disease, hyperthyroidism
	Agitation, dehydration
Treatments[3,10,14-16]	In the psychiatric unit: Withdraw antipsychotics, monitor temperature, pulse, BP
	In the medical/A&E unit: Rehydration, bromocriptine + dantrolene, sedation with benzodiazepines, artificial ventilation if required
	L-dopa and carbamazepine have also been used, among many other drugs. Consider ECT for treatment of psychosis
Restarting antipsychotics[10,14,17]	Antipsychotic treatment will be required in most instances and rechallenge is associated with acceptable risk
	Stop antipsychotics for at least 5 days, preferably longer. Allow time for symptoms and signs to resolve completely
	Begin with very small dose and increase very slowly with close monitoring of temperature, pulse and blood pressure. CK monitoring may be used, but is controversial
	Consider using an antipsychotic structurally unrelated to that associated with NMS or a drug with low dopamine affinity (quetiapine or clozapine)
	Avoid depots and high potency conventional antipsychotics

References

1. Gurrera RJ. Sympathoadrenal hyperactivity and the etiology of neuroleptic malignant syndrome. *American Journal of Psychiatry* 1999; **156**: 169–180.
2. Bristow MF, Kohen D. How 'malignant' is the neuroleptic malignant syndrome? In early mild cases it may not be malignant at all. *BMJ* 1993; **307**: 1223–1224.
3. Guzé BH, Baxter LR. Neuroleptic malignant syndrome. *New England Journal of Medicine* 1995; **313**: 163–165.
4. Hasan S, Buckley P. Novel antipsychotics and the neuroleptic malignant syndrome: a review and critique. *American Journal of Psychiatry* 1998; **155**: 1113–1116.
5. Sierra-Biddle D, Herran A, Diez-Aja S *et al.* Neuroleptic malignant syndrome and olanzapine. *Journal of Clinical Psychopharmacology* 2000; **20**: 704–705.
6. Stanley AK, Hunter J. Possible neuroleptic malignant syndrome with quetiapine. *British Journal of Psychiatry* 2000; **176**: 497.
7. Gallarda T, Olié J-P. Neuroleptic malignant syndrome in a 72-year-old-man with Alzheimer's disease: a case report and review of the literature. *European Neuropsychopharmacology* 2000; **10**(Suppl. 3): 357.
8. June R, Yunus M, Gossman W. Neuroleptic malignant syndrome associated with nortriptyline. *American Journal of Emergency Medicine* 1999; **17**: 736–737.
9. Young C. A case of neuroleptic malignant syndrome and serotonin disturbance. *Journal of Clinical Psychopharmacology* 1997; **17**: 65–66.
10. Levenson JL. Neuroleptic malignant syndrome. *American Journal of Psychiatry*, 1985; **142**: 1137–1145.
11. Hermesh H, Manor I, Shiloh R *et al.* High serum creatinine kinase level: possible risk factor for neuroleptic malignant syndrome. *Journal of Clinical Psychopharmacology* 2002; **22**: 252–256.
12. Spivak B, Gonen N, Mester R *et al.* Neuroleptic malignant syndrome associated with abrupt withdrawal of anticholinergic agents. *International Clinical Psychopharmacology* 1996; **11**: 207–209.
13. Spivak B, Weizman A, Wolovick L *et al.* Neuroleptic malignant syndrome during abrupt reduction of neuroleptic treatment. *Acta Psychiatrica Scandinavica* 1990; **81**: 168–169.
14. Olmsted TR. Neuroleptic malignant syndrome: guidelines for treatment and reinstitution of neuroleptics. *Southern Medical Journal* 1988; **81**: 888–891.
15. Shoop SA, Cernek PK. Carbidopa/levodopa in the treatment of neuroleptic malignant syndrome (letter). *Annals of Pharmacotherapy* 1997; **31**: 119.
16. Terao T. Carbamazepine in the treatment of neuroleptic malignant syndrome (letter). *Biological Psychiatry* 1999; **45**: 378–382.
17. Wells AJ, Sommi RW, Chrismon ML. Neuroleptic rechallenge after neuroleptic malignant syndrome: case report and literature review. *Drug Intelligence and Clinical Pharmacy* 1988; **22**: 475–480.

Antipsychotic-induced weight gain

Antipsychotics have long been recognised as weight-inducing agents. Suggested mechanisms include $5HT_{2C}$ antagonism, H_1 antagonism, hyperprolactinaemia and increased serum leptin (leading to leptin desensitisation)[1–3]. There is no evidence that drugs exert any direct metabolic effect: weight gain seems to result from increased food intake and, in some cases, reduced energy expenditure[4]. Risk of weight gain appears to be related to clinical response[5] and may also have a genetic basis[6].

All available antipsychotics have been associated with weight gain, although mean weight gained varies substantially between drugs. With all drugs, some patients gain no weight. Assessment of relative risk is made difficult by the poor quality of available data and the scarcity of long-term data. The following table suggest approximate relative risk of weight gain and mean weight gain (based on two systematic reviews[7,8]).

(See also page 73 for advice of treating drug-induced weight gain and page 27 for switching strategies.)

Table Drug-induced weight gain

Drug	Risk/extent of weight gain
Clozapine Olanzapine	**High**
Zotepine Thioridazine	**Moderate/high**
Chlorpromazine Quetiapine Risperidone	**Moderate**
Amisulpride Aripiprazole Haloperidol Trifluoperazine Ziprasidone	**Low**

References

1. McIntyre RS, Mancini DA, Basile VS. Mechanisms of antipsychotic-induced weight gain. *Journal of Clinical Psychiatry* 2001; **62**(Suppl. 23): 23–29.
2. Herran A, Garcia-Unzueta MT, Amado JA *et al.* Effects of long-term treatment with antipsychotics on serum leptin levels. *British Journal of Psychiatry* 2001; **179**: 59–62.
3. Monteleone P, Fabrazzo M, Tortorella A *et al.* Pronounced early increase in circulating leptin predicts lower weight gain during clozapine treatment. *Journal of Clinical Psychopharmacology* 2002; **22**: 424–426.
4. Virkkunen M, Wahlbeck K, Rissanen A *et al.* Decrease of energy expenditure causes weight increase in olanzapine treatment – a case study. *Pharmacopsychiatry* 2002; **35**: 124–126.
5. Czobor P, Volavka J, Sheitman B *et al.* Antipsychotic-induced weight gain and therapeutic response: a differential association. *Journal of Clinical Psychopharmacology* 2002; **22**: 244–251.
6. Basile VS, Masellis M, McIntyre RS *et al.* Genetic dissection of atypical antipsychotic-induced weight gain: novel preliminary data on the pharmacogenetic puzzle. *Journal of Clinical Psychiatry* 2001; **62**(Suppl. 23): 45–66.
7. Allison DB, Mentore JL, Moonseong H *et al.* Antipsychotic-induced weight gain: a comprehensive research synthesis. *American Journal of Psychiatry* 1999; **156**: 1686–1696.
8. Taylor DM, McAskill R. Atypical antipsychotics and weight gain – a systematic review. *Acta Psychiatrica Scandinavica* 2000; **101**: 416–432.

Treatment of drug-induced weight gain

Weight gain is socially disabling and confers important changes in cardiac mortality. Prevention and treatment are therefore matters of clinical urgency.

At present, treatment of drug-induced weight gain is not well informed by published data. Where weight gain is particularly associated with an individual drug then, where possible, switching to a drug with a lower potential for weight gain seems a sensible option. Note, however, that the effects of switching are poorly researched; clinical experience suggests that weight loss following switching is uncommon but that a reduction in the rate of weight gain can be expected.

Table Treatment of drug-induced weight gain: a summary of available data		
Intervention	**Comments**	**References**
Behavioural modification – diet and exercise	Involve nutritionist where possible	1,2
	Outcome highly variable – patient's motivation is predictor of success	
Switch to drug less likely to cause weight gain	Few data	3 (see page 72)
	Most psychotropics are weight-neutral or weight-gaining, so weight loss is unlikely	
Topiramate up to 150 mg daily	Causes sedation and is (rarely) linked to confusion and cognitive impairment Developing evidence base to support its use in drug-induced weight gain	4–7
Orlistat 120 mg tds pc	Reliable effect in obesity when combined with hypocalorific diet. Adverse effects socially undesirable	8,9
	Limited data suggest it does not affect pharmacokinetics of psychotropics	
Sibutramine 10–15 mg daily	Serotonergic drug associated with mania and anxiety. Hypertension may also be problematic. No studies in drug-induced weight gain	10
Metformin 500 mg tds	Possibly effective. Reduces plasma glucose	11
Reboxetine 4 mg daily	May attenuate olanzapine-induced weight gain	12
Methylcellulose 1500 mg before food	Anecdotal reports of good outcome. Rather unpalatable. No published evidence in drug-induced weight gain	
H₂ antagonists	Equivocal data	10
Fluoxetine	Probably not effective	10
Phenylpropanolamine	Probably not effective	13

Where switching is not an option, then behavioural methods are probably the treatment of first choice. The basis of these methods is the reduction in energy intake (via reduced intake of fat and sugar) and increase in energy expenditure. In the latter case, simply altering daily activity or travel arrangements is probably sufficient (walking instead of catching the bus, for example). The basic message is 'eat a little less, exercise a little more; keep doing it'. If possible, a nutritionist should be involved.

Behavioural methods may be used alongside pharmacological interventions. The table on page 73 summarises available data on the treatment of drug-induced weight gain.

References

1. Pendlebury J, Ost D. Cromwell house weight management programme for patients with severe enduring mental illness: preliminary results. Poster presented at ECNP Annual Congress. Barcelona, Spain, 5–9 October, 2002.
2. Cohen S, Glazewski R, Khan S *et al.* Weight gain with risperidone among patients with mental retardation: effect of calorie restriction. *Journal of Clinical Psychiatry* 2001; **62**: 114–116.
3. Gilbert J, Leal C, Bovio H *et al.* Switching to quetiapine in schizophrenic patients with antipsychotic-induced weight gain. Poster presented at the 15th European College of Neuropsychopharmacology Congress, Barcelona, Spain, 5–9 October, 2002.
4. Dursun SM, Devarajan S. Clozapine weight gain plus topiramate weight loss. *Canadian Journal of Psychiatry* 2000; **45**: 198.
5. Levy E, Margolese HC, Chouinard G. Topiramate produced weight loss following olanzapine-induced weight gain in schizophrenia. *Journal of Clinical Psychiatry* 2002; **63**: 1045.
6. Van Ameringen M, Mancini C, Campbell M *et al.* Topiramate treatment for SSRI-induced weight gain in anxiety disorders. *Journal of Clinical Psychiatry* 2002; **63**: 981–984.
7. Appolinario J C, Fontenelle L F, Papelbaum M *et al.* Topiramate use in obese patients with binge eating disorder: an open study. *Canadian Journal of Psychiatry* 2002; **47**: 271–273.
8. Sjostrom L, Rissanen A, Andersen T *et al.* Randomised placebo-controlled trial of orlistat for weight loss and prevention of weight regain in obese patients. *Lancet* 1998; **352**: 167–172.
9. Hilger E, Quiner S, Ginzel MD *et al.* The effect of orlistat on plasma levels of psychotropic drugs in patients with long-term psychopharmacotherapy. *Journal of Clinical Psychopharmacology* 2002; **22**: 68–70.
10. Werneke U, Taylor D, Sanders TAB. Options for pharmacological management of obesity in patients treated with atypical antipsychotics. *International Clinical Psychopharmacology* 2002; **17**: 145–159.
11. Morrison JA, Cottingham EM, Barton BA. Metformin for weight loss in pediatric patients taking psychotropic drugs. *American Journal of Psychiatry* 2002; **159**: 655–657.
12. Poyurovsky M, Isaacs I, Fuchs C *et al.* Reboxetine attenuates olanzapine-induced weight gain in schizophrenia patients. A double-blind placebo-controlled study. Poster presented at ECNP Annual Congress. Barcelona, Spain, 5–9 October, 2002.
13. Borovicka MC, Fuller MA, Konicki PE *et al.* Phenylpropanolamine appears not to promote weight loss in patients with schizophrenia who have gained weight during clozapine treatment. *Journal of Clinical Psychiatry* 2002; **63**: 345–348.

Psychotropic-related QT prolongation

Introduction

Many psychotropic drugs are associated with ECG changes and it is possible that certain drugs are linked to serious ventricular arrhythmias and sudden cardiac death. Specifically, some agents are linked to prolongation of the cardiac QT interval, a risk factor for the ventricular arrhythmia torsade de pointes, which is occasionally fatal. Recent case control studies have suggested that the use of some antipsychotics is associated with an increase in the rate of sudden cardiac death[1,2]. Overall risk, however, remains extremely low.

ECG monitoring of drug-induced changes in a mental health trust is complicated by a number of factors. Psychiatrists may have limited expertise in ECG interpretation, for example. (Self-reading, computerised ECG devices are available and to some extent compensate for some lack of expertise.) In addition, ECG machines may not be as readily available in all clinical areas as they are in general medicine. Also, time for ECG determination may not be available in many areas (e.g. outpatients). Lastly, ECG determination may be difficult to perform in acutely disturbed, physically uncooperative patients.

ECG monitoring of all patients is therefore impracticable and, given that risks are probably very small, of dubious benefit. This section sets out a pragmatic strategy for risk reduction and should be seen as guidance on minimising the *possible* risk associated with some drugs.

QT prolongation

- The cardiac QT interval (usually as QTc – QT corrected for heart rate) is a useful, but imprecise indicator of risk of Torsade de Pointes and of increased cardiac mortality[3]. Different correction factors and methods may give markedly different values[4].

- There is considerable controversy over the exact association between QTc and risk of arrhythmia. Very limited evidence suggests that risk is exponentially related to the extent of prolongation beyond normal limits (440 ms for men; 470 ms for women), although there are well-known exceptions which appear to disprove this theory[5]. Rather stronger evidence links QTc values over 500 ms to a clearly increased risk of arrhythmia[6].

- QTc measurements and evaluation are complicated by:
  - difficulty in determining the end of the T wave, particularly where U waves are present (this applies both to manual and self-reading ECG machines)[6];
  - normal physiological variation in QTc interval: QT varies with gender, time of day, food intake, alcohol intake, menstrual cycle, ECG lead, etc.[4,5];
  - variation in the extent of drug-induced prolongation of QTc because of changes in plasma levels. QTc prolongation is most prominent at peak drug plasma levels and least obvious at trough levels[4,5].

Other ECG changes

Other reported drug-induced changes include atrial fibrillation, giant P waves, T-wave changes, and heart block[5]. These occur much less commonly than QTc changes (with the possible exception of changes in T-wave morphology).

Quantifying risk

Drugs are categorised here according to data available on their effects on the cardiac QTc interval (as calculated using Bazett's correction formula). 'No-effect' drugs are those with which QTc prolongation has not been reported either at therapeutic doses or in overdose. 'Low-effect' drugs are those for which severe QTc prolongation has been reported *only* following overdose or where only small average increases (<10 ms) have been observed at clinical doses. 'Moderate-effect' drugs are those which have been observed to prolong QTc by >10 ms on average when given at normal clinical doses or where ECG monitoring is officially recommended in some circumstances. 'High-effect' drugs are those for which extensive average QTc prolongation (usually >20 ms at normal clinical doses) has been noted or where ECG monitoring is mandated by the manufacturer's data sheet.

Note that effect on QTc may not necessarily equate to risk of torsade de pointes or sudden death, although this is often assumed. Note also that categorisation is inevitably approximate given the problems associated with QTc measurements.

Table Psychotropics – effect on QTc[4,5,7]

No effect	Moderate effect
Amisulpride	Chlorpromazine
Aripiprazole	Quetiapine
Olanzapine	Ziprasidone
Sulpiride	Zotepine
	TCAs
SSRIs (except citalopram)	
Reboxetine	
Nefazodone	**High effect**
Mirtazapine	Any intravenous antipsychotic
MAOIs	Thioridazine
	Pimozide
Carbamazepine	Sertindole
Gabapentin	
Lamotrigine	Any drug or combination of drugs used in doses
Valproate	exceeding recommended maximum
Benzodiazepines	**Unknown effect**
	Flupentixol
	Loxapine
Low effect	Pipothiazine
Clozapine	Trifluoperazine
Haloperidol	Zuclopenthixol
Risperidone	
	Anticholinergic drugs (procyclidine, benzhexol, etc.)
Citalopram	
Venlafaxine	
Trazodone	
Lithium	

Other risk factors

A number of physiological/pathological factors are associated with an increased risk of QT changes and of arrhythmia (Table 1) and many non-psychotropic drugs are linked to QT prolongation (Table 2)[6].

Table I Physiological risk factors for QTc prolongation and arrhythmia

Cardiac
Long QT syndrome
Bradycardia
Ischaemic heart disease
Myocarditis
Myocardial infarction
Left ventricular hypertrophy

Metabolic
Hypokalaemia
Hypomagnesaemia
Hypocalcaemia

Others
Extreme physical exertion
Stress or shock
Anorexia nervosa
Extremes of age – children and elderly may be more susceptible to QT changes
Female gender

Note: Hypokalaemia-related QTc prolongation is more commonly observed in acute psychotic admissions[8].

Table 2 Non-psychotropics associated with QT prolongation

Antibiotics	Antiarrhythmics
Erythromycin	Quinidine
Clarithromycin	Disopyramide
Ampicillin	Procainamide
Co-trimoxazole	Sotalol
Pentamidine	Amiodarone
(Some 4 quinolones affect QTc – see manufacturers' literature)	Bretylium
Antimalarials	**Others**
Chloroquine	Amantadine
Mefloquine	Cyclosporin
Quinine	Diphenhydramine
	Hydroxyzine
	Nicardipine
	Tamoxifen

Note: β_2 agonists and sympathomimetics may provoke torsade de pointes in patients with prolonged QTc.

ECG monitoring recommendations

Generally, prescribing should be such that the need for ECG monitoring is minimised: alternative drugs are usually available and so ECG monitoring should be avoided whenever possible.

Table   ECG monitoring recommendations (*authors' opinion*)

	No other risk factors	Physiological/ pathological risk factors*	When co-administered with other QT-prolonging drugs**
'No-effect' drugs	None	None	None
'Low-effect' drugs	None	None	Baseline ECG, then 6-monthly, consider referral to cardiologist
'Moderate-effect' drugs	None	Correct if possible, if not baseline ECG, then 6 monthly, consider referral to cardiologist	Avoid or refer to cardiologist
'High-effect' drugs	Baseline ECG then 6-monthly, consider referral to cardiologist	Correct if possible, if not – avoid	Avoid
'Unknown-effect' drugs	None	Correct if possible if not – baseline ECG then 6-monthly, consider referral to cardiologist	Avoid or refer to cardiologist

Notes

* Many conditions necessitate close cardiac monitoring, regardless of drugs prescribed. Recommendations in this column therefore represent additional requirements to those already mandated by the patient's condition.

** Defined as any drug in Table 2 on page 77 or psychotropics of moderate or high effect. The use of some of these drugs may necessitate cardiac monitoring. Recommendations in this column therefore represent *additional* requirements to those already mandated by the use of these drugs alone.

Actions to be taken

- **QTc**   **<440 ms (men) or <470 ms (women)**
  No action required unless abnormal T-wave morphology – consider referral to cardiologist if in doubt.
- **QTc**   **>440 ms (men) or >470 ms (women) but <500 ms**
  Consider switch to drug of lower effect; reperform ECG and consider referral to cardiologist.
- **QTc**   **>500 ms**
  Stop suspected causative drug(s) and switch to drug of lower effect; refer to cardiologist immediately.
- **Abnormal T-wave morphology**
  Review treatment. Consider switch to drug of lower effect. Refer to cardiologist immediately.

Metabolic inhibition

The effect of drugs on QTc interval is plasma level-dependent. Drug interactions are therefore important, especially when metabolic inhibition results in increased plasma levels of the drug affecting QTc. Commonly used metabolic inhibitors include fluvoxamine, fluoxetine, paroxetine, nefazodone and valproate. This is a complex area with an expanding data base. See page 154 for further information on drug interactions.

Other cardiovascular risk factors

The risk of drug-induced arrhythmia and sudden cardiac death with psychotropics is very small with a few drugs and probably non-existent with many others. Of much greater concern are other patient-related risk factors for cardiovascular disease. These include smoking, obesity and impaired glucose tolerance and present a much greater risk to patient mortality than the uncertain outcome of QT changes. See relevant sections for discussion of these problems.

References

1. Reilly JG, Ayis SA, Ferrier IN *et al.* Thioridazine and sudden unexplained death in psychiatric in-patients. *British Journal of Psychiatry* 2002; **180**: 515–522.
2. Ray WA, Meredith S, Thapa PB *et al.* Antipsychotics and the risk of sudden cardiac death. *Archives of General Psychiatry* 2001; **58**: 1161–1167.
3. Malik M, Camm AJ. Evaluation of drug-induced QT interval prolongation. Implications for drug approval and labelling. *Drug Safety* 2001; **24**(5): 323–351.
4. Haddad PM, Anderson IM. Antipsychotic-related QTc prolongation, torsade de pointes and sudden death. *Drugs* 2002; **62**: 1649–1671.
5. Taylor DM. Antipsychotics and QT prolongation. *Acta Psychiatrica Scandinavica* 2003; **107**: 85–95.
6. Botstein P. Is QT interval prolongation harmful? A regulatory perspective. *American Journal of Cardiology* 1993; **72**(6): 50B–52B.
7. Glassman AH, Bigger JT. Antipsychotic drugs – prolonged QTc interval, torsade de pointes and sudden death. *American Journal of Psychiatry* 2001; **158**: 1774–1782.
8. Hatta K, Takahashi T, Nakamura H *et al.* Prolonged QT interval in acute psychotic patients. *Psychiatry Research* **94**: 279–285.

Antipsychotics, diabetes and impaired glucose tolerance

Schizophrenia

Schizophrenia seems to be associated with relatively high rates of insulin resistance and diabetes[1,2] – an observation that pre-dates the discovery of effective antipsychotics[3,4].

Typical antipsychotics

Phenothiazine derivatives have long been associated with impaired glucose tolerance and diabetes[5]. Diabetes prevalence rates have been reported to have substantially increased following the introduction and widespread use of conventional drugs[6]. Prevalence of impaired glucose tolerance seems to be higher with aliphatic phenothiazines than with fluphenazine or haloperidol[7]. Hyperglycaemia has also been reported with other conventional drugs, such as loxapine[8].

Atypical antipsychotics

Clozapine

Clozapine has been strongly linked to hyperglycaemia, impaired glucose tolerance and diabetic ketoacidosis[9]. The risk of diabetes appears to be higher with clozapine than with conventional drugs, especially in younger patients[10,11], although this is not a consistent finding[12].

As many as a third of patients may develop diabetes after 5 years of treatment[13]. Most cases of diabetes are noted in the first 6 months of treatment and some occur within one month[14]. Death from ketoacidosis has also been reported[14]. Diabetes associated with clozapine is not necessarily linked to obesity or to family history of diabetes[9].

Clozapine appears to increase plasma levels of insulin in a clozapine level-dependent fashion[15]. It has been shown to be more likely than typical drugs to increase plasma glucose and insulin following oral glucose challenge[16].

Olanzapine

Like clozapine, olanzapine has been strongly linked to impaired glucose tolerance, diabetes and diabetic ketoacidosis[17]. Risk of diabetes has also been reported to be higher than with typical drugs[18], again with a particular risk in younger patients[11]. The timecourse of development of diabetes has not been established but impaired glucose tolerance seems to occur even in the absence of obesity and family history of diabetes[9]. Olanzapine may be more diabetogenic than risperidone[19].

It appears that olanzapine is associated with plasma levels of glucose and insulin higher than those seen with conventional drugs (after oral glucose load)[16].

Risperidone

Risperidone has been linked mainly in case reports to impaired glucose tolerance[20], diabetes[21] and ketoacidosis[22]. The number of reports of such adverse effects is substantially smaller than with either clozapine or olanzapine. At least one study has suggested that changes in fasting glucose are significantly less common with risperidone than with olanzapine[19].

Risperidone seems no more likely than typical drugs to be associated with diabetes[11,18], although there may be an increased risk in patients under 40 years of age[11]. Risperidone has, however, been observed to affect adversely fasting glucose and plasma glucose (following glucose challenge) compared with those seen in healthy volunteers (but not compared with patients taking typical drugs)[16].

Quetiapine

Like risperidone, quetiapine has been linked to cases of new-onset diabetes and ketoacidosis[23]. Again, the number of reports is much less than with olanzapine or clozapine. Quetiapine appears to be more likely than conventional drugs to be associated with diabetes[11]. Inexplicably, quetiapine may ameliorate clozapine-related diabetes when given in conjunction with clozapine[24].

Other atypicals

At the time of publication there were no published reports of glucose homeostasis problems with amisulpride, ziprasidone, zotepine, aripiprazole or sertindole. This should not be taken to indicate that these drugs are not associated with diabetes: there have been no studies specifically establishing their safety in this respect.

Monitoring

Diabetes is a growing problem in western society and has a strong association with obesity, (older) age, (lower) educational achievement and with certain racial groups[25,26]. Diabetes markedly increases cardiovascular mortality, largely as a consequence of atherosclerosis[27]. Intervention to reduce plasma glucose levels and minimise other risk factors (obesity, hypercholesterolaemia) is therefore essential[28].

All patients on all antipsychotics should be closely monitored (see pages 30–34). All should undergo baseline and six-monthly glycosylated haemoglobin tests. With clozapine and olanzapine plasma glucose should be performed at one month to rule out severe, acute effects. HbA_{1C} needs to be estimated 3-monthly.

Table IGT and diabetes – summary of monitoring	
Drug	*Monitoring*
Clozapine and olanzapine	Baseline and 3-monthly HbA_{1C}. Plasma glucose after one month
	Consider oral glucose tolerance test (OGTT)
All other antipsychotics	Baseline and 6-monthly HbA_{1C}
	OGTT if fasting glucose suggests IGT

References

1. Schimmelbusch WH, Mueller PS, Sheps J. The positive correlation between insulin resistance and duration of hospitalization in untreated schizophrenia. *British Journal of Psychiatry* 1971; **118**: 429–36.
2. Waitzkin L. A survey of unknown diabetes in a mental hospital: 1. Men under age fifty. *Diabetes* 1966; **15**: 97–104.
3. Kasanin J. The blood sugar curve in mental disease. *Archives of Neurological Psychiatry* 1926; **16**: 414–419.
4. Braceland FJ, Meduna LJ, Vaichulis JA. Delayed action of insulin in schizophrenia. *American Journal of Psychiatry* 1945; **102**: 108–110.
5. Arneson GA. (1964) Phenothiazine derivatives and glucose metabolism. *Journal of Neuropsychiatry* 1964; **5**: 181.
6. Lindenmayer J-P, Nathan A-M, Smith RC. Hyperglycemia associated with the use of atypical antipsychotics. *Journal of Clinical Psychiatry* 2001; **62**(Suppl. 23): 30–38.
7. Keskiner A, el-Toumi A, Bousquet T. Psychotropic drugs, diabetes and chronic mental patients. *Psychosomatics* 1973; **14**: 176–81.
8. Tollefson G, Lesar T. Nonketotic hyperglycemia associated with loxapine and amoxapine: case report. *Journal of Clinical Psychiatry* 1983; **44**: 347–348.
9. Mir S, Taylor D. Atypical antipsychotics and hyperglycaemia. *International Clinical Psychopharmacology* 2001; **16**: 63–74.
10. Lund BC, Perry PJ, Brooks JM *et al*. Clozapine use in patients with schizophrenia and the risk of diabetes, hyperlipidemia, and hypertension: a claims-based approach. *Archives of General Psychiatry* 2001; **58**: 1172–1176.
11. Sernyak MJ, Leslie DL, Alarcon RD *et al*. Association of diabetes mellitus with use of atypical neuroleptics in the treatment of schizophrenia. *American Journal of Psychiatry* 2002; **159**: 561–566.
12. Wang PS, Glynn RJ, Ganz DA *et al*. Clozapine use and risk of diabetes mellitus. *Journal of Clinical Psychopharmacology* 2002; **22**: 236–243.
13. Henderson DC, Cagliero E, Gray C *et al*. Clozapine, diabetes mellitus, weight gain, and lipid abnormalities: a five-year naturalistic study. *American Journal of Psychiatry* 2000; **157**: 975–981.
14. Koller E, Schneider B, Bennett K *et al*. Clozapine-asociated diabetes. *American Journal of Medicine* 2001; **111**: 716–723.
15. Melkersson KI, Hulting A-L, Brismar KE. Different influences of classical antipsychotics and clozapine on glucose-insulin homeostasis in patients with schizophrenia or related psychoses. *Journal of Clinical Psychiatry* 1999; **60**: 783–791.
16. Newcomer JW, Haupt DW, Fucetola R *et al*. Abnormalities in glucose regulation during antipsychotic treatment of schizophrenia. *Archives of General Psychiatry* 2002; **59**: 337–345.
17. Wirshing DA, Spellberg BJ, Erhart SM *et al*. Novel antipsychotics and new onset diabetes. *Biological Psychiatry* 1998; **44**: 778–783.
18. Koro CE, Fedder DO, L'Italien GJ *et al*. Assessment of independent effect of olanzapine and risperidone on risk of diabetes among patients with schizophrenia: population based nested case-control study. *BMJ* 2002; **325**: 243–245.
19. Meyer JM. A retrospective comparison of weight, lipid, and glucose changes between risperidone- and olanzapine-treated inpatients: metabolic outcomes after 1 year. *Journal of Clinical Psychiatry* 2002; **63**: 425–433.
20. Mallya A, Chawla P, Boyer SK *et al*. Resolution of hyperglycemia on risperidone discontinuation: a case report. *Journal of Clinical Psychiatry* 2002; **63**: 453–454.
21. Wirshing DA, Pierre JM, Eyeler J *et al*. Risperidone-associated new-onset diabetes. *Biological Psychiatry* 2001; **50**: 148–149.
22. Hine TJ, Pitchford NJ, Kingdom FAA *et al*. Diabetic ketoacidosis associated with risperidone treatment? *Psychomasomatics* 2000; **41**: 369–371.
23. Henderson DC. Atypical antipsychotic-induced diabetes mellitus: how strong is the evidence? *CNS Drugs* 2002; **16**: 77–89.
24. Reinstein MJ, Sirotovskaya LA, Jones LE. Effect of clozapine-quetiapine combination therapy on weight and glycaemic control. *Clinical Drug Investigation* 1999; **18**: 99–104.
25. Mokdad AH, Ford ES, Bowman BA *et al*. The continuing increase of diabetes in the U.S. *Diabetes Care* 24: 412.
26. Mokdad AH, Ford ES, Bowman BA *et al*. Diabetes trends in the U.S: 1990–1998. *Diabetes Care* 2000; **23**: 1278.
27. Beckman JA, Creager MA, Libby P. Diabetes and atherosclerosis epidemiology, pathophysiology, and management. *JAMA* 2002; **287**: 2570–2581.
28. Haupt DW, Newcomer JW. Hyperglycemia and antipsychotic medications. *Journal of Clinical Psychiatry* 2001; **62**(Suppl. 27).

Antipsychotics and sexual dysfunction

Primary sexual disorders are common, although reliable normative data are lacking[1]. Reported prevalence rates vary depending on the method of data collection (low numbers with spontaneous reports, increasing with confidential questionnaires and further still with direct questioning[2]). Physical illness, psychiatric illness, substance misuse and prescribed drug treatment can all cause sexual dysfunction[2].

Baseline sexual functioning should be determined if possible (questionnaires may be useful) because sexual function can impact on quality of life and affect compliance with medication (sexual dysfunction is one of the major causes of treatment dropout[3]. Complaints of sexual dysfunction may also indicate progression or inadequate treatment of underlying medical or psychiatric conditions. It may also be due to drug treatment and intervention may greatly improve quality of life[4].

The human sexual response

There are 4 phases of the human sexual response, as detailed in the table below[2,5-7].

Table	The human sexual response
Desire	• Related to testosterone levels in men • Possibly increased by dopamine and decreased by prolactin • Psychosocial context and conditioning significantly affect desire
Arousal	• Influenced by testosterone in men and oestrogen in women • Other potential mechanisms include: central dopamine stimulation, modulation of the cholinergic/adrenergic balance, peripheral α_1 agonism and nitric oxide • Physical pathology such as hypertension or diabetes can have a significant effect
Orgasm	• May be related to oxytocin • Inhibition of orgasm may be caused by an increase in serotonin activity, as well as α_1 blockade
Resolution	• Occurs passively after orgasm
Note: Many other hormones and neurotransmitters may interact in a complex way at each phase	

Effects of psychosis

There is a paucity of research about sexual dysfunction in psychosis, particularly in women[8]. Women with psychosis are known to have reduced fertility[9]. People with psychosis are less able to develop good psychosexual relationships and, for some, treatment with an antipsychotic can improve sexual functioning[10]. Assessment of sexual functioning can clearly be difficult in someone who is psychotic.

Effects of antipsychotic drugs

Sexual dysfunction has been reported as a side-effect of all antipsychotics[4], and up to 45% of people taking typical antipsychotics experience sexual dysfunction[11]. Individual susceptibility varies and all effects are reversible. Antipsychotics decrease dopaminergic transmission, which in itself can decrease libido but may also increase prolactin levels via negative feedback. This can cause amenorrhoea in women and a lack of libido, breast enlargement and galactorrhoea in both men and women[12]. Anticholinergic effects can cause disorders of arousal[13] and drugs that block peripheral α_1 receptors cause particular problems with erection and ejaculation in men[4]. These principles can be used to predict the sexual side-effects of different antipsychotic drugs (see table below).

Table	Sexual adverse effects of antipsychotics
Drug	**Type of problem**
Phenothiazines	• Hyperprolactinaemia and anticholinergic effects. Reports of delayed orgasm at lower doses followed by normal orgasm but without ejaculation at higher doses[8]. • Most problems occur with thioridazine (which can also reduce testosterone levels)[14] • Priapism has been reported with thioridazine and chlorpromazine (probably due to α_1 blockade)[15,16]
Thioxanthenes	• Arousal problems and anorgasmia[11]
Haloperidol	• Similar problems to the phenothiazines[17] but anticholinergic effects reduced[15]
Olanzapine	• Possibly less sexual dysfunction due to relative lack of prolactin-related effects[17] • Priapism reported rarely[18]
Risperidone	• Potent elevator of serum prolactin • Less anticholinergic • Specific peripheral α_1 adrenergic blockade leads to a moderately high reported incidence of ejaculatory problems such as retrograde ejaculation[19,20] • Priapism reported rarely[8]
Sulpiride/amisulpride	• Potent elevators of serum prolactin[11]
Quetiapine	• No effect on serum prolactin[21]
Clozapine	• Significant α_1 adrenergic blockade and anticholinergic effects[22]. No effect on prolactin[23] • Probably fewer problems than with typical antipsychotics[24]

Treatment

Before attempting to treat sexual dysfunction, a thorough assessment is essential to determine the most likely cause. Assuming that physical pathology has been excluded, the following principles apply.

Spontaneous remission may occasionally occur[8]. The most obvious first step is to decrease the dose or discontinue the offending drug where appropriate. The next step is to switch to a different drug that is less likely to cause the specific sexual problem experienced (see table above). If this fails or is not practicable, 'antidote' drugs can be tried: for example, cyproheptadine (a $5HT_2$ antagonist at doses of 4–16 mg/day) has been used to treat SSRI-induced sexual dysfunction but sedation is a common side-effect[25]. Amantadine, buproprion, buspirone, bethanechol and yohimbine have all been used with varying degrees of success but have a number of unwanted side-effects and interactions with other drugs (see opposite).

Table Remedial treatments for psychotropic-induced sexual dysfunction

Drug	Pharmacology	Potential treatment for	Side-effects
Alprostadil[1,6]	Prostaglandin	Erectile dysfunction	Pain, fibrosis, hypotension, priapism.
Amantadine[1,27]	Dopamine agonist	Prolactin-induced reduction in desire and arousal (dopamine increases libido and facilitates ejaculation)	Return of psychotic symptoms, GI effects, nervousness, insomnia
Bethanechol[28]	Cholinergic or cholinergic potentiation of adrenergic neurotransmission	Anticholinergic induced arousal problems and anorgasmia (from TCAs, antipsychotics,etc)	Nausea and vomiting, colic, bradycardia, blurred vision, sweating
Bromocriptine[4]	Dopamine agonist	Prolactin induced reduction in desire and arousal	Return of psychotic symptoms, GI effects
Bupropion[29]	Noradrenaline and dopamine reuptake inhibitor	SSRI-induced sexual dysfunction (evidence poor)	Concentration problems, reduced sleep, tremor
Buspirone[25]	$5HT_{1a}$ partial agonist	SSRI induced sexual dysfunction, particularly decreased libido and anorgasmia	Nausea, dizziness, headache
Cyproheptadine[1,25,30]	$5HT_2$ antagonist	Sexual dysfunction caused by increased serotonin transmission (eg SSRIs), particularly anorgasmia	Sedation and fatigue. Reversal of the therapeutic effect of antidepressants
Sildenafil[6,31-33]	Phosphodiesterase inhibitor	Erectile dysfunction of any aetiology Anorgasmia in women	Mild headaches, dizziness
Yohimbine[1,6,34-36]	Central and peripheral α_2 adrenoceptor antagonist	SSRI-induced sexual dysfunction, particularly erectile dysfunction, decreased libido and anorgasmia (evidence poor)	Anxiety, nausea, fine tremor, increased BP, sweating, fatigue

Drugs such as sildenafil (Viagra) or alprostadil (Caverject) are only effective in the treatment of erectile dysfunction. In the UK they are available for prescription by GPs for a limited number of medical indications, not including psychosis or antipsychotic-induced impotence[26]. The psychological approaches used by sexual dysfunction clinics may be difficult for clients with mental health problems to engage in[4].

References

1. Baldwin DS, Thomas SC, Birtwistle J. Effects of antidepressant drugs on sexual function. *International Journal of Psychiatry in Clinical Practice* 1997; **1**: 47–58.
2. Pollack MH, Reiter S, Hammerness P. Genitourinary and sexual adverse effects of psychotropic medication. *International Journal of Psychiatry in Medicine* 1992; **22**: 305–327.
3. Montejo AL, Llorca G, Izquierdo JA *et al*. Incidence of sexual dysfunction associated with antidepressant agents: a prospective multicentre study of 1022 patients. *Journal of Clinical Psychiatry* 2001; **62**: 10–20.
4. Segraves RT. Effects of psychotropic drugs on human erection and ejaculation. *Archives of General Psychiatry* 1989; **46**: 275–284.
5. Stahl SM. The psychopharmacology of sex. Part 1. Neurotransmitters and the 3 phases of the human sexual response. *Journal of Clinical Psychiatry* 2001; **62**: 80–81.
6. Garcia-Reboll L, Mulhall JP, Goldstein I. Drugs for the treatment of impotence. *Drugs and Aging* 1997; **11**: 140–151.
7. DeGroat WC, Booth AM. Physiology of male sexual functioning. *Annals of Internal Medicine* 1980; **92**: 329–331.
8. Clayton DO, Shen WW. Psychotropic drug-induced sexual function disorders. *Drug Safety* 1998; **19**: 299–312.
9. Howard LM, Kumar C, Leese M *et al*. The general fertility rate in women with psychotic disorders. *American Journal of Psychiatry* 2002; **159**: 991–997.
10. Aizenberg D, Zemishlany Z, Dorfman-Etrog P *et al*. Sexual dysfunction in male schizophrenic patients. *Journal of Clinical Psychiatry* 1995; **56**: 137–141.
11. Smith S, O'Keane V, Murray R. Sexual dysfunction in patients taking conventional antipsychotic medication. *British Journal of Psychiatry* 2002; **181**: 49–55.
12. Meltzer HY, Casey DE, Garver DL *et al*. Adverse effects of the atypical antipsychotics. *Journal of Clinical Psychiatry* 1998; **59**(Suppl.12): 17–22.
13. Aldridge SA. Drug-induced sexual dysfunction. *Clinical Pharmacy* 1982; **1**: 141–147.
14. Kotin J, Wilbert DE, Verburg D *et al*. Thioridazine and sexual dysfunction. *American Journal of Psychiatry* 1976; **133**: 82–85.
15. Mitchell JE, Popkin MK. Antipsychotic drug therapy and sexual dysfunction in men. *American Journal of Psychiatry* 1982; **139**: 633–637.
16. Thompson JW, Ware MR, Blashfield RK. Psychotropic medication and priapism: a comprehensive review. *Journal of Clinical Psychiatry* 1990; **51**: 430–433.
17. Crawford A, Beasley C, Tollefson G. The acute and long term effect of olanzapine compared with placebo and haloperidol on serum prolactin concentrations. *Schizophrenia Research* 1997; **26**: 41–54.
18. Olanzapine SPC.
19. Tran PV, Hamilton SH, Kuntz AJ. Double-blind comparison of olanzapine versus risperidone in the treatment of schizophrenia and other psychotic disorders. *Journal of Clinical Psychopharmacology* 1997; **17**: 407–418.
20. Raja M. Risperidone-induced absence of ejaculation. *Journal of Clinical Psychopharmacology* 1999; **14**: 317–319.
21. Peuskens J, Link CGG. A comparison of quetiapine and chlorpromazine in the treatment of schizophrenia. *Acta Psychiatrica Scandinavica* 1997; **96**: 265–273.
22. Coward DM. General pharmacology of clozapine. *British Journal of Psychiatry* 1992; **160**(Suppl. 17): 5–11.
23. Meltzer HY, Goode DJ, Schyve PM *et al*. Effect of clozapine on human serum prolactin levels. *American Journal of Psychiatry* 1979; **136**: 1550–1555.
24. Aizenberg D, Modai I, Landa A *et al*. Comparison of sexual dysfunction in male schizophrenic patients maintained on treatment with classical antipsychotics versus clozapine. *Journal of Clinical Psychiatry* 2001; **62**: 541–544.
25. Rothschild AJ. Sexual side-effects of antidepressants. *Journal of Clinical Psychiatry* 2000; **61**: 28–36.
26. Health Service Circular (1999) 177.
27. Valevski A, Modai I, Zbarski E *et al*. Effect of amantadine on sexual dysfunction in neuroleptic-treated male schizophrenic patients. *Clinical Neuropharmacology* 1998; **21**: 355–357.
28. Gross MD. Reversal by bethanechol of sexual dysfunction caused by anticholinegic antidepressants. *American Journal of Psychiatry* 1982; **139**: 1193–1294.
29. Masand PS, Ashton AK, Gupta S *et al*. Sustained-release bupropion for selective serotonin reuptake inhibitor-induced sexual dysfunction: a randomised, double blind, placebo controlled, parallel group study. *American Journal of Psychiatry* 2001; **158**: 805–807.
30. Lauerma H. Successful treatment of citalopram-induced anorgasmia by cyproheptadine. *Acta Psychiatrica Scandinavica* 1996; **93**: 69–70.
31. Nurnberg HG, Hensley PL, Lauriello J *et al*. Sildenafil for women patients with antidepressant-induced sexual dysfunction. *Psychiatric Services* 1999; **50**: 1076–1078.
32. Salerian AJ, Deibler WE, Vittone BJ *et al*. Sildenafil for psychotropic-induced sexual dysfunction in 31 women and 61 men. *Journal of Sexual and Marital Therapy* 2000; **26**: 133–140.
33. Nurnberg HG, Hensley PL, Gelenberg AJ *et al*. Treatment of antidepressant-associated sexual dysfunction with sildenafil: a randomized controlled trial. *JAMA* 2003; **289**: 56–64.
34. Jacobsen FM. Fluoxetine-induced sexual dysfunction and an open trial of yohimbine. *Journal of Clinical Psychiatry* 1992; **53**: 119–122.
35. Michelson D, Kociban K, Tamura R *et al*. Mirtazapine, yohimbine or olanzapine augmentation therapy for serotonin reuptake-associated female sexual dysfunction: a randomised, placebo controlled trial. *Journal of Psychiatric Research* 2002; **36**: 147–152.
36. Woodrum ST, Brown CS. Management of SSRI-induced sexual dysfunction. *Annals of Pharmacotherapy* 1998; **32**: 1209–1215.

Antipsychotics: relative adverse effects – a rough guide

Drug	Sedation	Extra-pyramidal	Anti-cholinergic	Hypotension	Prolactin elevation
Amisulpride	–	+	–	–	+++
Aripiprazole	–	+/–	–	–	–
Benperidol	+	+++	+	+	+++
Chlorpromazine	+++	++	++	+++	+++
Clozapine	+++	–	+++	+++	–
Flupentixol	+	++	++	+	+++
Fluphenazine	+	+++	++	+	+++
Haloperidol	+	+++	+	+	+++
Loxapine	++	+++	+	++	+++
Olanzapine	++	+/–	+	+	+
Perphenazine	+	+++	+	+	+++
Pimozide	+	+	+	+	+++
Pipothiazine	++	++	++	++	+++
Promazine	+++	+	++	++	++
Quetiapine	++	–	+	++	–
Risperidone	+	+	+	++	+++
Sertindole	–	–	–	+++	+/–
Sulpiride	–	+	–	–	+++
Thioridazine	+++	+	+++	+++	++
Trifluoperazine	+	+++	+/–	+	+++
Ziprasidone	+	+/–	–	+	+/–
Zotepine	+++	+	+	++	++ +
Zuclopenthixol	++	++	++	+	+++

Key: +++ High incidence/ severity   ++ Moderate
        + Low   – Very low

Note: the table above is made up of approximate estimates of relative incidence and/or severity, based on clinical experience, manufacturers' literature and published research. This is a rough guide – see individual sections for more precise information.

chapter 3

Bipolar disorder

Valproate

Valproate is available in the UK in three forms: sodium valproate (Epilim) and valproic acid (Convulex), licensed for the treatment of epilepsy and semisodium valproate (Depakote), licensed for the acute treatment of mania (NB: not for prophylaxis). Both semisodium and sodium valproate are metabolised to valproic acid, which is apparently responsible for the pharmacological activity of all three preparations. Clinical studies of the treatment of affective disorders variably use sodium valproate, semisodium valproate, 'valproate' or valproic acid. The great majority have used valproate semisodium.

Randomised controlled trials (RCTs) have shown valproate to be effective in the treatment of mania[1,2]. Approximately 50% of patients respond during the acute phase[1]. Freeman *et al.*[2] found lithium to be more effective overall than valproate, while Swann *et al.*[3] found that patients who had depressive symptoms at baseline were more likely to respond to valproate than lithium. Patients who have experienced 10 or more episodes of mania may also respond better to valproate (as semisodium) than lithium[4], although this study may have preselected lithium-resistant patients. In a further double-blind, placebo-controlled study of valproate in 36 patients who had failed to respond to or could not tolerate lithium, the median decrease in Young Mania Rating Scale scores was 54% in the valproate group and 5% in the placebo group[5]. Open studies suggest that valproate may be effective in bipolar depression.

Although open-label studies suggest that valproate is effective in the prophylaxis of bipolar affective disorder[6,7] only one RCT has been published to date[8]. No difference was found between lithium, valproate semisodium and placebo in the primary outcome measure: time to any mood episode, although divalproex was superior to lithium and placebo on some secondary outcome measures. This study could be criticised for including patients who were 'not ill enough' and for not lasting 'long enough' (1 year). Valproate is sometimes used to treat aggressive behaviour of variable aetiology[9].

Plasma levels

Valproate has a complex pharmacokinetic profile, following a three-compartment model and showing protein-binding saturation. Plasma level monitoring is supposedly, therefore, of more limited use than with carbamazepine or lithium. A dose of at least 1000 mg/day and a serum level of at least 50 mg/l may be robustly associated with response[10]. Achieving therapeutic plasma levels rapidly using a loading dose regimen is well tolerated but not proven to provide a more rapid response in the treatment of mania[11]. (This study was not powered to detect any difference in efficacy.) Plasma levels can perhaps more reliably detect non-compliance or predict or confirm toxicity.

Adverse effects[12]

Sodium valproate causes both hyperammonaemia and gastric irritation, which can sometimes lead to intense nausea. Lethargy and confusion can occasionally occur with starting doses of above 200–300 mg bd. Weight gain can be significant[13], particularly when valproate is used in conjunction with clozapine. Hair loss with curly regrowth, and peripheral oedema can also occur. Sodium valproate may very rarely cause fulminant hepatic failure[14]. All cases reported to date have occurred in children, often receiving multiple anticonvulsants and with family histories of hepatic problems. It would seem wise to evaluate clinically any patient with raised LFTs and to also monitor other markers of hepatic function such as albumin and prothrombin time. Valproate can cause hyperandrogenism in women and polycystic ovaries[15]. It is also associated with thrombocytopenia, leucopenia, red cell hypoplasia and pancreatitis. Most side-effects of valproate are dose-related (peak plasma level-related) and increase in frequency and severity when the plasma level is >100 mg/l. The once-daily 'chrono' form of sodium valproate does not produce as high peaks as the conventional forms of valproate and may be better tolerated. There is also a suggestion that valproate semisodium may be better tolerated in some.

Interactions with other drugs[16,17]

Valproate is highly protein-bound (up to 94%): other drugs that are highly protein-bound can displace valproate from albumin and precipitate toxicity (e.g. *aspirin*[18]). Other, less strongly protein-bound drugs, can be displaced by valproate leading to higher free levels and increased therapeutic effect or toxicity (e.g. *warfarin*). Valproate is hepatically metabolised: drugs that inhibit CYP enzymes can increase valproate levels (e.g. *erythromycin, fluoxetine* and *cimetidine*). Valproate can increase the plasma levels of some drugs, possibly by inhibition/competitive inhibition of their metabolism. Examples include *TCAs* (particularly clomipramine[19]), *lamotrigine*[20] and *phenobarbitone.*

Pharmacodynamic interactions also occur: The anticonvulsant effect of valproate is antagonised by drugs that lower the seizure threshold (e.g. antipsychotics and antidepressants). Weight gain can be exacerbated by other drugs that have this effect (eg antipsychotics, particularly clozapine and olanzapine).

References

1. Bowden CL, Brugger AM, Swann AC *et al.* Efficacy of divalproex sodium vs lithium and placebo in the treatment of mania. *Journal of the American Medical Association* 1994; **271**: 918–924.
2. Freeman TW, Clothier JL, Pazzaglia P. A double-blind comparison of valproate and lithium in the treatment of acute mania. *American Journal of Psychiatry* 1992; **149**: 108–111.
3. Swann AC, Bowden CL, Morris D *el al.* Depression during mania: treatment response to lithium or divalproex. *Archives of General Psychiatry* 1997; **54**: 37–42.
4. Swann AC, Bowden CL, Calabrese JR. Differential effect of number of previous episodes of affective disorder on response to lithium or divalproex in acute mania. *American Journal of Psychiatry* 1999; **156**: 1264–1266.
5. Pope HG, McElroy SL, Keck PE *et al.* Valproate in the treatment of acute mania: a placebo-controlled study. *Archives of General Psychiatry* 1991; **48**: 62–68.
6. Calabrese JR, Delucchi GA. Spectrum of efficacy of valproate in 55 patients with rapid-cycling bipolar disorder. *American Journal of Psychiatry* 1990; **147**: 431–434.
7. McElroy SL, Keck PE, Pope HG. Sodium valproate: its use in primary psychiatric disorders. *Journal of Clinical Psychopharmacology* 1987; **7**: 16–24.
8. Bowden CL, Calabrese JR, McElroy SL *et al.* A randomised, placebo-controlled 12-month trial of divalproex and lithium in the treatment of outpatients with bipolar 1 disorder. *Archives of General Psychiatry* 2000; **57**: 481–489.
9. Lindenmayer JP, Kotsaftis A.Use of sodium valproate in violent and aggressive behaviours: a critical review. *Journal of Clinical Psychiatry* 2000; **61**: 123–128.
10. Taylor D, Duncan D. Doses of carbamazepine and valproate in bipolar affective disorder. *Psychiatric Bulletin* 1997; **21**: 221–223.
11. Hirschfeld RMA, Allen MH, McEvoy JP. Safety and tolerability of oral loading divalproex sodium in acutely manic bipolar patients. *Journal of Clinical Psychiatry* 1999; **60**: 815–818.
12. Summary of Product Characteristics for sodium valproate, semi sodium valproate and valproic acid. Data Sheet Compendium.
13. Vanina Y, Podolskaya A, Sedky K *et al.* Body weight changes associated with psychopharmacology. *Psychiatric Services* 2002; **53**: 842–847.
14. Rimmer EM, Richens A. An update on sodium valproate. *Pharmacotherapy* 1985; **5**: 171–184.
15. Piontec CM, Wisner KL (2000). Appropriate clinical management of women taking valproate. *Journal of Clinical Psychiatry* **61**: 161–163.
16. Spina E, Perucca E. Clinical significance of pharmacokinetic interactions between antiepileptic and psychotropic drugs. *Epilepsia* 2002; **43**: 37–44.
17. Patsalos PN, Froscher W, Pisani F *et al.* The importance of drug interactions in epilepsy therapy. *Epilepsia* 2002; **43**: 365–385.
18. Goulden KJ, Dooley JM, Camfield PR *et al.* Clinical valproate toxicity induced by acetylsalicylic acid. *Neurology* 1987; **37**: 1392–1394.
19. Fehr C, Grunder G, Hiemke C *et al.* Increase in serum clomipramine concentrations caused by valproate. *Journal of Clinical Psychopharmacology* 2000; **20**: 493–494.
20. Morris R, Black A, Lam E *et al.* Clinical study of lamotrigine and valproic acid in patients with epilepsy: using a drug interaction to advantage? *Therapeutic Drug Monitoring* 2000; **22**: 656–660.

Lithium

History

The use of lithium in medicine goes back some 150 years, and the most significant developments are listed below[1]:

1845–1860:	Lithium was used in the treatment of gout.
1865–1880:	Mania and melancholia were incorporated into the group of gouty diseases and were therefore treated with lithium-containing salts.
1880:	Carl Lange described periodic depression (thought to be another gouty disease) and treated patients prophylactically for many years with 'alkaline salts', resulting in the ingestion of 5–25 mmol lithium/day, although he never recognised lithium as the active ingredient of these salts.
1920s:	A Danish psychiatrist, H.J.Schou, described the same depressive illness as Carle Lange but was against the latter's prophylactic therapy of alkaline salts, thus ending an era. Ironically his son, Mogens Schou, later emerged as a major advocate of lithium therapy.
Early 1950s:	Lithium salts were used widely in the USA as a salt substitute in cardiac patients, with disastrous results, leading to the discovery of their renal toxicity, especially in sodium-depleted patients. Around the same time, John Cade first used lithium to treat various psychiatric disorders; he noted a very good response in manic patients and some improvement in patients with schizophrenia. Many of these patients showed signs of lithium toxicity (the pharmacokinetics of lithium were not fully understood).
Early 1970s:	A double-blind discontinuation study was published by Hartigan Baastrup, which demonstrated beyond doubt the efficacy of lithium therapy. Standardised testing of serum lithium was also introduced around this time.
1977:	A paper was published which showed that long-term lithium treatment might induce slight, chronic, irreversible kidney damage with accompanying reduction of renal concentrating ability. The acceptable therapeutic range for lithium has fallen steadily since, in order to maximise therapeutic response while minimising unwanted side-effects. It is now accepted as being 0.6–1.0 mmol/l, with the lower part of the range being appropriate for prophylaxis and for elderly patients, and the upper part being appropriate for acute treatment and the prophylaxis of unstable bipolar affective disorder. Interestingly, lithium salts are still freely available in some parts of the world as remedies for rheumatoid and gouty diseases.

Use

Lithium is widely used for the prophylaxis and treatment of mania and hypomania, recurrent depression and bipolar affective disorder. Its use in the treatment of acute mania[2] is limited by the fact that it usually takes at least a week to achieve a response[3] and that the co-administration of high doses of potent antipsychotics may increase the risk of neurological side-effects. It can also be difficult to achieve therapeutic serum levels rapidly and monitoring can be problematic if the patient is unco-operative.

Lithium and antidepressants are probably equally effective in the prophylaxis of recurrent depressive illness[4]. Lithium is a useful addition to an antidepressant in a patient with an acute depressive episode that is proving difficult to treat[3].

Lithium is also used in the prophylaxis of bipolar affective disorder where it reduces both the number and the severity of relapses[2,5], while also offering some protection against antidepressant-induced hypomania. It is accepted clinical practice to consider starting treatment with a mood sta-biliser if two episodes of mania or depression have occurred in a 3-year period[3]. Although numerous factors have been studied in an attempt to identify patients who are likely to respond to lithium, an empirical trial is still the best predictor of long-term outcome. Relapse within one year of starting lithium prophylaxis is highly suggestive of a poor long-term response. Clinical features associated with a favourable response include marked psychomotor retardation and endogenous and psychotic features. In addition, some evidence points to the previous pattern of illness as a predictor of response to lithium[6]: patients whose illness shows a pattern of mania followed by depression fol-lowed by a euthymic interval, or those whose illness shows an irregular pattern, are more likely to respond to lithium prophylaxis than those who show a pattern of depression –mania – euthymia or have a rapidly cycling illness (4 or more episodes/year)[7].

Intermittent treatment with lithium may worsen the natural course of bipolar illness (a much greater than expected incidence of manic relapse is seen in the first few months after discontinuing lithium[8,9]). This has led to recommendations that lithium treatment should not be started unless there is a clear intention to continue it for at least 3 years[10]. This advice has obvious implications for initiating lithium treatment against a patient's will (or in someone known to be non-compliant) during a period of acute illness. The risk of relapse may be reduced by decreasing the dose of lithium gradually over a period of one month[11]. Intermittent treatment with lithium does not seem to have the same detrimental effect on the course of unipolar depressive illness.

It is estimated that 15% of those with bipolar illness take their own life. Mortality from physical illness is also increased[12]. Chronic treatment with lithium reduces mortality from suicide to the same level as that seen in the general population[7,13,14]. There is no convincing evidence that mortal-ity from other causes is altered.

Lithium is used in combination with antipsychotics in the treatment of schizo-affective illness[15], and is also used to treat aggressive[16] and self-mutilating behaviour and in steroid-induced psychosis[17]. The neuropharmacology of lithium[18] is not clearly understood but its therapeutic effect is thought to be related, among other things, to its ability to block neuronal calcium channels, and its effects on GABA pathways. The efficacy of lithium does not go unchallenged. For a review, see Moncrieff[19].

Plasma levels

Lithium is rapidly absorbed from the gastrointestinal tract, but has a long distribution phase. Blood should ideally be taken 12 hours after the last dose was administered. Pharmacokinetic data show that the level, for any given individual, is reproducible if blood is taken 10–14 hours postdose (for once-daily dosing with modified-release preparations)[20].

On average, the serum level can be expected to fall by 0.2 mmol/l between 12 and 24 hours postdose[21].

Lithium should be started at a dose of 400 mg at night: lower in the elderly or in renal impairment. The serum level should be measured after 5–7 days, and then weekly until the desired level has been achieved. Once the serum level is stable, it should be checked 3–6 monthly: more often if problems are suspected or the patient is elderly or is co-prescribed interacting drugs. Full guidance on monitoring can be found on pages 100–101. Serum levels of 0.6–1.0 mmol/l are usually aimed for, although in some individuals further benefit can be gained by going slightly higher[22]. A re-analysis of the original lithium clinical trials cast doubt on this 'conventional wisdom': the authors con-cluded that the absolute level used for maintenance may be less important than the rapid reduction in serum lithium level that occurred in these trials when patients were switched from one treatment group to another[23]. Children and adolescents may require higher serum levels than adults to ensure that an adequate brain concentration is achieved[24].

Formulations of lithium

There is no significant difference in the pharmacokinetics of the two most widely prescribed brands of lithium: Priadel and Camcolit[3]. Not all preparations are bio-equivalent, however, and care must be taken to make sure that the patient receives the same preparation each time a new prescription is supplied.

● Lithium carbonate 400 mg tablets each contain 10.8 mmol lithium.

● Lithium citrate 564 mg tablets each contain 6 mmol lithium. Lithium citrate liquid is available in two strengths; it should be administered twice daily:
  – 5.4 mmol/5 ml equivalent to 200 mg lithium carbonate.
  – 10.8 mmol/5 ml equivalent to 400 mg lithium carbonate.

Lack of clarity over which preparation is intended when prescribing can lead to the patient receiving a subtherapeutic or toxic dose.

Adverse effects

Side-effects tend to be directly related to plasma levels and their frequency increases dramatically at levels above 1 mmol/l. Mild gastrointestinal symptoms can occur when therapy is initiated and are usually transient. Fine hand tremor may occur, as may mild thirst and polyuria. Polyuria may occur more frequently with twice-daily dosing[25]. Propranolol can be useful in the treatment of lithium-induced tremor. Certain skin conditions, such as psoriasis and acne, can be aggravated by lithium therapy.

In the longer term hypothyroidism may occur, although this should not be a reason for stopping lithium treatment: thyroxine replacement therapy is indicated. TFTs usually return to normal when lithium is discontinued. The risk of developing hypothyroidism is probably very much higher than is commonly believed, particularly in middle-aged women (prevalence up to 20%[26]). There is a strong case for testing for thyroid autoantibodies in this group before starting lithium (to better estimate risk) and for measuring TFTs more frequently in the first year of treatment[26]. Lithium treatment also increases the risk of hyperparathyroidism and patients receiving long-term lithium should have their serum calcium level monitored[27].

Some patients complain that lithium 'curbs creativity' or produces 'mental dulling'. A study of artists and writers found that for the majority creativity actually increased with lithium treatment, because of thoughts and actions being more organised. A small minority reported diminished creativity (those who felt inspired by high mood)[28].

The long-term complication that has received the most attention is nephrotoxicity. A small reduction in glomerular filtration rate is seen in 20% of patients[20]. In the vast majority of patients this effect is benign[29]. A very small number of lithium-treated patients may develop interstitial nephritis. Lithium can also cause a reduction in urinary concentrating capacity (nephrogenic diabetes insipidus – hence occurrence of thirst and polyuria), which is reversible in the short-to-medium term but may be irreversible after long-term treatment (>15 years)[20,29].

Lithium toxicity

Toxic effects reliably occur at levels >1.5 mmol/l and usually consist of gastrointestinal effects (increasing anorexia, nausea and diarrhoea) and CNS effects (muscle weakness, drowsiness, ataxia, coarse tremor and muscle twitching). Above 2 mmol/l increased disorientation and seizures are seen, which can progress to coma and death. In the presence of more severe symptoms, osmotic diuresis or forced alkaline diuresis should be initiated (*Note:* not thiazide or loop diuretics under any circumstances). Above 3 mmol/l, peritoneal or haemodialysis is often used[30]. These plasma levels are only a guide and individuals can vary in their susceptibility to symptoms of toxicity.

Before prescribing lithium

Before prescribing lithium, renal, cardiac and thyroid function should be checked[20]. Women of childbearing age should be advised to use reliable contraception. Patients should be informed about symptoms of toxicity: why they might occur and what to do. Bouts of vomiting/diarrhoea or any form of dehydration will lead to sodium depletion and therefore to increased plasma lithium levels. Similarly, a salt-free diet is contraindicated. It is also wise to ensure that the patient is aware of the importance of maintaining an adequate fluid balance and of the need not to double today's dose because yesterday's was forgotten. Basic information about lithium and how to minimise the risk of toxicity is contained in the *Patient Information Leaflet*. This can be found inside each box of lithium tablets.

Interactions with other drugs

Because of lithium's relatively narrow therapeutic index, interactions with other drugs can be very important. The most commonly encountered interactions are with:

Diuretics, which can increase serum lithium levels markedly by reducing its clearance. Thiazides are the worst culprits, while loop diuretics are somewhat safer. Initial thiazide diuresis is accompanied by the loss of sodium. This loss is compensated for within a few days by an increase in sodium reabsorption in the proximal tubule. As the kidney cannot differentiate between sodium and lithium at this site, it follows that there is also an increase in lithium reabsorption, leading to decreased renal clearance.

Non-steroidal anti-inflammatories (NSAIDs), which can increase serum lithium levels by up to 40%[31]. The mechanism of this interaction is not clearly understood, although it is thought to be related to the effects of NSAIDs on fluid balance, and is particularly important if PRN NSAIDs are added to a long-standing regular prescription of lithium. Lithium toxicity secondary to NSAID coprescription has led to legal cases where substantial damages have been awarded against psychiatrists. One case in 1999 was settled for £600,000[32]. Some NSAIDs can be obtained without a prescription. Patients should be aware of the potential interaction.

Haloperidol: following the famous publication by Cohen[33] reporting severe neurotoxicity, widespread anxiety set in about using the combination of lithium and haloperidol. It is important to put this interaction into perspective; if the lithium levels are in the therapeutic range (0.6–1.0 mmol/l) and the haloperidol dose is not increased rapidly to heroic heights, the chance of inducing a toxic state is very low indeed. Haloperidol and lithium is a widely prescribed and very useful combination.

Carbamazepine, which in combination with lithium has been reported to cause neurotoxic reactions. Again, higher (>1 mmol/l) plasma lithium levels were involved than are now thought acceptable, and most of the references state that a previous neurotoxic reaction to lithium alone is a risk factor! Carbamazepine and lithium are often combined in patients with refractory illness[35].

SSRIs have been linked to an increased incidence of CNS toxicity when used with lithium. Although the mechanism of this interaction is not completely understood, it is likely to be mediated through serotonin pathways. It is prudent to be aware and to check lithium levels soon after starting treatment with an SSRI (although it must be noted that some reports claim neurotoxic reactions in the absence of raised lithium levels). Clinical experience has shown this combination to be useful and any interaction rare[36].

ACE inhibitors decrease the excretion of lithium. They can also precipitate renal failure, so extra care is needed in monitoring both serum creatinine and lithium, if these drugs are prescribed together. Care is also required with **angiotensin 2 antagonists**[37] (losartan, valsartan, candesartan, eprosartan, irbesartan and telmisartan).

Summary table – lithium

Indications	Mania, hypomania; prophyaxis in bipolar disorder and recurrent depression. Also effective in schizo-affective disorder and aggression
Pre-lithium work-up	ECG, thyroid function tests, renal function tests (serum creatinine and urea), U&Es
Monitoring	Start at 400 mg once daily (200 mg in the elderly). Plasma level after 5–7 days, then every 5–7 days until the required level is reached (0.6–1.0 mmol/l)). Once stable, check level every 3–6 months. Check thyroid function every 6 months
Stopping	Slowly reduce over at least one month

References

1. Amdisen A. Historical origins. In: Johnson FN (ed). *Depression & Mania: modern lithium therapy*. Oxford: IRL Press, 1987, Chapter 6, pp. 24–28.
2. Cookson J. Lithium: balancing risks and benefits. *British Journal of Psychiatry* 1997; 178: 120–124.
3. Ferrier IN, Tyrer SP, Bell AJ. Lithium therapy. *Advances in Psychiatric Treatment* 1995; 1: 102–110.
4. Goodwin GM. Lithium treatment and prophylaxis in unipolar depression: a meta-analysis. *British Journal of Psychiatry* 1991; 158: 666–675.
5. Tondo L, Baldessarini RJ, Floris G. Long term clinical effectiveness of lithium maintenance treatment in types 1 and 11 bipolar disorder. *British Journal of Psychiatry* 2001; 178(Suppl. 41): 184–190.
6. Souza FGM, Goodwin GM. Episode sequence in bipolar disorder and response to lithium treatment. *American Journal of Psychiatry* 1991; 148: 1237–1239.
7. Tondo L, Hennen J, Baldessarini RJ. Lower suicide risk with long-term lithium treatment in major affective illness: a meta-analysis. *Acta Psychiatrica Scandinavica* 2001; 103: 163–172.
8. Faedda GL, Loudon JB. Rapid recurrence of mania following abrupt discontinuation of lithium. *Lancet* 1988; ii: 15–17.
9. Suppes T, Baldessarini R, Faedda GL *et al*. Risk of recurrence following discontinuation of lithium treatment for bipolar disorder. *Archives of General Psychiatry* 1991; 48: 1082–1085.
10. Goodwin GM. Recurrence of mania after lithium withdrawal. *British Journal of Psychiatry* 1994; 164: 149–152.
11. Baldessarine RJ, Tondo L, Faeda GL *et al*. Effects of the rate of discontinuing lithium maintenance treatment in bipolar disorders. *Journal of Clinical Psychiatry* 1996; 57: 441–448.
12. Harris EC, Barraclough B. Excess mortality of mental disorder. *British Journal of Psychiatry* 1998; 173: 11–53.
13. Schou M, Mult HC. Forty years of lithium treatment. *Archives of General Psychiatry* 1997; 54: 9–13.
14. Stat PR, Frank E, Kostelnik B. Suicide attempts in patients with bipolar 1 disorder during acute and maintenance phases of intensive treatment with pharmacotherapy and adjunctive psychotherapy. *American Journal of Psychiatry* 2002; 159: 1160–1164.

15. Jefferson JW. Lithium: the present and the future. *Journal of Clinical Psychiatry* 1990; **51**(Suppl.): 4–8.
16. Tyrer SP. Lithium and treatment of aggressive behaviour. *European Neuropsychopharmacology* 1994; 4: 234–236.
17. Falk WE, Mahnke MW, Poskanzer DC. Lithium prophylaxis with corticotropin-induced psychosis. *JAMA* 1979; **241**: 1011–1012.
18. Peet M, Pratt JP. Lithium. Current status in psychiatric disorder. *Drugs* 1993; **46**: 7–17.
19. Moncrieff J. Lithium: evidence reconsidered. *British Journal of Psychiatry* 1997; **171**: 113–119.
20. Using lithium safely. *Drug & Therapeutics Bulletin* 1999; **37**: 22–24.
21. *Priadel: psychiatrist's handbook.* Delandale Laboratories, 1986.
22. Gelenberg AJ, Kane JM, Keller MB *et al.* Comparison of standard and low serum levels of lithium for maintenance treatment of bipolar disorder. *New England Journal of Medicine* 1989; **21**: 1489–1493.
23. Perlis RH, Sachs GS, Lafer B. Effect of abrupt change from standard to low serum levels of lithium: a re-analysis of double-blind lithium maintenance data. *American Journal of Psychiatry* 2002; **159**: 1155–1159.
24. Moore CM, Demopulos CM, Henry ME. Brain-to-serum lithium ratio and age: an in vivo magnetic resonance spectroscopy study. *American Journal of Psychiatry* 2002; **159**: 1240–1242.
25. Bowen RC, Grof P, Grof E. Less frequent lithium administration and lower urine volume. *American Journal of Psychiatry* 1991; **148**: 189–192.
26. Johnson EM, Eagles JM. Lithium associated clinical hypothyroidism: prevalence and risk factors. *British Journal of Psychiatry* 1999; **175**: 336–339.
27. Bendz H, Sjodin I, Toss G *et al.* Hyperparathyroidism and long-term lithium therapy – a cross-sectional study and the effect of lithium withdrawal. *Journal of Internal Medicine* 1996; **240**: 357–365.
28. Muller-Oerlinghausen B. Mental functioning. In: Johnson FN (ed). *Depression & Mania: modern lithium therapy*. Oxford: IRL Press, 1987, Chaper 68, pp. 246–252.
29. Gitlin M. Lithium and the kidney: an updated review. *Drug Safety* 1999; **20**: 231–243.
30. Tyrer SP. Lithium intoxication: appropriate treatment. *CNS Drugs* 1996; **6**: 426–439.
31. Reimann IW, Diener U, Frolich C. Indomethacin but not aspirin increases plasma lithium ion levels. *Archives of General Psychiatry* 1983; **40**: 283–286.
32. Nicholson J, Fitzmaurice B. Monitoring patients on lithium – a good practice guideline. *Psychiatric Bulletin* 2002; **26**: 348–351.
33. Cohen WJ, Cohen NH. Lithium carbonate, haloperidol and irreversible brain damage. *JAMA* 1974; **230**: 1283–1287.
34. Goldney RD, Spence ND. Safety of the combination of lithium and neuroleptic drugs. *American Journal of Psychiatry* 1996; **143**: 882–884.
35. Freeman MP, Stoll AL. Mood stabiliser combinations: a review of efficacy and safety. *American Journal of Psychiatry* 1998; **155**: 12–22.
36. Hawley CJ, Loughlin PJ, Quick SJ *et al.* Efficacy, safety and tolerability of combined administration of lithium and selective serotonin reuptake inhibitors: a review of the current evidence. *International Clinical Psychopharmacology* 2000; **15**: 197–206.
37. Zwanger P, Marcuse A, Boerner RJ. Lithium intoxication after administration of AT$_1$ blockers. *Journal of Clinical Psychiatry* 2001; **62**: 208–209.

Further reading

Schou M. Lithium prophylaxis: myths and realities. *American Journal of Psychiatry* 1989; **146**: 573–576.
Young AH. Treatment of bipolar affective disorder. *BMJ* 2000; **321**: 1302–1303.
Various. Lithium in the treatment of manic-depressive illness: an update. Proceedings of a meeting. *Journal of Clinical Psychiatry* 1998: **59**(Suppl. 6).

Carbamazepine

Carbamazepine is primarily used as an anticonvulsant in the treatment of Grand Mal and focal seizures. It is also used in the management of trigeminal neuralgia and, in the UK, is licensed for the prophylaxis of bipolar illness in patients who do not respond to lithium. Carbamazepine monotherapy is effective in acute mania[1], with open studies showing a response rate of 50–60%[2]. It is probably as effective as lithium[3] (direct comparative studies have not been powered to detect a difference[4]). Carbamazepine also appears to usefully augment the effects of antipsychotics in acute mania[5].

Open studies also suggest that monotherapy is effective in bipolar depression[6]: carbamazepine has a similar molecular structure to TCAs, but without possessing their ability to induce mania in bipolar depression. Carbamazepine may also usefully augment antidepressants or other mood stabilisers in refractory unipolar depression[7,8]. Although carbamazepine is generally considered to be as effective as lithium in the prophylaxis of bipolar illness[9], several published studies report a very low response rate and high drop-out rate[3,10]. It is also 'perceived wisdom' that carbamazepine is more effective than lithium in rapid cycling illness (4 or more episodes/year). Although some evidence supports this view[11], negative studies have also been published[12].

There are also reports of carbamazepine being successful in treating aggressive behaviour in patients with schizophrenia[13]. This is apparently not a result of its anticonvulsant effect, as patients with normal EEGs may respond. A trial of carbamazepine is often thought worthwhile, as a last resort, in various psychiatric illnesses (such as panic disorder, borderline personality disorder and episodic dyscontrol syndrome) where no other drug is specifically indicated. The literature consists primarily of case reports and open case series. Carbamazepine is also used in the management of alcohol withdrawal symptoms[14], although the high doses required initially are often poorly tolerated.

Plasma levels

When used as an anticonvulsant the therapeutic range is stated as being 4–12 mg/l, although the supporting evidence is not strong. A dose of at least 600 mg/day and a serum level of at least 7 mg/l seem to be required in affective illness[15], although some studies do not support this view[16].

Carbamazepine serum levels vary significantly within a dosage interval. It is important to sample at a point in time where levels are likely to be reproducible for any given individual. The most appropriate way of monitoring is to take a trough level before the first dose of the day. Carbamazepine is an hepatic-enzyme inducer that induces its own metabolism as well as that of other drugs. An initial plasma half-life of around 30 hours is reduced to around 12 hours on chronic dosing. For this reason, plasma levels should be checked 2–4 weeks after an increase in dose to ensure that the desired level is still being obtained.

The published clinical trials that demonstrate the efficacy of carbamazepine as a mood stabiliser used doses that are significantly higher (usually in the order of 800–1200 mg/day) than those prescribed in everyday UK clinical practice[17].

Adverse effects

The main problems encountered with carbamazepine therapy are dizziness, drowsiness, ataxia and nausea. They can be largely avoided by starting with a low dose and increasing it slowly. Around 3% of patients treated with carbamazepine develop a generalised erythematous rash. Serious dermatological reactions can rarely occur (e.g. toxic epidermal necrolysis). Hyponatraemia can also be a problem.

Carbamazepine can induce a chronic low white blood cell (WBC) count. Many patients treated with carbamazepine have a WBC count at the lower end of the normal range, which rises on discontinuing treatment. One patient in 20,000 develops agranulocytosis and/or aplastic anaemia[18]. Raised ALP and GGT are, potentially, a sign of a hypersensitivity reaction to carbamazepine (a GGT of up to twice normal is common and should not cause concern). Normally, it would be recommended that therapy should be withdrawn, as this can progress to a multi-system hypersensitivity reaction (mainly manifesting itself as various skin reactions and a low WBC count, along with raised ALP and GGT), which can in turn lead to hepatitis. Fatalities have been reported. There is no clear timescale for these events, so it must not be assumed that raised LFTs for 6 months with no other clinical complications will not produce problems in the future. FBC and LFTs should be monitored in patients on long-term therapy.

Interactions with other drugs[19-21]

Carbamazepine is a potent inducer of hepatic cytochrome P450 enzymes and is metabolised by CYP3A4. Plasma levels of most **antidepressants**, most **antipsychotics, benzodiazepines,** some **cholinesterase inhibitors, methadone, thyroxine, theophylline, oestrogens**[22] and other steroids may be reduced by carbamazepine, resulting in treatment failure. Drugs that inhibit CYP3A4 will increase carbamazepine plasma levels and may precipitate toxicity. Examples include cimetidine, diltiazem, verapamil, dextropropoxyphene, erythromycin and SSRIs.

Pharmacodynamic interactions also occur: The anticonvulsant activity of carbamazepine is reduced by drugs that lower the seizure threshold (e.g. antipsychotics and antidepressants), the potential for carbamazepine to cause neutropenia may be increased by other drugs that have the potential to depress the bone marrow (e.g. clozapine) and the risk of hyponatraemia may be increased by other drugs that can deplete sodium (e.g. diuretics). Neurotoxicity has been reported with lithium and carbamazepine combinations[23]. This is rare. There are many complex interactions with other anticonvulsant drugs. The latest edition of the *British National Formulary* should be checked before prescribing anticonvulsant polypharmacy (see also page 201).

As carbamazepine is structurally similar to the TCAs, in theory it should not be given within 14 days of discontinuing a MAOI. Most side-effects of carbamazepine are dose-related (peak plasma level-related), and increase in frequency and severity when the plasma level is >12 mg/l (also this varies substantially from patient to patient). Side-effects can be minimised by using the slow-release preparation.

For references see page 102.

Table Mood stabilisers – brief details

Drug	Dose	Precautions
Lithium	Start on low (400 mg/day) dose Plasma levels to be monitored every 5–7 days until level is between 0.6–1.0 mmol/l Once level is stable, check levels every 3–6 months or if drug interaction is suspected All samples must be taken 12 hours postdose	**Renal function** U&Es before commencing lithium. Excreted through kidney exclusively and potentially nephrotoxic. Change in body salt concentration can affect levels Significant proportion develop **hypothyroidism**: TFT before starting & at 6-monthly intervals. Treat with thyroxine
Carbamazepine	Usual starting dose 200 mg bd, slowly increased until dose 600–1000 mg/day is achieved. MR preparation possibly better tolerated Target range 8–12 mg/l Sample at trough Induces own metabolism: monitor every 2–4 weeks until stable then every 3–6 months	Early **leucopenia** usually transient and benign but later occurring falls in white cells may be serious. Warn patient about fever, infections etc: Need baseline and regular FBCs every 2 weeks for first 2 months, then every 3–6 months Carbamazepine **toxicity**: severe diplopia, nausea, ataxia, sedation
Valproate	Commence on 500 mg MR daily (Epilim) or 250 mg tds (Depakote), then increase until plasma levels reach 50–100 mg/l Trough samples required MR prep may be given once daily, Depakote twice or three times daily	Check renal and hepatic function at baseline, then 6-monthly Full blood count at baseline, then 6-monthly
Lamotrigine	Dose as mood stabiliser not certain, likely to be similar to that used in epilepsy (50–200 mg/day) As dose depends on concomitant medication, see manufacturer's information	Monitor patient for **rash** – more likely to occur in children, with concomitant valproate or if dose started too high or increased too quickly. Most rashes occur within 8 weeks of starting therapy
Topiramate	Dose not yet clear, but suggest starting at 25 mg a day and increasing weekly by 25 mg to a maximum of 200 mg/day. Slow rate of increase if adverse effects troublesome	Monitor for signs **of visual disturbance** (stop topiramate immediately and refer) and **cognitive decline** (slow rate of dose increase)

100

Contraindications	Side effects	Drug interactions
Pregnancy (see page 207) **Breast-feeding**: avoid (see page 214) **Renal impairment** (may be given if close monitoring practicable) Thyroidopathies Sick sinus syndrome	Thirst, polyuria GI upset Tremor (may treat with propranolol) Diabetes insipidus – may inhibit ADH (must maintain fluid intake) Acne Muscular weakness Cardiac arrhythmias Weight gain common (?related to thirst and intake of high calorie drinks) Hypothyroidism	**Antipsychotics** – all antipsychotics may increase lithium's neurotoxicity but this is rarely observed in practice. **Diltiazem/verapamil** may also rarely be linked to neurotoxicity. **Diuretics** (thiazides): increase lithium concentration. **ACE inhibitors**: toxicity **NSAIDs**: all cause toxicity except aspirin and sulindac. Low-dose ibuprofen usually safe. **Alcohol**: increases peak lithium concentration **Xanthines**: increase lithium excretion **NaCl**: increases lithium excretion
Pregnancy (see page 208) Breast-feeding (see page 214)	Drowsiness, ataxia, diplopia, nausea Agranulocytosis – 1 in 20,000 Aplastic anaemia – 1 in 20,000 Transient leucopenia in about 10% in first 2 months Hypersensitivity – hepatitis SIADH Rashes – may be serious Toxic epidermal necrolysis in 1 in 20,000, monitor carefully throughout treatment; ask patient to report immediately any rash accompanied by fever/malaise	**Antipsychotics**: may add to CNS effects (drowsiness, ataxia, etc.) **Lithium:** CNS effects and increased risk of side effects of both drugs. **Ca^{++} channel blockers**: CNS effects. **MAOIs**: Need 2 weeks washout ?Toxicity with '**flu vaccine** Enzyme inducer: affects many other drugs, including **phenytoin** and oral contraceptives. Also decreases **tricyclic and antipsychotic** plasma levels. See page 201.
Pregnancy (see page 208) Breast-feeding (see page 214) Hepatic disease	*Commonly:* Nausea, vomiting and mild sedation Moderate weight gain Hair loss *Rarely:* Ataxia and headache Thrombocytopenia and platelet dysfunction Pancytopenia Pancreatitis	Complex interactions with other **anticonvulsants**: need to consult neurologist (see also page 201) Potentiates activity of **aspirin** and **warfarin** May increase **MAOI** and **TCA** levels Increases **lamotrigine** levels
Pregnancy (see page 208) Hepatic impairment	Rash, ataxia, diplopia, headache, vomiting	**Valproate** increases levels of lamotrigine Lamotrigine may increase levels of the active **carbamazepine epoxide metabolite**
Pregnancy – consult drug information services Breast-feeding	Nausea, weight loss, abdominal pain More rarely, confusion, impaired concentration, memory impairment, emotional lability, ataxia	Additive CNS effects with other anticonvulsants May increase levels of phenytoin

References

1. Vasudev K, Goswami U, Kohli K. Carbamazepine and valproate monotherapy: feasibility, relative safety and efficacy, and therapeutic drug monitoring in manic disorder. *Psychopharmacology* 2000; **150**:15–23.
2. Chou JC-Y. Recent advances in treatment of acute mania. *Journal of Clinical Psychopharmacology* 1991; **11**: 3–21.
3. Keck PE, McElroy SL, Strakowski SM. Anticonvulsants and antipsychotics in the treatment of bipolar disorder. *Journal of Clinical Psychiatry* 1998; **59**(Suppl. 6): 74–81.
4. Small JG, Klapper MH, Milstein V. Carbamazepine compared with lithium in the treatment of mania. *Archives of General Psychiatry* 1991; **48**: 915–921.
5. Klein E, Bental E, Lerer B. Carbamazepine and haloperidol vs placebo and haloperidol in excited psychoses. *Archives of General Psychiatry* 1984; **48**: 915–921.
6. Dilsaver SC, Swann SC, Chen YW *et al*. Treatment of bipolar depression with carbamazepine: results of an open study. *Biological Psychiatry* 1996; **40**: 935–937.
7. Cullen M, Mitchell P, Brodaty H. Carbamazepine for treatment-resistant melancholia. *Journal of Clinical Psychiatry* 1991; **52**: 472–476.
8. Kramlinger KG, Post RM. The addition of lithium to carbamazepine: antidepressant efficacy in treatment resistant depression. *Archives of General Psychiatry* 1989; **46**: 794–800.
9. Davis JM, Janicak PG, Hogan DM. Mood stabilisers in the prevention of recurrent affective disorders: a meta-analysis. *Acta Psychiatrica Scandinavica* 1999; **100**: 406–417.
10. Post RM, Leverich GS, Rosoff AS. Carbamazepine prophylaxis in refractory affective disorders: a focus on long-term follow-up. *Journal of Clinical Psychopharmacology* 1990; **10**: 318–327.
11. Joyce PR. Carbamazepine in rapid cycling bipolar affective disorder. *International Clinical Psychopharmacology* 1988; **3**: 123–129.
12. Okuma T. Effects of carbamazepine and lithium on affective disorders. *Neuropsychobiology* 1993; **27**: 138–145.
13. Brieden T, Ujeyl M, Naber D. Psychopharmacological treatment of aggression in schizophrenic patients. *Pharmacopsychiatry* 2002; **35**: 83–89.
14. Malcolm R, Myrisk H, Roberts J. The effects of carbamazepine and lorazepam on single versus multiple previous alcohol withdrawals in an outpatient randomised trial. *Journal of General Internal Medicine* 2002; **17**: 349–355.
15. Taylor D, Duncan D. Doses of carbamazepine and valproate in bipolar affective disorder. *Psychiatric Bulletin* 1997; **21**: 221–223,
16. Simhandl C, Denk E, Thau K. The comparative efficacy of carbamazepine low and high serum level and lithium carbonate in the prophylaxis of affective disorders. *Journal of Affective Disorders* 1993; **28**: 221–231.
17. Taylor DM, Starkey K, Ginary S. Prescribing and monitoring of carbamazepine and valproate – a case note review. *Psychiatric Bulletin* 2000; **24**: 174–177.
18. Kaufman DW, Kelly JP, Jurgelon JM. Drugs in the aetiology of agranulocytosis and aplastic anaemia. *European Journal of Haematology* 1996; **60**(Suppl.): 23–30.
19. Spina E, Perucca E. Cinical significance of pharmacokinetic interactions between antiepileptic and psychotropic drugs. *Epilepsia* 2002; **43**: 37–44.
20. Patsalos PN, Froscher W, Pisani F *et al*. The importance of drug interactions in epilepsy therapy. *Epilepsia* 2002; **43**: 365–385.
21. Ketler TA, Post RM, Worthington K. Principles of clinically important drug interactions with carbamazepine. Part 1. *Journal of Clinical Psychopharmacology* 1991; **11**: 198–203.
22. Crawford P. Interactions between antiepileptic drugs and hormonal contraception. *CNS Drugs* 2002; **16**: 263–272.
23. Shula S, Godwin CD, Long LEB. Lithium–carbamazepine neurotoxicity and risk factors. *American Journal of Psychiatry* 1984; **141**: 1604–1606.

Treatment of acute mania or hypomania

The table below illustrates a suggested treatment plan for mania occurring in patients with known bipolar disorder. (For patients with *de novo* manic or hypomanic symptoms that may not be related to bipolar disorder (e.g. drug-induced), the use of antipsychotics with benzodiazepines is preferred.)

Table	Suggested treatment plan	
Step	**Recommendation**	**Comments**
1	**Combine mood-stabiliser* with antipsychotic** (see page 105)	– Use plasma level monitoring to optimise mood-stabiliser[1] – Withdraw any antidepressant[2]
2	**Add benzodiazepine**	– Suggest lorazepam[3] up to 4 mg daily or clonazepam[4] up to 2 mg daily** – Assess over 2–3 days – Withdraw if not effective or after reduction in symptoms
3	**Consider other putative anti-manic agents or strategies** For example: – combinations of mood-stabilisers[2] – clozapine[5,6] (dosing as for schizophrenia) – topiramate[7,8] up to 200 mg/day	– Variable support in literature – Clozapine has good record in refractory mania

* Suggested *starting* doses:
Lithium 400 mg MR daily
Carbamazepine 200 mg MR BD
Valproate – *Epilim Chrono* 500 mg daily or *Depakote* 250 mg tds
(Valproate 'loading' (20 mg/kg/day valproate semisodium) is also effective[9,10] and may have a more rapid onset of action)
** Many centres use higher doses of benzodiazepines (e.g. up to 8 mg/day clonazepam/lorazepam)

Other drugs that may have activity in mania include lamotrigine[11] (up to 200 mg/day), gabapentin[12,13] (up to 2400 mg/day) and phenytoin[14] (300–400 mg/day). None is widely used in practice and considerable doubt surrounds their efficacy (e.g. a controlled trial of gabapentin suggested no effect[15]). Lithium may be somewhat less effective in mixed states[16] or where there is substance misuse[17]. The use of ECT should be considered for refractory acute mania.

References

1. Taylor DM, Duncan D. Doses of carbamazepine and valproate in bipolar affective disorder. *Psychiatry Bulletin* 1997; **21**: 221–223.
2. American Psychiatric Association. Practice guideline for the treatment of patients with bipolar disorder. *American Journal of Psychiatry* 1994; **151**: 1–36.
3. Modell JG, Lenox RH, Weiner S. Inpatient clinical trial of lorazepam for the management of manic agitation. *Journal of Clinical Psychopharmacology* 1985; **5**: 109–113.
4. Sachs GS, Rosenbaum JF, Jones J. Adjunctive clonazepam for maintenance treatment of bipolar affective disorder. *Journal of Clinical Psychopharmacology* 1990; **10**: 42–47.
5. Mahmood T, Devlin M, Silverstone T. Clozapine in the management of bipolar and schizoaffective manic episodes resistant to standard treatment. *Australian NZ Journal of Psychiatry* 1997; **31**: 424–426.
6. Green AI, Tohen M, Patel JK *et al.* Clozapine in the treatment of refractory psychotic mania. *American Journal of Psychiatry* 2000; **157**: 982–986.
7. Grunze HCR, Normann C, Langosch J *et al.* Antimanic efficacy of topiramate in 11 patients in an open trial with an of-off-on design. *Journal of Clinical Psychiatry* 2001; **62**: 464–468.

8. Lakshmi NY, Kuusmakar V, Calabrese JR *et al.* Third generation anticonvulsants in bipolar disorder: a review of efficacy and summary of clinical recommendations. *Journal of Clinical Psychiatry* 2002; **63**: 275–283.
9. McElroy SL, Keck PE, Stanton SP *et al.* A randomized comparison of divalproex oral loading versus haloperidol in the initial treatment of acute psychotic mania. *Journal of Clinical Psychiatry* 1996; **57**: 142–146.
10. Hirschfeld RMA, Allen MH, McEvoy JP *et al.* Safety and tolerability of oral loading divalproex sodium in acutely manic bipolar patients. *Journal of Clinical Psychiatry* 1999; **60**: 815–818.
11. Calabrese JR, Bowden CL, McElroy SL *et al.* Spectrum of activity of lamotrigine in treatment-refractory bipolar disorder. *American Journal of Psychiatry* 1999; **156**: 1019–1023.
12. Macdonald KJ, Young LT. Newer antiepileptic drugs in bipolar disorder. *CNS Drugs* 2002; **16**: 549–562.
13. Cabras PL, Hardoy MJ, Hardoy MC *et al.* Clinical experience with gabapentin in patients with bipolar or schizoaffective disorder: results of an open-label study. *Journal of Clinical Psychiatry* 1999; **60**: 245–248.
14. Mishory A, Yaroslavsky Y, Bersudsky Y *et al.* Phenytoin as an antimanic anticonvulsant: a controlled study. *American Journal of Psychiatry* 2000; **157**: 463–465.
15. Pande AC, Crockatt JG, Janney CA *et al.* Gabapentin in bipolar disorder: a placebo-controlled trial of adjunctive therapy. *Bipolar Disorders* 2000; **2**(3 Pt 2): 249–255.
16. Swann AC, Secunda SK, Katz MM *et al.* Lithium treatment of mania: clinical characteristics, specificity of symptom change, and outcome. *Psychiatry Research* 1986; **18**: 127–141.
17. Goldberg JF, Garnò JL, Leon AC *et al.* A history of substance abuse complicates remission from acute mania in bipolar disorder. *Journal of Clinical Psychiatry* 1999; **60**: 733–740.

Further reading

Joffe RT, Macqueen GM, Marriott M *et al.* Induction of mania and cycle acceleration in bipolar disorder: effect of different classes of antidepressant. *Acta Psychiatrica Scandinavica* 2002; **105**: 427–430.

Table Drugs for acute mania – relative costs (March 2003)

Drug	Cost for 30 days' treatment	Comments
Lithium (Priadel) 800 mg/day	£2.95	Add cost of plasma level monitoring
Carbamazepine (Tegretol Retard) 800 mg/day	£11.08	Self-induction complicates acute treatment
Sodium valproate (Epilim Chrono) 1500 mg/day	£18.19	Not licensed for mania, but may be given once daily
Valproate semisodium (Depakote) 1500 mg/day	£72.19	Licensed for mania, but given twice or three times daily
Haloperidol (Serenace) 10 mg/day	£8.81	Most widely used typical antipsychotic
Olanzapine (Zyprexa) 15 mg/day	£156.79	Only licensed atypical

Antipsychotics in bipolar disorder

Typical antipsychotics have long been used in mania and several studies support their use in a variety of hypomanic and manic presentations[1–3]. Their effectiveness seems to be enhanced by the addition of a mood stabiliser[4,5]. In the longer-term treatment of bipolar disorder, typicals are widely used (presumably as prophylaxis)[6] but robust supporting data are absent[7]. The observation that typical antipsychotics may induce depression and tardive dyskinesia in bipolar patients militates against their long-term use[7,8].

Among atypical antipsychotics, olanzapine has been most robustly evaluated and is licensed in the UK for the treatment of mania. Olanzapine is more effective than placebo in mania[9,10], and at least as effective as valproate semisodium[11] and lithium[12]. As with typical drugs, olanzapine may be most effective when used in combination with a mood-stabiliser[13]. Preliminary data suggest olanzapine may offer benefits in longer-term treatment[14,15] but it is not formally licensed as prophylaxis.

Clozapine seems to be effective in refractory bipolar conditions, including refractory mania[16–18]. Risperidone has also shown efficacy in mania[19], particularly in combination with a mood-stabiliser[20,21]. Data relating to quetiapine[22,23] and amisulpride[24] are scarce.

References

1. Prien R, Point P, Caffey E *et al.* Comparison of lithium carbonate and chlorpromazine in the treatment of mania. *Archives of General Psychiatry* 1972; **26**: 146–153.
2. Sachs G, Grossman F, Nassir G *et al.* Combination of a mood stabilizer with risperidone or haloperidol for treatment of acute mania: a double-blind, placebo-controlled comparison of efficacy and safety. *American Journal Psychiatry* 2002; **159**: 1146–1154.
3. McElroy S, Keck P, Stanton S *et al.* A randomized comparison of divalproex oral loading versus haloperidol in the initial treatment of acute psychotic mania. *Journal of Clinical Psychiatry* 1996; **57**: 142–146.
4. Chou J, Czobor P, Owen C *et al.* Acute mania: haloperidol dose and augmentation with lithium or lorazepam. *Journal of Clinical Psychopharmacology* 1999; **19**: 500–505.
5. Small JG, Kellams JJ, Milstein *et al.* A placebo-controlled study of lithium combined with neuroleptics in chronic schizophrenia patients. *American Journal of Psychiatry* 1975; **132**: 1315–1317.
6. Soares J, Barwell M, Mallinger A *et al.* Adjunctive antipsychotic use in bipolar patients: an open 6-month prospective study following an acute episode. *Journal of Affective Disorders* 1998; **56**: 1–8.
7. Keck P, McElroy S, Strakowski S. Anticonvulsants and antipsychotics in the treatment of bipolar disorder. *Journal of Clinical Psychiatry* 1998; **59**(Suppl. 6): 74–81.
8. Tohen M, Zarate C. Antipsychotic agents and bipolar disorder. *Journal of Clinical Psychiatry* 1998; **59**(Suppl. 1): 38–49.
9. Tohen M, Sanger T, Mcelroy S *et al.* Olanzapine versus placebo in the treatment of acute mania. *American Journal of Psychiatry* 1999; **156**: 702–709.
10. Tohen M, Jacobs T, Grundy S *et al.* Efficacy of olanzapine in acute bipolar mania. *Archives of General Psychiatry* 2000; **57**: 841–849.
11. Tohen M, Barker R, Altshuler L *et al.* Olanzapine versus Divalproex in the treatment of acute mania. *American Journal of Psychiatry* 2002; **159**: 1011–1017.
12. Berk M, Ichim I, Brook S. Olanzapine compared to lithium in mania: a double-blind randomised controlled trial. *International Clinical Psychopharmacology* 1999; **13**: 339–343.
13. Tohen M, Chengappa R, Suppes T *et al.* Efficacy of olanzapine in combination with valproate or lithium in the treatment of mania in patients partially non responsive to valproate or lithium monotherapy. *Archives of General Psychiatry* 2002; **69**: 62–69.
14. Sanger T, Grundy S, Gibson J *et al.* Long-term olanzapine therapy in the treatment of bipolar I disorder: an open-label continuation phase study. *Journal of Clinical Psychiatry* 2001; **62**: 273–280.
15. Vieta E, Reinares M, Corbella B *et al.* Olanzapine as long-term adjunctive therapy in treatment-resistant bipolar disorder. *Journal of Clinical Psychopharmacology* 2001; **21**: 469–473.
16. Calabrese J, Kimmel S, Woysville *et al.* Clozapine for treatment-refractory mania. *American Journal of Psychiatry* 1996; **153**: 759–764.
17. Green A, Tohen M, Patel J *et al.* Clozapine in the treatment of refractory psychotic mania. *American Journal of Psychiatry* 2000; **157**: 982–986.
18. Calabrese J, Kimmel S, Woysville *et al.* Clozapine in treatment-refractory mood disorders. *Journal of Clinical Psychiatry* 1994; **55**: 91–93.

19. Segal J, Berk M, Brook S. Risperidone compared with both lithium and haloperidol in mania: A double-blind randomised controlled trial. *Clinical Neuropharmacology* 1998; **21**: 176–180.
20. Sachs G, Grossman F, Nassir G *et al.* Combination of a mood stabiliser with risperidone or haloperidol for treatment of acute-mania: a double-blind, placebo-controlled comparison of efficacy and safety. *American Journal of Psychiatry* 2002; **159**: 1146–1154.
21. Vieta E, Herraiz M, Parramon G *et al.* Risperidone in the treatment of mania: efficacy and safety results from a large multicentre, open study in Spain. *Journal of Affective Disorders* 2002; **72**: 15–19.
22. Ghaemi N, Katzow J. The use of quetiapine for treatment-resistant bipolar disorder: a case series. *Annals of Clinical Psychiatry* 1999; **11**: 137–140.
23. Sachs G, Mullen JA, Devine NA *et al.* Quetiapine versus placebo as adjunct to mood stabilizer for the treatment of acute bipolar mania. AstraZeneca Pharmaceuticals. Presented at the 15th Congress of the European College of Neuropsychopharmacology, October 5–9 2002, Barcelona, Spain.
24. Pariante C, Orru M, Carpinello B *et al.* Multiple sclerosis and major depression resistant to treatment. Case of a patient with antidepressive therapy induced mood disorder associated with manic features (Italian). *Clinica Therapeutica* 1995; **146**: 449–452.

Rapid-cycling bipolar affective disorder

Rapid-cycling is usually defined as bipolar disorder in which 4 or more episodes of (hypo)mania or depression occur in a 12-month period. It is generally thought to be less responsive to drug treatment than non-rapid-cycling bipolar illness[1]. The following algorithm for treatment of rapid-cycling is based on rather limited data from a very few studies. In practice, response to treatment is often idiosyncratic: individuals sometimes show dramatic improvement only on one particular treatment. This may reflect the fact that spontaneous or drug-related remissions seem to occur in around a third of rapid-cyclers[2].

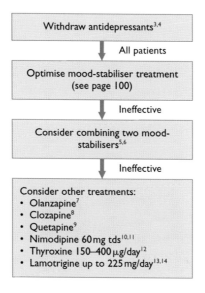

Withdraw antidepressants[3,4]

↓ All patients

Optimise mood-stabiliser treatment (see page 100)

↓ Ineffective

Consider combining two mood-stabilisers[5,6]

↓ Ineffective

Consider other treatments:
- Olanzapine[7]
- Clozapine[8]
- Quetapine[9]
- Nimodipine 60 mg tds[10,11]
- Thyroxine 150–400 μg/day[12]
- Lamotrigine up to 225 mg/day[13,14]

Notes

- Take a detailed history and consider precipitants of mood change that might be predicted or controlled (e.g. thyroid dysfunction, external stressors, life events).
- Choice of 'other treatments' is dependent on individual patient factors – there are no comparative data to suggest which treatments might be more effective.
- Lamotrigine may be treatment of choice for depressive episodes in rapid cycling – it is effective treatment and prophylaxis but does not induce mania.

References

1. Calabrese JR, Shelton MD, Rapport DJ *et al.* Current research on rapid cycling bipolar disorder and its treatment. *Journal of Affective Disorders* 2001; **67**: 241–255.
2. Koukopoulos A, Sani G, Koukopoulos AE *et al.* Duration and stability of the rapid-cycling course: a long-term personal follow-up of 109 patients. *Journal of Affective Disorders* 2003; **73**: 75–85.
3. Wehr TA, Goodwin FK. Can antidepressants cause mania and worsen the course of affective illness? *American Journal of Psychiatry* 1987; **144**: 1403–1411.
4. Altshuler LL, Post RM, Leverich GS. Antidepressant-induced mania and cycle acceleration: a controversy revisited. *American Journal of Psychiatry* 1995; **152**: 1130–1138.
5. Calabrese JR, Woyshville, MJ. A medication algorithm for treatment of bipolar rapid cycling? *Clinical Psychiatry* 1995; **56**(Suppl. 3): 11–18.
6. Taylor DM, Duncan D. Treatment options for rapid-cycling bipolar affective disorder. *Psychiatric Bulletin* 1996; **20**: 601–603.

7. Sanger TM, Tohen M, Vieta E *et al.* Olanzapine in the acute treatment of bipolar I disorder with a history of rapid cycling. *Journal of Affective Disorders* 2003; **73**: 155–161.
8. Calabrese JR, Meltzer HY, Markovitz PJ. Clozapine prophylaxis in rapid cycling bipolar disorder. *Journal of Clinical Psychopharmacology* 1991; **11**: 396–397.
9. Vieta E, Parramon G, Padrell E *et al.* Quetiapine in the treatment of rapid cycling bipolar disorder. *Bipolar Disorders* 2002; **4**: 335–340.
10. Goodnick PJ. Nimodipine treatment of rapid cycling bipolar disorder. *Journal of Clinical Psychiatry* 1995; **56**: 330.
11. Pazzagila PJ, Post RM, Ketter TA *et al.* Preliminary controlled trial of nimodipine in ultra-rapid cycling affective dysregulation. *Psychiatry Research* 1993; **49**: 257–272.
12. Bauer MS, Whybrow PC. Rapid cycling bipolar affective disorder. *Archives of General Psychiatry* 1990; **47**: 435–440.
13. Fatemi SH, Rapport DJ, Calabrese JR *et al.* Lamotrigine in rapid-cycling bipolar disorder. *Journal of Clinical Psychiatry* 1997; **58**: 522–527.
14. Calabrese JR, Suppes T, Bowden CL *et al.* A double-blind, placebo-controlled, prophylaxis study of lamotrigine in rapid-cycling bipolar disorder. *Journal of Clinical Psychiatry* 2000; **61**: 841–850.

chapter 4

Depression and anxiety

Antidepressant drugs – tricyclics*

Tricyclic	Licensed indication	Licensed doses (elderly doses not included)	Main adverse effects	Major interactions	Approx. half-life (h)	Cost (£)
Amitriptyline	Depression Nocturnal enuresis in children	30–200 mg/day 7–10 yr: 10–20 mg 11–16 yr: 25–50 mg at night for max. 3 months	Sedation, often with hangover; postural hypotension; tachycardia/arrhythmias; dry mouth, blurred vision, constipation, urinary retention	SSRIs (except citalopram), phenothiazines, cimetidine – ↑ plasma levels of TCAs Alcohol Antimuscarinics Antipsychotics (esp. pimozide/thioridazine) MAOIs	9–25 18–96 Active metabolite (nortriptyline)	0.04/50 mg
Clomipramine	Depression Phobic & obsessional states Adjunctive treatment of cataplexy associated with narcolepsy	10–250 mg/day 10–150 mg/day 10–75 mg/day	As for amitriptyline	As for amitriptyline	19–37 54–77 Active metabolite (desmethyl-clomipramine)	0.14/50 mg
Dosulepin (dothiepin)	Depression	75–225 mg/day	As for amitriptyline	As for amitriptyline	11–40 22–60 Active metabolite (desmethyldosulepin)	0.15/75 mg
Doxepin	Depression	10–300 mg/day (up to 100 mg as a single dose)	As for amitriptyline	As for amitriptyline	8–25 28–52 Active metabolite (desmethyldoxepin)	0.05/50 mg

110

Drug	Indication	Dose			Half-life (h)	mg
Imipramine	Depression	10–200 mg/day (up to 100 mg as a single dose; up to 300 mg in hospital patients)	As for amitriptyline but less sedative	As for amitriptyline	4–18 12–24 Active metabolite (desipramine)	0.04/25 mg
	Nocturnal enuresis in children	7 yr: 25 mg 8–11 yr: 25–50 mg >11 yr: 50–75 mg at night for max. 3 months				
Lofepramine	Depression	140–210 mg/day	As for amitriptyline but less sedative/anticholinergic/ cardiotoxic	As for amitriptyline	1.5–6 12–24 Active metabolite (desipramine)	0.18/70 mg
Nortriptyline	Depression	30–150 mg/day	As for amitriptyline but less sedative/anticholinergic/ hypotensive Constipation may be problematic	As for amitriptyline	18–96	0.25/25 mg
	Nocturnal enuresis in children	7 yr: 10 mg 8–11 yrs: 10–20 mg >11 yr: 25–35 mg at night for max. 3 months				
Trimipramine	Depression	30–300 mg/day	As for amitriptyline but more sedative	As for amitriptyline Safer with MAOIs than other tricyclics	7–23	0.30/50 mg

* For full details refer to the manufacturer's information

Antidepressant drugs – SSRIs*

SSRI	Licensed indication	Licensed doses (elderly) doses are not included	Main adverse effects	Major interactions	Approx. half-life (h)	Cost (£)
Citalopram	Depression – treatment of the initial phase & as maintenance therapy against potential relapse or recurrence Panic disorder +/– agoraphobia	20–60 mg/day 10 mg for one week, increasing up to 60 mg/day	Nausea, vomiting, dyspepsia, abdominal pain, diarrhoea, rash, sweating, agitation, anxiety, headache, insomnia, tremor, sexual dysfunction (male & female), hyponatraemia, cutaneous bleeding disorders. Discontinuation symptoms may occur. See pages 148 et seq.	Not a potent inhibitor of cytochrome enzymes. MAOIs – avoid. Avoid – St Johns Wort. Caution with alcohol (although no interaction seen)/ NSAIDs/ tryptophan/ warfarin.	33 Has weak active metabolites	0.57/20 mg Drops 0.72/ 16 mg/8 drops (= 20 mg tab)
Escitalopram	Depression Panic disorder +/– agoraphobia	10–20 mg/day 5 mg/day for one week, increasing up to 20 mg/day	As for citalopram	As for citalopram	~30 Has weak active metabolites	0.57/10 mg
Fluoxetine	Depression +/– anxiety OCD Bulimia nervosa Premenstrual dysphoric disorder	20 mg/day 20–60 mg/day 60 mg/day 20 mg/day	As for citalopram but insomnia and agitation more common. Rash may occur more frequently. May alter insulin requirements.	Inhibits CYP2D6, CYP3A4. Increases plasma levels of some antipsychotics/ some benzos/carbamazepine/ cyclosporin/ phenytoin/ tricyclics MAOIs – never. Avoid: selegiline/ St John's wort/ terfenadine. Caution – alcohol (although no interaction seen)/NSAIDs/ tryptophan/warfarin	2–3 days 4–16 days Active metabolite (norfluoxetine)	0.26/20 mg (generic – BNF) Liquid 0.95/20 mg/5 ml
Fluvoxamine	Depression OCD	100–300 mg/day bd if >100 mg 100–300 mg/day bd if >100 mg	As for citalopram but nausea more common	Inhibits CYP1A2/ 2C9/ 3A4. Increases plasma levels of some benzos/carbamazepine/ciclosporin/ methadone/olanzapine/phenytoin/ propranolol/ theophylline/ some tricyclics/ warfarin. MAOIs – never Avoid – astemizole/ cisapride/ terfenadine Caution: alcohol/ lithium/ NSAIDs/St John's wort/ tryptophan/warfarin	17–22	0.63/100 mg

	Indication	Dose	Adverse effects	Interactions	Half-life (hours)	Cost/dose
Paroxetine	Depression +/– anxiety	20–50 mg/day	As for citalopram but antimuscarinic effects and sedation more common. Extrapyramidal symptoms more common, but rare. Discontinuation symptoms common – withdraw slowly	Potent inhibitor of CYP2D6. Increases plasma level of some antipsychotics/ tricyclics. MAOIs – never. Avoid: St John's wort. Caution: alcohol/lithium/ NSAIDs/tryptophan/ warfarin	15–2 (non-linear kinetics)	0.59/20 mg Liquid 1.38/20 mg/10 ml
	OCD	20–60 mg/day				
	Panic disorder +/– agoraphobia	10–50 mg/day				
	Social phobia	20–50 mg/day				
	PTSD	20–50 mg/day				
	Generalised anxiety disorder	20 mg/day				
Sertraline	Depression +/– anxiety and prevention of relapse or recurrence of depression +/– anxiety	50–200 mg/day	As for citalopram	Inhibits CYP2D6 (more likely to occur at doses ≥100 mg/day). Increases plasma levels of some antipsychotics/ tricyclics. Avoid: St John's wort. Caution: alcohol (although no interaction seen)/lithium/ NSAIDs/ tryptophan/ warfarin	~ 26 Has a weak active metabolite	0.95/100 mg (0.58/50 mg)
	OCD (under specialist supervision in children)	50–200 mg/day (adults) 6–12 yr: 25–50 mg/day, may be increased in steps of 50 mg to 200 mg/day 13–17 yr: 50–200 mg/day				
	PTSD in women	25–50 mg/day				

* For full details refer to the manufacturer's information

Antidepressant drugs – MAOIs*

MAOI	Licensed indication	Licensed doses (elderly doses are not) included	Main adverse effects	Major interactions	Approx. half-life (h)	Cost (£)
Isocarboxazid	Depression	30 mg/day in single or divided doses, increased after 4 weeks to max. 60 mg/day for 4–6 weeks 10–40 mg/day maintenance	Postural hypotension, dizziness, drowsiness, insomnia, headaches, oedema, anticholinergic adverse effects, nervousness, paraesthesia, weight gain, hepatotoxicity, leucopenia, hypertensive crisis	Tyramine in food, sympathomimetics, alcohol, opioids, antidepressants, levodopa, 5HT$_1$ agonists	36	0.53/10 mg
Phenelzine	Depression	15 mg tds – qid (hospital patients: max. 30 mg tds). Consider reducing to lowest possible maintenance dose	As for isocarboxazid but more postural hypotension, less hepatotoxicity	As for isocarboxazid. Probably safest of MAOIs and is the one that should be used if combinations are considered	1.5	0.20/15 mg
Tranylcypromine	Depression	10 mg bd Doses >30 mg/day under close supervision only Usual maintenance: 10 mg/day Last dose no later than 3 pm	As for isocarboxazid but insomnia, nervousness, hypertensive crisis more common than with other MAOIs; hepatotoxicity less common Mild dependence as amphetamine-like structure	As for isocarboxazid but interactions more severe. Never use in combination therapy with other antidepressants	2.5	0.05/10 mg

114

| Moclobemide (Reversible inhibitor of MAO-A) | Depression | 150–600 mg/day bd after food | Sleep disturbances, nausea, agitation, confusion Hypertension reported – may be related to tyramine ingestion | Tyramine interactions rare and mild but possible if high doses (>600 mg/day) used or if large quantities of tyramine ingested CNS excitation/depression with dextromethorphan/ pethidine Avoid: clomipramine/levodopa/ selegiline/sympathomimetics/ SSRIs Caution with fentanyl/morphine/tricyclics Cimetidine – use half dose of moclobemide | 2–4 | 0.33/150 mg |
| | Social phobia | 300–600 mg/day bd after food Last dose before 3 pm | | | | |

* For full details refer to the manufacturer's information

Antidepressant drugs – others*

Antidepressant	Licensed indication	Licensed doses (Elderly doses are not included)	Main adverse effects	Major interactions	Approx. half-life (h)	Cost (£)
Mianserin	Depression	30–90 mg daily	Sedation, rash; rarely: blood dyscrasias, jaundice, arthralgia No anticholinergic effects Sexual dysfunction uncommon Low cardiotoxicity	Other sedatives, alcohol MAOIs: avoid Effect on hepatic enzymes unclear, so caution is required	10–20 2-desmethyl-mianserin is major metabolite (?activity)	0.17/30 mg
Mirtazapine	Depression	15–45 mg/day	Increased appetite, weight gain, drowsiness, oedema, dizziness, headache, ?blood dyscrasias Nausea/sexual dysfunction are relatively uncommon	Minimal effect on CYP2D6/1A2/3A Caution: alcohol/sedatives	20–40 25 Active metabolite (demethyl-mirtazapine)	0.82/30 mg
Nefazodone (now withdrawn in many countries)	Depression including depressive syndromes associated with anxiety or sleep disturbances	100–300 mg bd	Dizziness, postural hypotension, somnolence, nausea, paraesthesias, liver toxicity. Visual trailing rarely Sexual dysfunction is uncommon	Potent inhibitor of CYP3A4. Increases plasma levels of some benzos/buspirone/carbamazepine/ciclosporin/digoxin/haloperidol/pimozide/tacrolimus/terfenadine. Avoid: MAOIs/pimozide/sibutramine/simvastatin. Fluoxetine increases plasma levels of mCPP (anxiogenic metabolite). Caution: alcohol (although no interaction seen)	2–4 (dose-dependent) Active metabolites: 2–4 (hydroxynefazo-done) 18–33 (desethyl-hydroxy) 4–9 (mCPP: minor)	0.30/200 mg

116

Reboxetine	Depression – acute & maintenance	4–6 mg bd	Insomnia, sweating, dizziness, dry mouth, constipation, tachycardia, urinary hesitancy Erectile dysfunction may occur rarely	Metabolised by CYP3A4 – avoid drugs inhibiting this enzyme (e.g. erythromycin/nefazodone/ketoconazole). Minimal effect on CYP2D6/3A4. MAOIs: avoid. No interaction with alcohol	13	0.32/4 mg
Trazodone	Depression +/– anxiety	150–300 mg/day (up to 600 mg/day in hospitalised patients) bd dosing above 300 mg/day	Sedation, dizziness, headache, nausea, vomiting, tremor, postural hypotension, tachyardia, priapism. Not anticholinergic, less cardiotoxic than tricyclics	Caution: sedatives/alcohol/other antidepressants/digoxin/phenytoin MAOIs: avoid	5–13 (biphasic)	0.40/100 mg Liquid 0.71/100 mg/ 10 ml
	Anxiety	75–300 mg/day			4-9 Active metabolite (mCPP)	
Venlafaxine	Depression +/– anxiety and prevention of relapse or recurrence of depression	75–375 mg/day (bd) with food 75–225 mg XL/day (od) with food	Nausea, insomnia, dry mouth, somnolence, dizziness, sweating, nervousness, headache, sexual dysfunction Elevation of blood pressure at higher doses. Discontinuation symptoms common – withdraw slowly	Metabolised by CYP2D6/3A4 – caution with drugs known to inhibit both isozymes. Minimal effects on CYP2D6. No effects on CYP1A2/2C9/3A4. MAOIs: avoid Caution: alcohol (although no interaction seen)/cimetidine/clozapine/warfarin	5	0.71/75 mg 0.86/75 mg XL
	Generalised anxiety disorder (XL prep only)	75 mg XL/day (discontinue if no response after 8 weeks)			11 Active metabolite (O-desmethyl-venlafaxine)	

* For full details refer to the manufacturer's information

Treatment of affective illness

Depression

Basic principles of prescribing in depression

- Discuss with the patient choice of drug and utility/availability of other, non-pharmacological treatments

- Discuss with the patient likely outcomes, e.g. gradual relief from depressive symptoms over several weeks

- Prescribe a dose of antidepressant (after titration, if necessary) that is likely to be effective

- Continue treatment for at least 4–6 months after resolution of symptoms

- Withdraw antidepressants gradually; always inform patients of the risk and nature of discontinuation symptoms

Drug treatment of depression

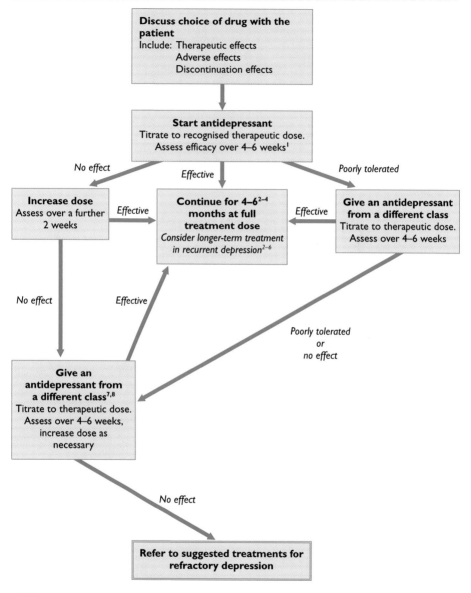

Discuss choice of drug with the patient
Include: Therapeutic effects
Adverse effects
Discontinuation effects

Start antidepressant
Titrate to recognised therapeutic dose.
Assess efficacy over 4–6 weeks[1]

No effect

Effective

Poorly tolerated

Increase dose
Assess over a further
2 weeks

Effective

Continue for 4–6[2–4] months at full treatment dose
Consider longer-term treatment in recurrent depression[2–6]

Effective

Give an antidepressant from a different class
Titrate to therapeutic dose.
Assess over 4–6 weeks

No effect

Effective

*Poorly tolerated
or
no effect*

Give an antidepressant from a different class[7,8]
Titrate to therapeutic dose.
Assess over 4–6 weeks,
increase dose as
necessary

No effect

Refer to suggested treatments for refractory depression

Notes
- Tools such as the Montgomery-Asberg depression rating scale and the Hamilton depression rating scale are recommended to assess drug effect.
- Switching between drug classes in cases of poor tolerability is not well supported by published studies but has a strong theoretical basis. In cases of non-response, there is some evidence that switching within a drug class can be effective[8,9], but switching between classes is, in practice, the most common option (see page 143).

119

References

1. Snow V, Lascher S, Mottur-Pilson C *et al.* Pharmacologic treatment of acute major depression and dysthymia. *Annals of Internal Medicine* 2000; **132**: 738–742.
2. Anderson IM, Nutt DJ, Deakin JFW. Evidence-based guidelines for treating depressive disorders with antidepressants: a revision of the 1993 British Association for Psychopharmacology guidelines. *Journal of Psychopharmacology* 2000; **14**: 3–19.
3. Crismon ML, Trivedi M, Pigott TA *et al.* The Texas medication algorithm project: report of the Texas consensus conference panel on medication treatment of major depressive disorder. *Journal of Clinical Psychiatry* 1999; **60**: 142–156.
4. Practice guideline for major depressive disorder in adults. *American Journal of Psychiatry* 1993; **150**: 1–26.
5. Kocsis JH, Friedman RA, Markowitz JC *et al.* Maintenance therapy for chronic depression. *Archives of General Psychiatry* 1996; **53**: 769–774.
6. Dekker J, de Jonghe F, Tuynman H. The use of anti-depressants after recovery from depression. *European Journal of Psychiatry* 2000; **14**: 207–212.
7. Nelson JC. Treatment of antidepressant nonresponders: augmentation or switch? *Journal of Clinical Psychiatry* 1998; **59**: 35–41.
8. Joffe RT. Substitution therapy in patients with major depression. *CNS Drugs* 1999; **11**: 175–180.
9. Thase ME, Feighner JP, Lydiard RB. Citalopram treatment of fluoxetine nonresponders. *Journal of Clinical Psychiatry* 2001; **62**: 683–687.

Further reading

Barbui C, Hotopf M. Amitriptyline v. the rest: still the leading antidepressant after 40 years of randomised controlled trials. *British Journal of Psychiatry* 2001; **178**: 129–144.

Smith D, Dempster C, Glanville J, Freemantle N, Anderson I. Efficacy and tolerability of venlafaxine compared with selective serotonin reuptake inhibitors and other antidepressants: a meta-analysis. *British Journal of Psychiatry* 2002; **180**: 396–404.

Recognised minimum effective doses – antidepressants

Tricyclics

Tricyclics	Unclear; at least 75–100 mg/day[1], possibly 125 mg/day[2]
Lofepramine	140 mg/day[3]

SSRIs

Citalopram	20 mg/day[4]
Escitalopram	10 mg/day[5]
Fluoxetine	20 mg/day[6]
Fluvoxamine	50 mg/day[7]
Paroxetine	20 mg/day[8]
Sertraline	50 mg/day[9]

Others

Mirtazapine	30 mg/day[10]
Moclobemide	300 mg/day[11]
Nefazodone	300 mg/day[12]
Reboxetine	8 mg/day[13]
Trazodone	150 mg/day[14]
Venlafaxine	75 mg/day[15]

References

1. Farukawa TA, McGuire H, Barbui C. Meta-analysis of effects and side effects of low dosage tricyclic antidepressants in depression: systematic review. *BMJ* 2002; **325**: 991–995
2. Donoghue J, Taylor DM. Suboptimal use of antidepressants in the treatment of depression. *CNS Drugs* 2000; **13**: 365–383
3. Lancaster SG, Gonzalez JP. Lofepramine – a review of its pharmacodynamic and pharmaco-kinetic properties, and therapeutic efficacy in depressive illness. *Drugs* 1989; **37**: 123–140.
4. Montgomery SA, Pedersen V, Tanghoj P *et al.* The optimal dosing regimen for citalopram – a meta-analysis of nine placebo-controlled studies. *International Clinical Psychopharmacology* 1994; **9**(Suppl. 1): 35–40
5. Burke WJ, Gergel I, Bose A. Fixed-dose trial of the single isomer SSRI escitalopram in depressed outpatients. *Journal of Clinical Psychiatry* 2002; **63**: 331–336.
6. Altamura AC, Montgomery SA, Wernicke JF. The evidence for 20 mg a day of fluoxetine as the optimal dose in the treatment of depression. *British Journal of Psychiatry* 1998; **153**(Suppl. 3): 109–112
7. Walczak DD, Apter JT, Halikas JA. The oral dose-effect relationship for fluvoxamine: a fixed-dose comparison against placebo in depressed outpatients. *Annals of Clinical Psychiatry* 1996; **8**: 139–151.
8. Dunner DL, Dunbar GC. Optimal dose regimen for paroxetine. *Journal of Clinical Psychiatry* 1992; **53**(Suppl. 2): 21–26.
9. Moon CA, Jago W, Wood K *et al.* A double-blind comparison of sertraline and clomipramine in the treatment of major depressive disorder and associated anxiety in general practice. *Journal of Psychopharmacology* 1994; **8**: 171–176.
10. Van-Moffaert M, De Wilde J, Vereecken A *et al.* Mirtazapine is more effective than trazodone: a double-blind controlled study in hospitalized patients with major depression. *International Clinical Psychopharmacology* 1995; **10**: 3–9.
11. Priest RG, Schmid-Burgk W. Moclobemide in the treatment of depression. *Review of Contemporary Pharmacotherapy* 1994; **5**: 35–43.
12. Fontaine R, Ontiveros A, Elie R *et al.* A double-blind comparison of nefazodone, imipramine and placebo in major depression. *Journal of Clinical Psychiatry* **55**: 234–241.
13. Schatzberg AF. Clinical efficacy of reboxetine in major depression. *Journal of Clinical Psychiatry* 2000; **61**(Suppl. 10): 31–38.
14. Brogden RN, Heel RC, Speight TM *et al.* Trazodone: a review of its pharmacological properties and therapeutic use in depression and anxiety. *Drugs* 1981; **21**: 401–429.
15. Feighner JP, Entsuah AR, McPherson MK. Efficacy of once-daily venlafaxine extended release (XR) for symptoms of anxiety in depressed outpatients. *Journal of Affective Disorder* 1998; **47**: 55–62

Antidepressant prophylaxis

First episode

A single episode of depression should be treated for 4–6 months after recovery (i.e. a total of 9 months in all)[1,2]. If antidepressant therapy is stopped immediately on recovery, 50% of patients will experience a return of their depressive symptoms[1].

Recurrent depression

Of those patients who have one episode of major depression, 50–85% will go on to have a second episode and 80–90% of those who have a second episode will go on to have a third[3]. Many factors are known to increase the risk of recurrence. These include: a family history of depression, recurrent dysthymia, concurrent non-affective psychiatric illness, chronic medical illness and social factors (e.g. lack of confiding relationships/psychosocial stressors). Some prescription drugs may precipitate depression[4]. Up to 15% of people with depression take their own life[3].

The figure below outlines the risk of recurrence for multiple-episode patients: those recruited to the study had already experienced at least 3 episodes of depression, with 3 years or less between episodes[5,6].

A meta-analysis of antidepressant continuation studies[7] concluded that continuing treatment with antidepressants reduces the odds of depressive relapse by around two-thirds, which is approximately equal to halving the absolute risk. This benefit persisted at 36 months and seemed to be similar across heterogeneous patient groups (first episode, multiple episode and chronic), although none of the studies included first-episode patients only. Specific studies in first-episode patients are required to confirm that treatment beyond 6–9 months confers additional benefit in this patient group.

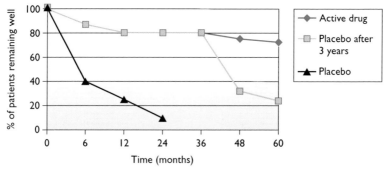

Dose for prophylaxis

Adults should receive the same dose as used for acute treatment, i.e. for most TCAs this should be at least 125 mg (see page 121). There is very limited evidence that lower doses are effective[8,9]. There is some evidence to support the use of lower doses in elderly patients: dothiepin 75 mg/day offers effective prophylaxis[8]. There is no evidence to support the use of lower than standard doses of SSRIs[10].

Relapse rates after ECT are similar to those after stopping antidepressants[11]. Antidepressant prophylaxis will be required, ideally with a different drug from the one that failed to get the patient well in the first instance, although good data in this area are lacking.

Key points that patients should know

- A single episode of depression should be treated for 6 months after recovery.
- The risk of recurrence of depressive illness is high and increases with each episode.
- Those who have had multiple episodes may require treatment for many years.
- The chances of staying well are greatly increased by taking antidepressants.
- Antidepressants are:
  - effective
  - not addictive
  - not known to lose their efficacy over time
  - not known to cause new long-term side-effects
- Medication needs to be continued at the treatment dose. If side-effects are intolerable, it may be possible to find a more suitable alternative.
- If the patient decides to stop their medication, this must not be done suddenly, as this may lead to unpleasant discontinuation effects (see page 148). The medication needs to be reduced slowly under the supervision of a doctor.

References

1. Loonen AJ, Peer PG, Zwanikken GJ. Continuation and maintenance therapy with antidepressive agents: meta-analysis of research. *Pharm Weekly Sci* 1991; **13**: 167–175.
2. Reimherr FW, Amsterdam JD, Quitkin FM. Optimal length of continuation therapy in depression: a prospective assessment during long-term fluoxetine treatment. *American Journal of Psychiatry* 1998; **155**: 1247–1253.
3. Forshall S, Nutt D. Maintenance pharmacotherapy of unipolar depression. *Psychiatric Bulletin* 1999; **23**: 370–373.
4. Patten SB, Love EJ. Drug-induced depression. *Psychotherapy & Psychosomatics* 1997; **66**: 63–73.
5. Frank E, Kupfer DJ, Perel JM *et al*. Three-year outcomes for maintenance therapies in recurrent depression. *Archives of General Psychiatry* 1990; **47**: 1093–1099.
6. Kupfer DJ, Frank E, Perel JM *et al*. Five-year outcome for maintenance therapies in recurrent depression. *Archives of General Psychiatry* 1992; **49**: 769–773.
7. Geddes JR, Carney SM, Davies C *et al*. Relapse prevention with antidepressant drug treatment in depressive disorders: a systematic review. *Lancet* 2003; **361**: 653–661.
8. Frank E, Kupfer DJ, Perel JM. Comparison of full dose versus half dose pharmacotherapy in the maintenance treatment of recurrent depression. *Journal of Affective Disorders* 1993; **27**: 139–145.
9. Old age depression interest group. How long should the elderly take antidepressants? A double-blind placebo controlled study of continuation/prophylaxis therapy with dothiepin. *British Journal of Psychiatry* 1993; **162**: 175–182.
10. Franchini L, Gasperini M, Perez J *et al*. Dose-response efficacy of paroxetine in preventing depressive recurrences: a randomised double-blind study. *Journal of Clinical Psychiatry* 1998; **59**: 229–232.
11. Nobler MS, Sackeim HA. Refractory depression and electroconvulsive therapy. In: Nolen WA, Zohar J, Roose SP *et al*. (eds). *Refractory depression: current strategies and future directions*. Chichester: John Wiley & Sons Ltd, 1994, pp. 69–81.

Further reading

Jackson GA, Maciver I. Psychiatrist's attitudes to maintenance drug treatment in depression. *Psychiatric Bulletin* 1999; **23**: 74–77.

Treatment of refractory depression – first choice

Table First choice: commonly used treatments generally well supported by published literature

Treatment	Advantages	Disadvantages	References
Add **lithium** Aim for plasma level of 0.4–0.6 mmol/l	• Well established • Effective in around half of cases • Well supported in the literature	• Sometimes poorly tolerated at higher plasma levels • Potentially toxic • Usually needs specialist referral • Plasma monitoring is essential	1–3
ECT	• Well established • Effective • Well supported in the literature	• Poor reputation in public domain • Necessitates general anaesthetic • Needs specialist referral	4,5
Venlafaxine (high dose) (>200 mg/day)	• Usually well tolerated • Can be initiated in primary care	• Limited support in literature • Nausea and vomiting more common • Discontinuation reactions common • Blood pressure monitoring essential	6–8
Add **tri-iodothyronine** (20–50 µg/day)	• Usually well tolerated • Moderate literature support	• TFT monitoring required • Usually needs specialist referral • Trials mainly support tricyclic augmentation • Danger of serotonin syndrome	9
Add **tryptophan** 2–3 g tds	• Usually well tolerated • Well researched	• Theoretical risk of eosinophilia–myalgia syndrome • Patient and prescriber must register with manufacturers • Data relate mainly to combination with tricyclics/MAOIs	10
Fluoxetine + olanzapine	• Usually well tolerated • Limited research but well conducted	• Expensive • Risk of weight gain • Limited clinical experience in UK	11–13

Note: Data relating to augmentation strategies in refractory depression are poor by evidence-based standards[14,15]. Recommendations are therefore partly based on clinical experience and expert consensus.

References

1. Fava M, Rosenbaum JF, McGrath PJ *et al.* Lithium and tricyclic augmentation of fluoxetine treatment. *American Journal of Psychiatry* 1994; **151**: 1372–1374
2. Dinan TG. Lithium augmentation in sertraline-resistant depression: a preliminary dose-response study. *Acta Psychiatrica Scandinavica* 1993; **88**: 300–301
3. Bauer M, Döpfmer S. Lithium augmentation in treatment-resistant depression: meta-analysis of placebo-controlled studies. *Journal of Clinical Psychopharmacology* 1999; **19**: 427–434
4. Folkerts HW, Michael N, Tölle R *et al.* Electroconvulsive therapy vs paroxetine in treatment-resistant depression – a randomized study. *Acta Psychiatrica Scandinavica* 1997; **96**: 334–342
5. Gonzalez-Pinto A, Gutierrez M, Gonzalez N *et al.* Efficacy and safety of venlafaxine-ECT combination in treatment-resistant depression. *Journal of Neuropsychiatry and Clinical Neuroscience* 2002; **14**: 206–209
6. Poiriere MF, Boyer P. Venlafaxine and paroxetine in treatment-resistant depression. *British Journal of Psychiatry* 1999; **175**: 12–16
7. Nierenberg AA, Feighner JP, Rudolph R *et al.* Venlafaxine for treatment-resistant unipolar depression. *Journal of Clinical Psychopharmacology* 1994; **14**: 419–423
8. Smith D, Dempster C, Glanville J *et al.* Efficacy and tolerability of venlafaxine compared with selective serotonin reuptake inhibitors and other antidepressants: a meta-analysis. *British Journal of Psychiatry* 2002; **180**: 396–404
9. Joffe RT, Singer W. A comparison of tri-iodothyronine and thyroxine in the potentiation of tricyclic antidepressants. *Psychiatry Research* 1990; **32**: 241–251
10. Smith S. Tryptophan in the treatment of resistant depression – a review. *Pharm Journal* 1998; **261**: 819–821
11. Dube S, Andersen S, Paul S *et al.* Meta-analysis of olanzapine/fluoxetine use in treatment-resistant depression. Presented at 15th European College of Neuropsychopharmacology, October 5–9, 2002, Barcelona, Spain.
12. Dube S, Andersen S, Paul S *et al.* Onset of action of olanzapine/fluoxetine combination for bipolar depression. Presented at 15th European College of Neuropsychopharmacology, October 5–9, 2002, Barcelona, Spain.
13. Corya S, Andersen S, Paul S *et al.* Safety meta-analysis of olanzapine/fluoxetine combination versus fluoxetine. Presented at 15th European College of Neuropsychopharmacology, October 5–9, 2002, Barcelona, Spain.
14. Lam R, Wan D, Cohen N *et al.* Combining antidepressants for treatment-resistant depression: a review. *Journal of Clinical Psychiatry* 2002; **63**: 685–693.
15. Stimpson N, Agrawal N, Lewis G. Randomised controlled trials investigating pharmacological and psychological interventions for treatment-refractory depression. Systematic review. *British Journal of Psychiatry* 2002; **181**: 284–294.

Treatment of refractory depression – 2nd choice

Table Second choice: less commonly used, variably supported by published evaluations

Treatment	Advantages	Disadvantages	References
Add **pindolol** (5 mg tds) (*Higher doses may be more robustly effective[1] but safety data lacking*)	● Well tolerated ● Well researched ● Can be initiated in primary care	● Literature somewhat contradictory ● Data relate mainly to acceleration of response (evidence is more compelling)	2,3
Add **dexamethasone** (4 mg daily for 4/7)	● Well tolerated ● Short course	● Little clinical experience ● Very limited literature support	4,5
Add or try **lamotrigine** (aim for 200 mg/day but lower doses may be effective)	● Probably effective	● Risk of rash ● Slow titration ● Sparse literature	6–9
High-dose tricyclics (e.g. imipramine 300 mg/day)	● Widely used (especially in USA) ● Inexpensive	● Danger of ECG abnormalities ● ECG monitoring essential	10
MAOI + TCA (e.g. trimipramine + phenelzine)	● Widely used in 1960s and 1970s ● Inexpensive	● Potential for dangerous interaction ● Becoming less popular	11
Add **buspirone**	● Apparently well tolerated ● Supported by a placebo-controlled study	● Limited clinical experience	12

References

1. Rabiner E, Bhagwagar Z, Gunn R *et al.* Pindolol augmentation of selective serotonin reuptake inhibitors:PET evidence that the dose used in clinical trials is too low. *American Journal Psychiatry* 2001; **158**: 2080–2082.
2. McAskill R, Mir S, Taylor D. Pindolol augmentation of antidepressant therapy. *British Journal of Psychiatry* 1998; **173**: 203–208.
3. Räsänen P, Hakko H, Tuhonen J. Pindolol and major affective disorders: a three-year follow-up study of 30,483 patients. *Journal Clinical Psychopharmacology* 1999; **19**: 297–302
4. Dinan TG, Lavelle E, Cooney J *et al.* Dexamethasone augmentation in treatment-resistant depression *Acta Psychiatrica Scandinavica* 1997; **95**: 58–61.
5. Bodani M, Sheehan B, Philpot M. The use of dexamethasone in elderly patients with antidepressant-resistant depressive illness. *Journal Psychopharmacology* 1999; **13**: 196–197
6. Calabrese JR, Bowden CL, Sachs GS. A double-blind placebo-controlled study of lamotrigine monotherapy in outpatients with bipolar I depression. *Journal of Clinical Psychiatry* 1999; **60**: 79–88.
7. Maltese TM. Adjunctive lamotrigine treatment for major depression. *American Journal of Psychiatry* 1999; **156**: 1833 (letter).
8. Normann C, Hummel B, Scharer L *et al.* Lamotrigine as adjunct to paroxetine in acute depression: a placebo-controlled, double-blind study. *Journal of Clinical Psychiatry* 2002; **63**: 337–344
9. Barbee J, Jamhour N. Lamotrigine as an augmentation agent in treatment-resistant depression. *Journal of Clinical Psychiatry* 2002; **63**: 737–741.
10. Malhi GS, Bridges PK. Management of resistant depression. *International Journal of Psychiatry in Clinical Practice* 1997; **1**: 269–276.
11. White K, Simpson G. The combined use of MAOIs and tricyclics. *Journal of Clinical Psychiatry* 1984; **45**: 67–69.
12. Appelberg B, Syvalahti E, Koskinen T. Patients with severe depression may benefit from buspirone augmentation of selective serotonin reuptake inhibitors: results from a placebo-controlled, randomized, double-blind, placebo, wash-in study. *Journal of Clinical Psychiatry* 2001; **62**: 448–452.

Treatment of refractory depression – other reported treatments

Table	Other reported treatments (may be worth trying, but limited published support)

Treatment	References
● Add bupropion 300 mg/day	1,2
● Add clonazepam 0.5–1.0 mg at night	3
● Add mirtazapine 15–30 mg ON	4,5
● Add modafinil 100–200 mg/day	6
● Add risperidone 0.5–1.0 mg/day	7,8
● Ketoconazole 400–800 mg/day	9
● Oestrogens (various regimes used)	10
● SSRI + TCA (e.g. citalopram 20 mg/day with amitriptyline 50 mg/day)	11
● Try S-adenosyl-l-methionine 400 mg/day im	12
● SSRI + reboxetine	13,14
● Add omega-3 fatty acid (EPA 1 g daily)	15

References

1. Fatemi SH, Emamian ES, Kist DA. Venlafaxine and bupropion combination therapy in a case of treatment-resistant depression. *Annals of Pharmacotherapy* 1999; **33**: 701–703.
2. Pierre JM, Gitlin MJ. Buproprion-tranylcypromine combination for treatment- refractory depression. *Journal of Clinical Psychiatry* 2000; **61**: 449–450.
3. Smith WT, Londborg PD, Glaudin V *et al*. Short-term augmentation of fluoxetine with clonazepam in the treatment of depression: a double-blind study. *American Journal of Psychiatry* 1998; **155**: 1339–1345.
4. Carpenter LL, Jocic Z, Hall JM *et al*. Mirtazapine augmentation in the treatment of refractory depression. *Journal of Clinical Psychiatry* 1999; **60**: 45–49.
5. Carpenter LL, Yasmin S, Price LH. A double-blind, placebo-controlled study of antidepressant augmentation with mirtazapine. *Biological Psychiatry* 2002; **51**(2): 183–188.
6. Menza MA, Kaufman KR, Castellanos A. Modafinil augmentation of antidepressant treatment in depression. *Journal of Clinical Psychiatry* 2000; **61**: 378–381.
7. Ostroff RB, Nelson JC. Risperidone augmentation of selective serotonin reuptake inhibitors in major depression. *Journal of Clinical Psychiatry* 1999; **60**: 256–259.
8. Stoll AL, Haura G. Tranylcypromine plus risperidone for treatment refractory major depression. *Journal of Clinical Psychopharmacology* 2000; **61**: 495–497 (letter).
9. Wolkowitz OM, Reus VI, Chan T *et al*. Antiglucocorticoid treatment of depression: double-blind ketoconazole. *Biological Psychiatry* 1999; **45**: 1070–1074.
10. Stahl SM. Basic psychopharmacology of antidepressants, Part 2: oestrogen as an adjunct to antidepressant treatment. *Journal Clinical Psychiatry* 1998; **59**(Suppl. 4): 15–24.

11. Taylor D. Selective serotonin reuptake inhibitors and tricyclic antidepressants in combination: interactions and therapeutic uses. *British Journal of Psychiatry* 1995; **167**: 575–580.

12. Pancheri P, Scapicchio P, Delle Chiaie R. A double-blind, randomized parallel-group, efficacy and safety study of intramuscular S-adenosyl-l-methionine, 1, 4-butanedisulphonate (SAMe) versus imipramine in patients with major depressive disorder. *International Journal of Neuropsychopharmacology* 2002; **5**: 287–294.

13. Dursun S, Devarajan S, Kutcher S. The 'dalhousie serotonin cocktail' for treatment-resistant major depressive disorder. *Journal of Psychopharmacology* 2001; **15**: 136–138

14. Devarajan S, Dursun S. Citalopram plus reboxetine in treatment-resistant depression. *Canadian Journal of Psychiatry* 2000; **45**: 489–490.

15. Peet M, Horrobin D. A dose ranging study of the effects of ethyl-eicosapentanoate in patients with ongoing depression despite apparently adequate treatment with standard drugs. *Archives of General Psychiatry* 2002; **59**: 913–919

Psychotic depression

The response to tricyclic antidepressants alone in patients with psychotic major depression (PMD) is poorer than in patients with non-psychotic major depression; one meta-analysis found rates to be 35% and 67%, respectively[1]. It is now well established from many studies that the response of PMD to a combination of an antipsychotic and a TCA is superior to either alone[2,3], although this is not entirely undisputed[4]. Amoxapine is a TCA that also has an antipsychotic-like pharmacological profile. While advocated by some as a single agent for PMD, this is based on one underpowered trial suggesting equal efficacy to a tricyclic/antipsychotic combination[5].

PMD is one of the indications for ECT; ECT is at least as effective as combined antidepressant/antipsychotic therapy[2,6] and may be more effective in psychotic than non-psychotic depression[7]. However, the usual caveats to ECT use apply, including contraindications, side-effects and the tendency to relapse.

There are fewer studies of newer antidepressants and atypical antipsychotics, either alone or in combination, specifically for PMD, although open studies suggest they are also efficacious[8]. However, preliminary reports from a recent large RCT show response rates of 56% for combined olanzapine and fluoxetine compared to 36% for olanzapine alone and 30% for placebo[9].

Long-term outcome is generally poorer for PMD than for simple depression.[10]

Novel approaches being developed include those based on antiglucocorticoid strategies; one small open study found rapid effects of the glucocorticoid receptor antagonist mifepristone[9].

There is no specific indication for other therapies or augmentation strategies in PMD over and above that for resistant depression or psychosis seen elsewhere.

References

1. Chan CH, Janicak PG, Davis JM, Altman E, Andriukaitis S, Hedeker D. Response of psychotic and nonpsychotic depressed patients to tricyclic antidepressants. *Journal of Clinical Psychiatry* 1987; **48**: 197–200.
2. Kroessler DK. Relative efficacy rates for therapies of delusional depression. *Convulsion Therapy* 1985; **1**: 173–182.
3. Spiker DG, Weiss JC, Dealy RS *et al.* The pharmacological treatment of delusional depression. *American Journal Psychiatry* 1985; **142**: 430–436.
4. Mulsant BH, Sweet RA, Rosen J *et al.* The double-blind randomized comparison of nortriptyline plus perphenazine versus nortriptyline plus placebo in the treatment of psychotic depression in late life. *Journal of Clinical Psychiatry* 2001; **62**: 597–604.
5. Anton RF, Burch EA. A comparison study of amoxapine vs amitriptyline plus perphenazine in the treatment of psychotic depression. *American Journal Psychiatry* 1990; **147**: 1203–1218.
6. Parker G, Roy K, Hadzi-Pavlovic D, Pedic F. Psychotic (delusional) depression: a meta-analysis of physical treatments. *Journal of Affective Disorders* 1992; **24**: 17–24.
7. Petrides G, Fink M, Husain MM *et al.* ECT remission rates in psychotic versus nonpsychotic depressed patients: a report from CORE. *Journal of ECT* 2001; **17**(4): 244–253.
8. Wheeler Vega JA, Mortimer AM, Tyson PJ, [Review] [115 refs] [Journal Article. Review. Review AO. Somatic treatment of psychotic depression: review and recommendations for practice. *Journal of Clinical Psychopharmacology* 2000; **20**: 504–519.
9. Corya S, Dube S, Anderson SW, *et al.* Olanzapine-fluoxetine combination for psychotic major depression. *International Journal of Neuropsychopharmacology* 2002; **5**(Suppl. 1): S144.
10. Flint A, Rifat S. Two-year outcome of psychotic depression in late life. *American Journal of Psychiatry* 1998; **155**: 178–183.
11. Belanoff JK, Rothschild AJ, Cassidy F, et al. An open label trial of C-1073 (mifepristone) for psychotic major depression. *Biological Psychiatry* 2002; **52**(5): 386–392.

ECT and psychotropics

The table below summarises the effect of various psychotropics on seizure duration during ECT. Note that there are few well-controlled studies in this area and so recommendations should be viewed with this in mind.

Drug	Effect on ECT seizure duration	Comments[1-9]
Benzodiazepines	Reduced	All may raise seizure threshold and so should be avoided where possible. Many are long acting and may need to be discontinued some days before ECT. Benzodiazepines may also complicate anaesthesia If sedation is required, consider hydroxyzine. If very long term and essential, continue and use higher stimulus
SSRIs	Minimal effect; small increase possible	Generally considered safe to use during ECT. Beware complex pharmacokinetic interactions with anaesthetic agents
Venlafaxine	Minimal effect	Limited data suggest no effect on seizure duration but possibility of increased risk of asystole with doses above 300 mg/day
TCAs	Possibly increased	Few data relevant to ECT but many TCAs lower seizure threshold. TCAs are associated with arrhythmias following ECT and should be avoided in elderly patients and those with cardiac disease. In others, it is preferable to continue TCA treatment during ECT. Close monitoring is essential. Beware hypotension
MAOIs	Minimal effect	Data relating to ECT very limited but long history of ECT use during MAOI therapy MAOIs probably do not effect seizure duration but interactions with sympathomimetics occasionally used in anaesthesia are possible and may lead to hypertensive crisis MAOIs may be continued during ECT but the anaesthetist must be informed. Beware hypotension
Lithium	Possibly increased	Conflicting data on lithium and ECT. The combination may be more likely to lead to delirium and confusion and some authorities suggest discontinuing lithium 48 hours before ECT. In the UK, ECT is often used during lithium therapy but starting with a low stimulus and with very close monitoring. The combination is generally well tolerated Note that lithium potentiates the effects of non-depolarising neuromuscular blockers such as suxamethonium
Antipsychotics	Possibly increased	Few published data but widely used. Phenothiazines and clozapine are perhaps most likely to prolong seizures and some suggest withdrawal before ECT. However, safe concurrent use has been reported. ECT and antipsychotics appear generally to be a safe combination
Anticonvulsants	Reduced	If used as a mood stabiliser, continue but be prepared to use higher energy stimulus. If used for epilepsy, their effect is to normalise seizure threshold. Interactions are possible. Valproate may prolong the effect of thiopental; carbamazepine may inhibit neuromuscular blockade
Barbiturates	Reduced	All barbiturates reduce seizure duration in ECT but are widely used as sedative anaesthetic agents Thiopental and methohexital may be associated with cardiac arrhythmias

For drugs known to lower seizure threshold, treatment is best begun with a low energy stimulus (50 mC). Staff should be alerted to the possibility of prolonged seizures and iv diazepam should be available. With drugs known to elevate seizure threshold, higher stimuli may, of course, be required. Methods are available to lower seizure threshold or prolong seizures[10], but discussion of these is beyond the scope of this book.

ECT frequently causes confusion, disorientation and, more rarely, delirium. Close observation is essential. Very limited data support the use of thiamine (200 mg daily) in reducing post ECT confusion[11].

References

1. Bazire S. *Psychotropic Drug Directory*. Dinton, Wilts: Quay Books Division, 2001.
2. Curran S, Freeman CP. ECT and drugs. In: Freeman CP (ed). *The ECT Handbook – the second report of the Royal College of Psychiatrists' special committee on ECT*. Henry Ling Ltd, Dorset Press 1995.
3. Jarvis MR, Goewert AJ, Zorumski CF. Novel antidepressants and maintenance electroconvulsive therapy. *Annals of Clinical Psychiatry* 1993; 4: 275–284
4. Kellner CH, Nixon DW, Bernstein HJ. ECT – drug interactions: a review. *Psychopharmacol Bulletin* 1991; 27: 595–609.
5. Maidment I. The interaction between psychiatric medicines and ECT. *Hospital Pharmacist* 1997; 4: 102–105.
6. Welch CA. Electroconvulsive therapy. In: Ciraulo DA, Shader RI, Greenblatt DJ, Creelman W (ed). *Drug Interactions in Psychiatry* 2nd edition. Williams & Wilkins, 1995.
7. Gonzalez-Pinto A, Gutierrez M, Gonzalez N *et al*. Efficacy and safety of venlafaxine-ECT combination in treatment-resistant depression. *Journal of Neuropsychiatry andClinical Neuroscience* 2002; 14: 206–209.
8. Naguib M, Koorn R. Interactions between psychotropics, anaesthetics and electroconvulsive therapy. *CNS Drugs* 2002; 16: 230–247.
9. Jha AK, Stein GS, Fenwick P. Negative interaction between lithium and electroconvulsive therapy – a case-control study. *British Journal of Psychiatry* 1996; 168: 241–243.
10. Datta C, Rai AK, Ilivicky HJ *et al*. Augmentation of seizure induction in electroconvulsive therapy: a clinical reappraisal. *Journal of ECT* 2002; 18: 118–125.
11. Linton CR, Reynolds MTP, Warner NJ. Using thiamine to reduce post-ECT confusion. *International Journal of Geriatric Psychiatry* 2002; 17: 189–192.

Antidepressant-induced hyponatraemia

Most antidepressants have been associated with hyponatraemia. The mechanism of this adverse effect is probably the syndrome of inappropriate secretion of anti-diuretic syndrome (SIADH). Hyponatraemia is a rare but potentially serious adverse effect of antidepressants, which demands careful monitoring, particularly in those patients at greatest risk (see table below).

Table   Risk factors[1–4]
Old age
Female sex
Low body weight
Some drug treatments *(e.g. diuretics, NSAIDs, carbamazepine, cancer chemotherapy)*
Reduced renal function *(especially acute and chronic renal failure)*
Medical co-morbidity *(e.g. hypothyroidism, diabetes, COPD, hypertension, head injury, CVA, various cancers)*
Warm weather (summer)

Antidepressants

No antidepressant has been shown *not* to be associated with hyponatraemia and most have a reported association[5]. It has been suggested that serotonergic drugs are relatively more likely to cause hyponatraemia[6,7], although this is disputed[8].

Monitoring

All patients taking antidepressants should be observed for signs of hyponatraemia (dizziness, nausea, lethargy, confusion, cramps, seizures). Serum sodium should be determined (at baseline, two and four weeks, then three-monthly[9]) for those at high risk of drug-induced hyponatraemia:

– Extreme old age (>80 years)
– History of hyponatraemia
– Co-therapy with other drugs known to be associated with hyponatraemia (as above)
– Reduced renal function (GFR < 50 ml/min)
– Medical co-morbidity (as above)

Treatment[10]

Withdraw antidepressant immediately (note risk of discontinuation effects which may complicate clinical picture)

- If serum sodium >125 mmol/l – monitor sodium daily until normal

- If serum sodium <125 mmol/l – refer to specialist medical care

Restarting treatment

- Consider ECT

- Prescribe a drug from a different class. Consider noradrenergic drugs such as reboxetine and lofepramine. Begin with a low dose, increasingly slowly, and monitor closely. If hyponatraemia recurs and continued antidepressant use is essential, consider water restriction and/or careful use of demeclocycline (see BNF).

Other psychotropics

Carbamazepine has a well-known association with SIADH. Note also that antipsychotic use has also been linked to hyponatraemia[11-13].

References

1. Spigset O, Hedenmalm K. Hyponatraemia in relation to treatment with antidepressants: a survey of reports in the World Health Organization data base for spontaneous reporting of adverse drug reactions. *Pharmacotherapy* 1997; 17: 348–352
2. Madhusoodanan S, Bogunovic OJ, Moise D *et al*. Hyponatraemia associated with psychotropic medications: a review of the literature and spontaneous reports. *Adverse Drug Reactions & Toxicological Reviews* 2002; 21: 17–29
3. Wilkinson TJ, Begg EJ, Winter AC *et al*. Risk factors with hyponatraemia with SSRIs assessed. *British Journal of Clinical Pharmacology* 1999; 47: 211–217
4. McAskill R, Taylor D. Psychotropics and hyponatraemia. *Psychiatry Bulletin* 1997; 21: 33–35
5. Thomas A, Verbalis JG. Hyponatraemia and the syndrome of inappropriate antidiuretic hormone secretion associated with drug therapy in psychiatric patients. *CNS Drugs* 1995; 5: 357–369
6. Movig KLL, Leufkens HGM, Lenderink AW *et al*. Serotonergic antidepressants associated with an increased risk for hyponatraemia in the elderly. *European Journal of Clinical Pharmacology* 2002; 58: 143–148
7. Movig KLL, Leufkens HGM, Lenderink AW *et al*. Association between antidepressant drug use and hyponatraemia: a case-control study. *British Journal of Clinical Pharmacology* 2002; 53: 363–369.
8. Kirby D, Ames D. Hyponatraemia and selective serotonin re-uptake inhibitors in elderly patients. *International Journal of Geriatric Psychiatry* 2001; 16: 484–493.
9. Arinzon ZH, Yehoshua AL, Fidelman ZG. Delayed recurrent SIADH associated with SSRIs. *The Annals of Pharmacotherapy* 2002; 36: 1175–1177.
10. Sharma H, Pompei P. Antidepressant-induced hyponatraemia in the aged. *Drugs & Aging* 1996; 8: 430–435.
11. Ohsawa H, Kishimoto T, Motoharu H *et al*. An epidemiological study on hyponatremia in psychiatric patients in mental hospitals in Nara Prefecture. *The Japanese Journal of Psychiatry and Neurology* 1992; 46: 883–889.
12. Leadbetter RA, Shutty MS. Differential effects of neuroleptics and clozapine on polydipsia and intermittent hyponatraemia. *Journal of Clinical Psychiatry* 1994; 55: 110–113.
13. Collins A, Anderson J. SIADH induced by two atypical antipsychotics. *International Journal of Geriatric Psychiatry* 2000; 15: 282–285.

Further reading

Management of antipsychotic drug-reduced SIADH. *Drug Therapy Perspectives* 1985; 6: 12–16.

Post-stroke depression

Post-stroke depression is a common problem seen in at least 30–40% of survivors of intracerebral haemorrhage[1,2]. Depression probably slows functional rehabilitation[3] but antidepressants may be beneficial through relieving depressive symptoms and allowing faster rehabilitation[4].

Prophylaxis

The high incidence of depression after stroke makes prophylaxis worthy of consideration. Nortriptyline and fluoxetine may prevent post-stroke depression[5] but data are very limited. Amitriptyline appears to prevent central post-stroke pain[6].

Treatment

Treatment is complicated by medical co-morbidity and by the potential for interaction with other co-prescribed drugs (especially warfarin). Contraindication to antidepressant treatment seems to be substantially more likely with tricyclics than with SSRIs[7]. Fluoxetine[8] and nortriptyline[9] are probably the most studied and seem to be effective. SSRIs and nortriptyline are widely recommended for post-stroke depression. Despite early fears, SSRIs seem not to increase risk of stroke[10].

Post-stroke depression – recommended drugs

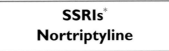

SSRIs*
Nortriptyline

* If patient is also taking warfarin, suggest citalopram[11]

References

1. Gainotti G, Antonucci G, Marra C et al. Relation between depression after stroke, antidepressant therapy, and functional recovery. *Journal of Neurology and Neurosurgical Psychiatry* 2001; 71: 258–261.
2. Hayee MA, Akhtar N, Haque A et al. Depression after stroke-analysis of 297 stroke patients. *Bangladesh Medical Research Council Bulletin* 2001; 27: 96–102.
3. Paolucci S, Antonucci G, Grasso MG et al. Post-stroke depression, antidepressant treatment and rehabilitation results: a case-control study. *Cerebrovascular Diseases* 2001; 12: 264–271.
4. Gainotti G, Marra C. Determinants and consequences of post-stroke depression. *Current Opinion in Neurology* 2002; 15: 85–89.
5. Narushima K, Kosier JT, Robinson RG. Preventing poststroke depression: a 12-week double-blind randomized treatment trial and 21-month follow-up. *Journal of Nergv Mental Diseases* 2002; 190: 296–303.
6. Lampl C, Yazdi K, Röper C. Amitriptyline in the prophylaxis of central poststroke pain: preliminary results of 39 patients in a placebo-controlled, long-term study. *Stroke* 2002; 33: 3030–3032.
7. Cole MG, Elie LM, McCusker J et al. Feasibility and effectiveness of treatments for post-stroke depression in elderly inpatients: systematic review. *Journal of Geriatric Psychiatry & Neurology* 2001; 14: 37–41.
8. Wiart L, Petit H, Joseph PA et al. Fluoxetine in early poststroke depression: a double-blind placebo-controlled study). *Stroke* 2000; 31: 1829–1832.
9. Robinson R, Schultz SK, Castillo C et al. Nortriptyline versus fluoxetine in the treatment of depression and in short-term recovery after stroke: a placebo-controlled, double-blind study. *American Journal of Psychiatry* 2000; 157: 351–359.
10. Bak S, Tsiropoulos I, Kjaersgaard JO et al. Selective serotonin reuptake inhibitors and the risk of stroke: a population-based case-control study. *Stroke* 2002; 33: 1465–1473.
11. Sayal KS, Duncan-McConnell DA, McConnell HW et al. Psychotropic interactions with warfarin. *Acta Psychiatrica Scandinavica* 2000; 102: 250–255.

Treatment of depression in the elderly

The prevalence of most physical illnesses increases with age. Many physical problems such as cardiovascular disease, chronic pain and Parkinson's disease are associated with a high risk of depressive illness[1]. The morbidity and mortality associated with depression are increased as the elderly are more physically frail and therefore more likely to suffer serious consequences from self-neglect (e.g. life-threatening dehydration or hypothermia) and immobility (e.g. venous stasis). Almost 20% of completed suicides occur in the elderly[2].

The elderly may take longer to respond to antidepressants than younger adults[3] and may require to be treated for longer periods overall. Flint & Rifat[4] found that, of a cohort of elderly people who had recovered from a first episode of depression and had received antidepressants for 2 years, 60% relapsed within 2 years if antidepressant treatment was withdrawn. Lower doses of antidepressants may be effective as prophylaxis. Dothiepin (dosulepin) 75 mg/day has been shown to be effective in this regard[5]. There is no evidence to suggest that the response to antidepressants is reduced in the physically ill[6], although outcome in the elderly in general is often suboptimal[7,8].

There is no ideal antidepressant. All are associated with problems (see table overleaf). Choice is determined by the individual clinical circumstances of each patient, particularly physical co-morbidity and concomitant medication (both prescribed and 'over the counter').

References

1. Katona C, Livingston G. Impact of screening old people with physical illness for depression. *Lancet* 2000; **356**: 91–92.
2. Cattell H, Jolley DJ. One hundred cases of suicide in elderly people. *British Journal of Psychiatry* 1995; **166**: 451–457.
3. Paykel ES, Raman R, Cooper Z *et al.* Residual symptoms after partial remission: an important outcome in depression. *Psychological Medicine* 1995; **25**: 1171–1180.
4. Flint AJ, Rifat SL. Recurrence of first-episode geriatric depression after discontinuation of maintenance antidepressants. *American Journal of Psychiatry* 1999; **156**: 943–945.
5. Old Age Depression Special Interest Group. How long should the elderly take antidepressants? A double blind placebo controlled study of continuation/prophylaxis therapy with dothiepin. *British Journal of Psychiatry* 1993; **162**: 175–182.
6. Evans M, Hammond M, Wilson K *et al.* Placebo-controlled treatment trial of depression in elderly physically ill patients. *International Journal of Geriatric Psychiatry* 1997; **12**: 817–824.
7. Heeren TJ, Derksen P, Heycop TH *et al.* Treatment, outcome and predictors of response in elderly depressed in-patients. *British Journal of Psychiatry* 1997; **170**: 436–440.
8. Tuma TA. Outcome of hospital-treated depression at 4.5 years: an elderly and a younger adult cohort compared. *British Journal of Psychiatry* 2000; **178**: 224–228.

Further reading

Movig KL, Leufkens HG, Lenderink AW. Serotonergic antidepressants associated with an increased risk of hyponatraemia in the elderly. *European Journal of Clinical Pharmacology* 2002; **58**: 143–148.

National Service Framework for Older People. London: Department of Health. (A whole supplement is dedicated to the use of medicines in older people.) 2001.

Pacher P, Ungvari Z. Selective serotonin reuptake inhibitor antidepressants increase the risk of falls and hip fractures in elderly people by inhibiting cardiovascular ion channels. *Medical Hypotheses* 2001; **57**: 469–471.

Spina E, Scordo MG. Clinically significant drug interactions with antidepressants in the elderly. *Drugs & Aging* 2002; **19**: 299–320.

Van Walraven C, Mamdani MM, Wells PS *et al.*. Inhibition of serotonin re-uptake by antidepressants and upper gastrointestinal bleeding in elderly patients: retrospective cohort study. *BMJ* 2001; **323**: 655–658.

Wilson K, Mottram P, Sivanranthan A *et al.* Antidepressants versus placebo for depressed elderly (Cochrane review). In: Cochrane Database of Systematic Reviews. Issue 2, 2002; Update Software.

Table Antidepressants and the elderly

	Anticholinergic side-effect (urinary retention, dry mouth, blurred vision, constipation)	Postural hypotension	Sedation
Older tricyclics	Variable: moderate with nortriptyline, imipramine & dosulepin (dothiepin). Marked with others	All can cause postural hypotension. Dosage titration is required	Variable: from minimal with imipramine to profound with trimipramine
Lofepramine	Moderate, although constipation/sweating can be severe	Can be a problem but generally better tolerated than the older tricyclics	Minimal
SSRIs	Dry mouth can be a problem with paroxetine	Much less of a problem, but an increased risk of falls is documented with SSRIs.	Can be a problem with paroxetine. Unlikely with the other SSRIs
Others	Minimal with mirtazapine and venlafaxine. Can be rarely a problem with reboxetine	Can be a problem with venlafaxine (as it can increase BP at higher doses)	Mirtazapine, mianserin and trazodone are sedative

Weight gain	Safety in overdose	Other side-effects	Drug interactions
All tricyclics can cause weight gain	Dothiepin & amitriptyline are the most toxic (seizures & cardiac arrhythmias)	Seizures, anticholinergic-induced cognitive impairment	Mainly pharmacodynamic: increased sedation with benzodiazepines, increased hypotension with diuretics, increased constipation with other anticholinergic drugs etc.
Few data, but lack of spontaneous reports may indicate less potential than the older tricyclics	Relatively safe	Raised LFTs	
Paroxetine & possibly citalopram may cause weight gain. Others are weight-neutral	Safe with the possible exception of citalopram (one minor metabolite is possibly cardiotoxic)	GI & headaches, hyponatraemia, increased risk of GI bleeds in the elderly, orofacial dyskinesias with paroxetine	Fluvoxamine, fluoxetine & paroxetine are potent inhibitors of several hepatic cytochrome enzymes (see page 154). Sertraline is safer and citalopram is the safest
Greatest problem is with mirtazapine	All are relatively safe	Insomnia and hypokalaemia with reboxetine	Nefazadone and, to a lesser extent, moclobemide and venlafaxine all inhibit CYP450 enzymes. Check for potential interactions. Reboxetine is safe

Cardiac effects of antidepressants

Drug	Heart rate	Blood pressure	QTc
Tricyclics[1,2]	Increase in heart rate	Postural hypotension	Prolongation of QTc interval
Lofepramine[1,3]	Modest increase in heart rate	Less decrease in postural blood pressure compared with other TCAs	Can possibly prolong QTc interval at higher doses (desipramine is main) metabolite
MAOIs[1]	Decrease in heart rate	Postural hypotension. Risk of hypertensive crisis	Unclear but may shorten QTc interval
Fluoxetine[4-6]	Small decrease in mean heart rate	Minimal effect on blood pressure	No effect on QTc interval
Paroxetine[7,8]	Small decrease in mean heart rate	Minimal effect on blood pressure	No effect on QTc interval
Sertraline[9,10]	Minimal effect on heart rate	Minimal effect on blood pressure	No effect on QTc interval
Citalopram[11]	Small decrease in heart rate	Slight drop in systolic blood pressure	No effect on QTc interval
Fluvoxamine[12]	Minimal effect on heart rate	Small drops in systolic blood pressure	No significant effect on QTc
Venlafaxine[13]	Marginally increased	Some increase in postural blood pressure. At higher doses increase in blood pressure	Possible prolongation in overdose
Mirtazapine[14]	Minimal change in heart rate	Minimal effect on blood pressure	No effect on QTc interval
Reboxetine[15,16]	Significant increase in heart rate	Marginal increase in both systolic and diastolic blood pressure. Postural decrease at higher doses	Unclear
Moclobemide[17,18]	Marginal decrease in heart rate	Minimal effect on blood pressure. Isolated cases of hypertensive episodes	No effect on QTc interval
Nefazodone[19]	Small decrease in heart rate	Reports of postural hypotension	No effect on QTc interval
Trazodone[1]	Decrease in heart rate more common, although increase can also occur	Can cause significant postural hypotension	Can prolong QTc interval

Note: SSRIs are generally recommended in cardiac disease but beware cytochrome-mediated interactions with co-administered cardiac drugs.

138

Arrhythmias	Conduction disturbance	Licensed restrictions post-MI	Comments
Class I anti-arrhythmic activity	Slows down cardiac conduction	CI in patients with recent MI	TCAs affect cardiac contractility. Some TCAs linked to. ischaemic heart disease. Association with sudden cardiac death
May occur at higher doses	Benign effect on cardiac conduction	CI in patients with recent MI	Less cardiotoxic than other TCAs. Reasons unclear
May cause arrhythmias and decrease LVF	No clear effect on cardiac conduction	Use with caution in patients with cardiovascular disease	
Few cases reported in literature	None	Caution. Clinical experience is limited	
None	None	General caution in cardiac patients	
None	None	None – probably drug of choice	Only antidepressants studied in patients with recent MI
None	None	Caution, although no ECG changes	Minor metabolite which may ↑ QTc interval
None	None	Caution	Limited changes in ECG have been observed
Some reports of cardiac arrhythmias	Rare reports of conduction abnormalities	Caution. Has not been evaluated in post-MI patients	
None	None	Caution in patients with recent MI	
Rhythm abnormalities may occur	Atrial and ventricular ectopic beats, especially in the elderly	Caution in patient with cardiac disease	
None	None	None	
Asymptomatic sinus bradycardia occasionally reported	Does not appear to alter cardiac conduction	Caution in patients with recent MI	
Several case reports of arrhythmias	May have a minimal effect on cardiac conduction	Care in patients with severe cardiac disease	May be arrhythmogenic in patients with pre-existing cardiac disease

References

1. Warrington SJ, Padgham C, Lader M. The cardiovascular effects of antidepressants. *Psychol Medicine* 1989; Suppl. 16 (monograph).
2. Hippisley-Cox J, Pringle M, Hammersley V *et al.* Antidepressants as a risk factor for ischaemic heart disease in primary care. *BMJ* 2001; **323**: 666–669.
3. Stern H, Konetschny J, Herrmann L *et al.* Cardiovascular effects of single doses of the antidepressants amitriptyline and lofepramine in healthy subjects. *Pharmacopsychiatry* 1985; **18**: 272–277.
4. Fisch C. Effect of fluoxetine on the electrocardiogram. *Journal of Clinical Psychiatry* 1985; **46**: 42–44.
5. Ellison ME, Milofsky JE, Ely E. Fluoxetine-induced bradycardia and syncope in two patients. *Journal of Clinical Psychiatry* 1990; **51**: 385–386.
6. Roose SP, Glassman AH, Attia E *et al.* Cardiovascular effects of Fluoxetine in depressed patients with heart disease. *American Journal of Psychiatry* 1998; **155**: 660–665.
7. Kuhs H, Rudolf GA. Cardiovascular effects of paroxetine. *Psychopharmacology* 1990; **102**: 379–382.
8. Roose SP, Laghrissi-Thode F, Kennedy JS *et al.* Comparison of paroxetine and nortriptyline in depressed patients with ischemic heart disease. *JAMA* 1998; **279**: 287–291.
9. Shapiro PA, Lespérance F, Frasure-Smith N *et al.* An open-label preliminary trial of sertraline for treatment of major depression after acute myocardial infarction (the SADHAT trial). *American Heart Journal* 1999; **137**: 1100–1106.
10. Glassman AH, O'Connor CM, Califf RM *et al.* Sertraline treatment of major depression in patients with acute MI or unstable angina. *JAMA* 2002; **288**: 701–709.
11. Rasmussen SL, Overø KF, Tanghøj P. Cardiac safety of citalopram: Prospective trials and retrospective analyses. *Journal of Clinical Psychopharmacology* 1999; **19**: 407–415.
12. Strik JJ, Honig A, Lousberg R *et al.* Cardiac side effects of two selective serotonin reuptake inhibitors in middle-aged and elderly patients. *International Clinical Psychopharmacology* 1998; **13**: 263–267.
13. ABPI. Venlafaxine SPC. *Compendium of Data Sheets and Summaries of Product Characteristics, 1999.*
14. Montgomery SA. Safety of mirtazapine: a review. *International Clinical Psychopharmacology* 1995; **10**(Suppl. 4): 37–45.
15. Mucci M. Reboxetine: a review of antidepressant tolerability. *Journal of Psychopharmacology* 1997; **11**(Suppl. 4): S33–S37.
16. Holm KJ, Spencer CM. Reboxetine: A review of its use in depression. *CNS Drugs* 1999; **12**: 65–83.
17. Moll E, Neumann N, Schmid-Burgk W *et al.* Safety and efficacy during long-term treatment with moclobemide. *Clinical Neuropharmacology* 1994; **17**(Suppl. 1): S74–S87.
18. Hilton S, Jaber B, Ruch R. Moclobemide safety: Monitoring a newly developed product in the 1990s. *Journal of Clinical Psychopharmacology* 1995; **15**(Suppl. 2): 76S–83S.
19. Robinson DS, Roberts LD, Smith JM *et al.* The safety profile of Nefazodone. *Journal of Clinical Psychiatry* 1996; **57**(Suppl. 2): 31–38.

Antidepressants and sexual dysfunction

Primary sexual disorders are common, although reliable normative data are lacking[1]. Reported prevalence rates vary depending on the method of data collection (low numbers with spontaneous reports, increasing with confidential questionnaires and further still with direct questioning)[1,2]. Physical illness, psychiatric illness, substance misuse and prescribed drug treatment can all cause sexual dysfunction[1,2]. Baseline sexual functioning should be determined, if possible (questionnaires may be useful), because sexual function can affect quality of life and compliance (sexual dysfunction is one of the major causes of treatment dropout[3]). Complaints of sexual dysfunction may also indicate progression or inadequate treatment of underlying medical or psychiatric conditions. It may also be the result of drug treatment and intervention may greatly improve quality of life[4]. The normal human sexual response is described on page 83.

Effects of depression

Both depression and the drugs used to treat it can cause disorders of desire, arousal and orgasm. The precise nature of the sexual dysfunction may indicate whether depression or treatment is the more likely cause. For example, 40–50% of people with depression report diminished libido and problems regarding sexual arousal in the month before diagnosis, compared with only 15–20% who experience orgasm problems prior to taking an antidepressant[5].

Effects of antidepressant drugs

Antidepressants can cause sedation, hormonal changes, disturbance of cholinergic/adrenergic balance, peripheral alpha-adrenergic antagonism, inhibition of nitric oxide and increased serotonin neurotransmission, all of which can result in sexual dysfunction[6]. Sexual dysfunction has been reported as a side-effect of all antidepressants, although rates vary (see table below). Individual susceptibility also varies and all effects are reversible.

Not all of the sexual side-effects of antidepressants are undesirable[1]: serotonergic antidepressants are effective in the treatment of premature ejaculation and may also be beneficial in paraphilias.

Table   Sexual adverse effects of antidepressant drugs

Drug	Approximate prevalence	Type of problem
Tricyclics[7–10]	30%	Decreased libido, erectile dysfunction, delayed orgasm, impaired ejaculation. Prevalence of delayed orgasm with clomipramine may be double that with other TCAs. Painful ejaculation reported rarely
Trazodone[3,11–13]	Unknown	Impaired ejaculation and both increases and decreases in libido reported. Used in some cases to promote erection. Priapism occurs in approximately 0.01%
MAOIs[3,14]	40%	Similar to TCAs, although prevalence may be higher[1] Moclobemide much less likely to cause problems than older MAOIs (4% v 40%)
SSRIs[3,15–18]	60–70%	Decreased libido and delayed orgasm. Paroxetine is associated with more erectile dysfunction and decreased vaginal lubrication than the other SSRIs. High prevalence with SSRIs may be due to selective reporting. Difficult to determine relative prevalence but there is evidence that ejaculatory delay is worse with paroxetine than citalopram[19] Penile anaesthesia has been reported rarely with fluoxetine
Venlafaxine[3]	70%	Decreased libido and delayed orgasm common. Erectile dysfunction less common
Mirtazapine[3,16]	25%	Decreased libido and delayed orgasm possible. Erectile dysfunction less common
Nefazodone[3,9]	10%	Low incidence of decreased libido and delayed orgasm. Erectile dysfunction uncommon
Reboxetine[20]	5–10%	Various abnormalities of orgasmic function

Treatment

Spontaneous remission occurs in approximately 10% of cases and partial remission in a further 11%[3]. If this does not happen, the dose may be reduced or the antidepressant discontinued where appropriate.

Drug 'holidays' or delayed dosing may be used[21]. This approach is problematic as the patient may relapse or experience antidepressant discontinuation symptoms. More logical is a switch to a different drug that is less likely to cause the specific sexual problem experienced (see table above). Note that amfebutamone (buproprion – not licensed for depression in UK) may have the lowest risk of sexual dysfunction[22] among newer antidepressants.

Adjunctive or 'antidote' drugs may also be used (see page 85 for further information).

References

1. Baldwin DS, Thomas SC, Birtwistle J. Effects of antidepressant drugs on sexual function. *International Journal of Psychiatry in Clinical Practice* 1997; **1**: 47–58.
2. Pollack MH, Reiter S, Hammerness P. Genitourinary and sexual adverse effects of psychotropic medication. *International Journal of Psychiatry in Medicine* 1992; **22**: 305–327.
3. Montejo AL, Llorca G, Izquierdo JA *et al.* Incidence of sexual dysfunction associated with antidepressant agents: a prospective multicentre study of 1022 outpatients. *Journal of Clinical Psychiatry* 2001; **62**(Suppl.3): 10–20.
4. Segraves RT. Effects of psychotropic drugs on human erection and ejaculation. *Archives of General Psychiatry* 1989; **46**: 275–284.
5. Kennedy SH, Dickens SE, Eisfeld BS *et al.* Sexual dysfunction before antidepressant therapy in major depression. *Journal of Affective Disorders* 1999; **56**: 201–208.
6. Clayton AH. Recognition and assessment of sexual dysfunction associated with depression. *Journal of Clinical Psychiatry* 2001; **62**: 5–9.
7. Harrison WM, Rabkin JG, Ehrhardt AA *et al.* Effects of antidepressant medication on sexual function: a controlled study. *Journal of Clinical Psychopharmacology* 1986; **6**: 144–149.
8. Beaumont G. Sexual side effects of clomipramine. *Journal of International Medical Research* 1977; **51**: 37–44.
9. Rickels K, Robinson DS, Schweizer E *et al.* Nefazodone: aspects of efficacy. *Journal of Clinical Psychiatry* 1995; **56**(Suppl. 6): 43–46.
10. Sovner R. Anorgasmia associated with imipramine but not desipramine: case report. *Journal of Clinical Psychiatry* 1983; **44**: 345–346.
11. Garbell N. Increased libido in women receiving trazodone. *American Journal of Psychiatry* 1986; **143**: 781–782.
12. Sullivan G. Increased libido in three men treated with trazodone. *Journal of Clinical Psychiatry* 1988; **49**: 202–203.
13. Thompson JW, Ware MR, Blashfield RK. Psychotropic medication and priapism: a comprehensive review. *Journal of Clinical Psychiatry* 1990; **51**: 430–433.
14. Lesko LM, Stotland NL, Segraves RT. Three cases of female anorgasmia associated with MAOIs. *American Journal of Psychiatry* 1982; **139**: 1353–1354.
15. Herman JB, Brotman AW, Pollack MH *et al.* Fluoxetine induced sexual dysfunction. *Journal of Clinical Psychiatry* 1990; **51**: 25–27.
16. Gelenberg AJ, Laukes C, McGahuey C *et al.* Mirtazepine substitution in SSRI-induced sexual dysfunction. *Journal of Clinical Psychiatry* 2000; **61**: 356–360.
17. Jacobsen FM. Fluoxetine-induced sexual dysfunction and an open trial of yohimbine. *Journal of Clinical Psychiatry* 1992; **53**: 119–122.
18. Lauerma H. Successful treatment of citalopram-induced anorgasmia by cyproheptadine. *Acta Psychiatrica Scandinavica* 1996; **93**: 69–70.
19. Waldinger MD, Zwinderman AH, Olivier B. SSRIs and ejaculation: a double-blind, randomized, fixed-dose study with paroxetine and citalopram. *Journal of Clinical Psychopharmacology* 2001; **21**: 556–560.
20. Haberfellner EM. Sexual dysfunction caused by reboxetine. *Pharmacopsychiatry* 2002; **35**: 77–78.
21. Rothschild AJ. Selective serotonin reuptake inhibitor-induced sexual dysfunction: efficacy of a drug holiday. *American Journal of Psychiatry* 1995; **152**: 1514–1516.
22. Clayton AH, Pradko JF, Croft HA *et al.* Prevalence of sexual dysfunction among newer antidepressants. *Journal of Clinical Psychiatry* 2002; **63**: 357–366.

Further reading

Fava M, Rankin M. Sexual functioning and SSRIs. *Journal of Clinical Psychiatry* 2002; **63**(Suppl. 5): 13–16.

Antidepressants – swapping and stopping

General guidelines

- All antidepressants have the potential to cause withdrawal phenomena. When taken continuously *for six weeks or longer,* antidepressants should not be stopped abruptly unless a serious adverse event has occurred (e.g. cardiac arrhythmia with a tricyclic). (See page 148.)

- When swapping from one antidepressant to another, abrupt withdrawal should usually be avoided. Cross-tapering is preferred, where the dose of the ineffective or poorly tolerated drug is slowly reduced while the new drug is slowly introduced.

Example		Week 1	Week 2	Week 3	Week 4
Withdrawing dosulepin	150 mg OD	100 mg OD	50 mg OD	25 mg OD	Nil
Introducing citalopram	Nil	10 mg OD	10 mg OD	20 mg OD	20 mg OD

- The speed of cross-tapering is best judged by monitoring patient tolerability. No clear guidelines are available, so caution is required.

- Note that the co-administration of some antidepressants, even when cross-tapering, is absolutely contra-indicated. In other cases, theoretical risks or lack of experience preclude recommending cross-tapering.

- In some cases cross-tapering may not be considered necessary. An example is when switching from one SSRI to another: their effects are so similar that administration of the second drug is likely to ameliorate withdrawal effects of the first. However, there is little firm evidence of this occurring.

- Potential dangers of simultaneously administering two antidepressants include pharmacodynamic interactions (serotonin syndrome, hypotension, drowsiness) and pharmacokinetic interactions (e.g. elevation of tricyclic plasma levels by some SSRIs).

Serotonin syndrome – symptoms[1,2]

Increasing severity

Restlessness
Diaphoresis
Tremor
Shivering
Myoclonus
Confusion
Convulsions
Death

- The advice given in the following table should be treated with caution and patients should be very carefully monitored when switching.

References

1. Sternbach H. The serotonin syndrome. *American Journal of Psychiatry* 1999; **148**: 705–713.
2. Mir S, Taylor D. Serotonin syndrome. *Psychiatry Bulletin* 1999; **23**: 742–747.

Table Antidepressants – swapping and stopping[*]

From \ To	MAOIs-hydrazines	Tranyl-cypromine	Tricyclics	Citalopram	Fluoxetine	Paroxetine
MAOIs-hydrazines	Withdraw and wait for 2 weeks	Withdraw and wait for 2 weeks	Withdraw and wait for 2 weeks	Withdraw and wait for 2 weeks	Withdraw and wait for 2 weeks	Withdraw and wait for 2 weeks
Tranyl-Cypromine	Withdraw and wait for 2 weeks	–	Withdraw and wait for 2 weeks	Withdraw and wait for 2 weeks	Withdraw and wait for 2 weeks	Withdraw and wait for 2 weeks
Tricyclics	Withdraw and wait for one week	Withdraw and wait for 1 week	Cross-taper cautiously	Halve dose and add citalopram then slow withdrawal[b]	Halve dose and add fluoxetine then slow withdrawal[b]	Halve dose and add paroxetine then slow withdrawal[b]
Citalopram	Withdraw and wait for one week	Withdraw and wait for 1 week	Cross-taper cautiously[b]	–	Withdraw then start fluoxetine at 10 mg/day	Withdraw and start paroxetine at 10 mg/day
Paroxetine	Withdraw and wait for 2 weeks	Withdraw and wait for 1 week	Cross- taper cautiously with very low dose of tricylic[b]	Withdraw and start citalopram	Withdraw then start fluoxetine	–
Fluoxetine[c]	Withdraw and wait 5–6 weeks	Withdraw and wait 5–6 weeks	Stop fluoxetine Start tricyclic at very low dose and increase very slowly	Stop fluoxetine Wait 4–7 days Start citalopram at 10 mg/day and increase slowly	–	Stop fluoxetine Wait 4–7 days, then start paroxetine 10 mg/day

[*] Note: Advice given in this table is partly derived from manufacturers' information and partly theoretical. Caution is required in every instance

Sertraline	Trazodone/ nefazodone	Moclobemide	Reboxetine	Venlafaxine	Mirtazapine
Withdraw and wait for 2 weeks	Withdraw and wait for 2 weeks	Withdraw and wait for 2 weeks[a]	Withdraw and wait for 2 weeks	Withdraw and wait for 2 weeks	Withdraw and wait for 2 weeks
Withdraw and wait for 2 weeks	Withdraw and wait for 2 weeks	Withdraw and wait for 2 weeks[a]	Withdraw and wait for 2 weeks	Withdraw and wait for 2 weeks	Withdraw and wait for 2 weeks
Halve dose and add sertraline then slow withdrawal[b]	Halve dose and add trazodone/ nefazodone, then slow withdrawal	Withdraw and wait at least one week	Cross-taper cautiously	Cross-taper cautiously, starting with venlafaxine 37.5 mg/day	Cross-taper cautiously
Withdraw and start sertraline at 25 mg/day	Withdraw before starting titration of trazodone/ nefazodone	Withdraw and wait at least 2 weeks	Cross-taper cautiously	Withdraw citalopram Start venlafaxine 37.5 mg/day and increase very slowly	Cross-taper cautiously
Withdraw and start sertraline at 25 mg/day	Withdraw before starting titration of trazodone/ nefazodone	Withdraw and wait at least 2 weeks	Cross-taper cautiously	Withdraw paroxetine Start venlafaxine 37.5 mg/day and increase very slowly	Cross-taper cautiously
Stop fluoxetine Wait 4–7 days, then start sertraline 25 mg/day	Stop fluoxetine Wait 4–7 days then start low dose trazodone/ nefazodone	Withdraw and wait at least 5 weeks	Withdraw Start reboxetine at 2 mg bd and increase cautiously	Withdraw Wait 4–7 days Start venlafaxine at 37.5 mg/day Increase very slowly	Withdraw and start mirtazapine cautiously

Table   Antidepressants – swapping and stopping[*] – (cont.)

From	To MAOIs-hydrazines	Tranyl-cypromine	Tricyclics	Citalopram	Fluoxetine	Paroxetine
Sertraline	Withdraw and wait for 2 weeks[a]	Withdraw and wait for 2 weeks	Cross-taper cautiously with very low dose of tricyclic[b]	Withdraw then start citalopram	Withdraw then start fluoxetine	Withdraw then start paroxetine
Trazodone/ nefazodone	Withdraw and wait at least one week	Withdraw and wait at least one week	Cross- taper cautiously with very low dose of tricyclic	Withdraw then start citalopram	Withdraw then start fluoxetine	Withdraw then start paroxetine
Moclobemide	Withdraw and wait 24 hours	Withdraw and wait 24 hours	Withdraw and wait 24 hours	Withdraw and wait 24 hours	Withdraw and wait 24 hours	Withdraw and wait 24 hours
Reboxetine	Withdraw and wait at least one week	Withdraw and wait at least one week	Cross-taper cautiously	Cross-taper cautiously	Cross- taper cautiously	Cross-taper cautiously
Venlafaxine	Withdraw and wait at least one week	Withdraw and wait at least one week	Cross-taper cautiously with very low dose of tricyclic[b]	Cross-taper cautiously Start with 10 mg/day	Cross-taper cautiously Start with 20 mg every other day	Cross-taper cautiously Start with 10 mg/day
Mirtazapine	Withdraw and wait for 1 week	Withdraw and wait for 1 week	Withdraw then start tricyclic	Withdraw then start citalopram	Withdraw then start fluoxetine	Withdraw then start paroxetine
Stopping[d]	Reduce over 4 weeks	Reduce over 4 weeks	Reduce over 4 weeks	Reduce over 4 weeks	At 20 mg/day, just stop At 40 mg/day, reduce over 2 weeks	Reduce over 4 weeks or longer, if necessary[e]

Notes

[a] Abrupt switching is possible but not recommended.

[b] Do not co-administer clomipramine and SSRIs or venlafaxine. Withdraw clomipramine before starting.

[c] Beware interactions with fluoxetine may still occur for 5 weeks after stopping fluoxetine because of long half-life.

[d] See general guidelines (page 148).

[e] Withdrawal effects seem to be more pronounced. Slow withdrawal over 1–3 months may be necessary.

Sertraline	Trazodone/ nefazodone	Moclobemide	Reboxetine	Venlafaxine	Mirtazapine
–	Withdraw before starting trazodone/ nefazodone	Withdraw and wait at least 2 weeks	Cross-taper cautiously	Withdraw. Start venlafaxine at 37.5 mg/day	Cross-taper cautiously
Withdraw then start sertraline	–	Withdraw and wait least 1 week	Withdraw, start reboxetine at 2 mg BD and increase cautiously	Withdraw. Start venlafaxine at 37.5/day	Cross-taper cautiously
Withdraw and wait 24 hours	Withdraw and wait 24 hours		Withdraw and wait 24 hours	Withdraw and wait 24 hours	Withdraw and wait 24 hours
Cross-taper cautiously	Cross-taper cautiously	Withdraw and wait at least 1 week	–	Cross-taper cautiously	Cross-taper cautiously
Cross-taper cautiously Start with 25 mg/day	Cross-taper cautiously	Withdraw and wait at least 1 week	Cross-taper cautiously	–	Cross-taper cautiously
Withdraw then start sertraline	Withdraw then start trazodone/ nefazodone	Withdraw and wait 1 week	Withdraw then start reboxetine	Withdraw then start venlafaxine	–
Reduce over 4 weeks	Reduce over 4 weeks	Reduce over 4 weeks	Reduce over four weeks	Reduce over 4 weeks or longer, if necessary°	Reduce over 4 weeks

Antidepressant discontinuation symptoms

What are discontinuation symptoms?

The term 'discontinuation symptoms' is used to describe symptoms experienced on stopping pre-scribed drugs that are not drugs of dependence. There is an important semantic difference between 'discontinuation' and 'withdrawal' symptoms – the latter implies addiction, the former does not. While this distinction is important for precise medical terminology, it may be irrelevant to patient experience. Discontinuation symptoms may occur after stopping many drugs, including antidepres-sants, and can often be explained in the context of 'receptor rebound'[1] – e.g. an antidepressant with potent anticholinergic side-effects may be associated with diarrhoea on discontinuation.

Discontinuation symptoms may be entirely new or similar to some of the original symptoms of the illness, and so cannot be attributed to other causes. They are experienced by at least a third of patients[2].

The onset is usually within 5 days of stopping treatment (depending on the half-life of the antide-pressant) or occasionally during taper or after missed doses[3,4] (short half-life drugs only). Symptoms can vary in form and intensity and occur in any combination. They are usually mild and self-limiting, but can occasionally be severe and prolonged. The perception of symptom severity is prob-ably made worse by the absence of forewarnings. Some symptoms are more likely with individual drugs.

Table Antidepressant discontinuation symptoms

	MAOIs	TCAs	SSRIs & related
Symptoms	**Common** Agitation, irritability, ataxia, movement disorders, insomnia, somnolence, vivid dreams, cognitive impairment, slowed speech, pressured speech **Occasionally** Hallucinations, paranoid delusions	**Common** Flu-like symptoms (chills, myalgia, excessive sweating, headache, nausea), insomnia, excessive dreaming **Occasionally** Movement disorders, mania, cardiac arrhythmias	**Common** Flu-like symptoms, 'shock-like' sensations, dizziness exacerbated by movement, insomnia, excessive (vivid) dreaming, irritability, crying spells **Occasionally** Movement disorders, problems with concentration and memory
Drugs most commonly associated with discontinuation symptoms	All Tranylcypromine is partly metabolised to amphetamine and is therefore associated with a true 'withdrawal syndrome'	Amitriptyline Imipramine	Paroxetine Venlafaxine

Clinical relevance[2]

The symptoms of a discontinuation reaction may be mistaken for a relapse of illness or the emergence of a new physical illness[5] leading to unnecessary investigations or reintroduction of the antidepressant. Symptoms may be severe enough to interfere with daily functioning and those who have experienced discontinuation symptoms may reason (perhaps appropriately) that antidepressants are 'addictive' and not wish to accept treatment.

Who is most at risk?[1,2,5]

Although anyone can experience discontinuation symptoms, the risk is increased in those prescribed short half-life drugs[3] (e.g. paroxetine, venlafaxine), particularly if they do not take them regularly. Two-thirds of patients prescribed antidepressants may skip a few doses from time to time[6]. The risk is also increased in those who have been taking antidepressants for 8 weeks or longer[7], those who have developed anxiety symptoms at the start of antidepressant therapy (particularly with SSRIs), those receiving other centrally-acting medication (e.g. antihypertensives, antihistamines, antipsychotics), children and adolescents and those who have experienced discontinuation symptoms before.

How to avoid[1,2,5]

Generally, antidepressant therapy should be discontinued over at least a 4-week period (this is not required with fluoxetine)[3]. The shorter the half-life of the drug, the more important that this rule is followed. The end of the taper may need to be slower as symptoms may not appear until the reduction in the total daily dosage of the antidepressant is (proportionately) substantial. Patients receiving MAOIs may need to be tapered over a longer period. Tranylcypromine may be particularly difficult to stop. At-risk patients (see above) may need a slower taper.

Many people suffer symptoms despite slow withdrawal. For these patients the option of abrupt withdrawal should be discussed. Some may prefer to face a week or two of intense symptoms rather than months of less severe discontinuation syndrome.

How to treat[2,5]

There are few systematic studies in this area. Treatment is pragmatic. If symptoms are mild, reassure the patient that these symptoms are not uncommon after discontinuing an antidepressant and will pass in a few days. If symptoms are severe, reintroduce the original antidepressant (or another with a longer half-life from the same class) and taper gradually while monitoring for symptoms.

Some evidence supports the use of anticholinergic agents in tricyclic withdrawal[8] and fluoxetine for symptoms associated with stopping clomipramine[9] or venlafaxine[10] – fluoxetine, having a longer plasma half-life, seems to be associated with a lower incidence of discontinuation symptoms than other similar drugs[11].

Key points that patients should know

- Antidepressants are not addictive (a survey of 2000 people across the UK conducted in 1991 found that 78% thought that antidepressants were addictive[12]). It is important to dispel this myth. In order for a drug to be addictive it must also fulfil certain other criteria including tolerance, escalating use, etc. This should be discussed. Note, however, that this semantic and categorical distinction may be lost on many people.

- Patients should be informed that they may experience discontinuation symptoms (and the most likely symptoms associated with the drug that they are taking) when they stop their antidepressant.

- Antidepressants should not be stopped abruptly. The dose should be tapered down over at least 4 weeks. Fluoxetine is an exception to this rule[3].

- Discontinuation symptoms may occur after missed doses if the antidepressant prescribed has a short half-life.

References

1. Antidepressant discontinuation syndrome: update on serotonin reuptake inhibitors. *Journal of Clinical Psychiatry* 1997; **58**(Suppl. 7): 3–40.
2. Lejoyeux M, Ades J, Mourad I. Antidepressant withdrawal syndrome: recognition, prevention and management. *CNS Drugs* 1996; **5**: 278–292.
3. Rosenbaum JF, Fava M, Hoog SL *et al*. Selective serotonin reuptake inhibitor discontinuation syndrome: a randomised controlled trial. *Biological Psychiatry* 1998; **44**: 77–88.
4. Michelson D, Fava M, Amsterdam J *et al*. Interruption of selective serotonin reuptake inhibitor treatment. *British Journal of Psychiatry* 2000; **176**: 363–368.
5. Haddad PM. Antidepressant discontinuation syndromes. *Drug Safety* 2001; **24**: 183–197.
6. Meijer WEE, Bouvy ML, Heerdink ER. Spontaneous lapses in dosing during chronic treatment with selective serotonin reuptake inhibitors. *British Journal of Psychiatry* 2001; **179**: 519–522.
7. Kramer JC, Klein DF, Fink M. Withdrawal symptoms following discontinuation of imipramine therapy. *American Journal of Psychiatry* 1961; **118**: 549–550.
8. Dilsaver SC, Feinberg M, Greden JF. Antidepressant withdrawal symptoms treated with anticholinergic agents. *American Journal of Psychiatry* 1983; **140**(2): 249–251.
9. Benazzi F. Fluoxetine for clomipramine withdrawal symptoms. *American Journal of Psychiatry* 1999; **156**(4): 661–662.
10. Giakas WJ, Davis JM. Intractable withdrawal from venlafaxine treated with fluoxetine. *Psychiatric Annals* 1997; **27**(2): 85–92.
11. Coupland NJ, Bell CJ, Potokar JP. Serotonin reuptake inhibitor withdrawal. *Journal of Clinical Psychopharmacology* 1996; **16**: 356–362.
12. Priest RG, Vize C, Roberts A *et al*. Lay people's attitudes to treatment of depression: results of opinion pole for Defeat Depression Campaign just before its launch. *BMJ* 1996; **313**: 858–859.

St John's wort

St John's wort (SJW) is the popular name for the plant *Hypericum perforatum*. It contains a combination of at least ten different components, including hypericins, flavonoids and xanthons[1]. Preparations of SJW are often unstandardised and this has complicated the interpretation of clinical trials.

The active ingredient and mechanism of action of SJW are unclear although many hypotheses have been proposed. At one time MAO inhibition was thought to be the most likely mechanism of action but more recent research has shown that this may account for only a small part of SJW's antidepressant effect[2]. Reuptake inhibition of both noradrenaline and serotonin has been demonstrated, as has the up-regulation of serotonin receptors[3]. At this time no firm conclusions can be drawn.

SJW is not a licensed preparation in the UK but is available as a herbal or complementary therapy. (It is licensed in Germany for the treatment of depression.)

Evidence for SJW in the treatment of depression

A number of trials have been published that look at the efficacy of SJW in the treatment of depression. They have been extensively reviewed[1,4,5] and most authors conclude that SJW may be effective in the treatment of mild-to-moderate depression. This conclusion is suitably cautious in view of the many limitations of the studies:

- The active component of SJW for treating depression has not yet been determined. The trials used different preparations of SJW which were standardised according to their total content of hypericins. However, recent evidence suggests that hypericins alone do not treat depression[6]. It is illogical to recommend a treatment where the dosage stated is not that of the active ingredient.

- None of the trials has lasted longer than eight weeks.

- SJW was often compared to subtherapeutic doses of standard antidepressants. Patients showed a surprisingly good response to low doses of TCAs used in the trials, which also brings into question the methodology of the studies. One, more recent, study found *Hypericum perforatum* to be as effective as imipramine 150 mg daily in the treatment of mild-to-moderate depression[7].

- SJW is often said to be much better tolerated than standard antidepressants. This is misleading, since only two trials have compared SJW to the newer antidepressants such as the SSRIs[8,9].

SJW may prove to be an effective and well-tolerated treatment for mild to moderate depression. However, until more trials are conducted to address the above points, we should continue to use antidepressants which are proven to be effective and whose long-term effects and possible interactions with other drugs have been determined.

Note also that SJW has been shown to be ineffective in the treatment of severe depression[10].

Adverse effects

The most common side-effects of SJW are dry mouth, nausea, constipation, fatigue, dizziness, headache and restlessness[4,5,7,11]. In addition, SJW contains a red pigment that can cause photosensitivity reactions[12]. In common with other antidepressant drugs, SJW has been known to precipitate hypomania in people with bipolar affective disorder[13].

Drug interactions

It is thought that SJW is an inducer of the hepatic cytochrome P450 system[14]. Studies have shown that SJW significantly reduces plasma concentrations of digoxin and indinavir[15,16] (a drug used in the treatment of HIV). There have also been a number of case reports where SJW has lowered the plasma concentrations of theophylline, cyclosporin, warfarin and the combined oral contraceptive pill and has led to treatment failure[14]. There is a theoretical risk that SJW may interact with some anticonvulsant drugs[17]. Serotonin syndrome has been reported when SJW was taken together with sertraline, paroxetine, nefazodone and the triptans[17,18] (a group of serotonin agonists used to treat migraine). SJW should not be taken with any drugs that have a predominantly serotonergic action.

Key points that patients should know

- The evidence so far available suggests that SJW may be effective in the treatment of mild (not severe) depression but we do not know enough about how much should be taken or what the side-effects are.

- The symptoms of depression can sometimes be caused by other physical or mental illness. It is important that these possible causes are investigated.

- SJW can interact with other medicines, resulting in serious side-effects. Some important drugs may be metabolised more rapidly and therefore become ineffective with serious consequences (e.g. increased viral load in HIV, reduced anticoagulant effect with warfarin leading to thrombosis).

- SJW is not suitable for some groups of people, including anyone who is severely depressed.

- It is always best to discuss with the doctor if any herbal or natural remedy is being taken or the patient is thinking of taking one.

Many people regard herbal remedies as 'natural' and therefore harmless[19]. They are not aware of the potential of such remedies for causing side-effects or interacting with other drugs. A small US study (n = 22) found that people tend to take SJW because it is easy to obtain alternative medicines and also because they perceive herbal medicines as being purer and safer than prescription medicines. Few would discuss this medication with their conventional healthcare provider[11]. Clinicians need to be proactive in asking patients if they use such treatments and try to dispel the myth that natural is the same as safe.

References

1. Linde K, Ramirez G, Mulrow CD *et al.* St John's wort for depression – an overview and meta-analysis of randomised controlled trials. *British Medical Journal* 1996; **313**: 253–258.
2. Colt JM. In vitro receptor binding and enzyme inhibition by *Hypericum perforatum* extract. *Psychopharmacology* 1997; **30**(Suppl. 2):108–112.
3. Muller WE, Rolli M, Schafer C *et al.* Effects of *Hypericum* extract (LI116) in biochemical models of antidepressant activity. *Psychopharmacology* 1997; **30**(Suppl. 2): 102–107.
4. Volz HP. Controlled clinical trials of *Hypericum* extracts in depressed patients – an overview. *Pharmacopsychiatry* 1997; **30**(Suppl. 2): 72–76.
5. Gaster B, Holroyd J. St Johns's wort for depression – a systematic review. *Archives of Internal Medicine* 2000; **160**: 152–156.
6. Teufel-Mayer R, Gleitz J. Effects of long-term administration of *Hypericum* extracts on the affinity and density of the central serotonergic 5HT1a and 5HT2a receptors. *Pharmacopsychiatry* 1997; **30**(Suppl. 2): 113–116.
7. Woelk H. Comparison of St John's wort and imipramine for treating depression: randomised controlled trial. *BMJ* 2000; **321**: 356–359.
8. Brenner R, Azbel V, Madhusoodanan S *et al.* Comparison of an extract of *Hypericum* (LI160) and sertraline in the treatment of depression: a double blind randomised pilot study. *Clinical Therapeutics* 2000; **22**: 411–419.
9. Behnke K, Jensen JS, Graubaum HJ et al. *Hypericum perforatum* versus fluoxetine in the treatment of mild to moderate depression. *Advances in Therapy* 2002; **19**: 43–52.
10. Davidson JRT, Gadde KM, Fairbank JA *et al.* Effect of *Hypericum perforatum* (St John's wort) in major depressive disorder: a randomised controlled trial. *JAMA* 2002; **287**: 1807–1814.
11. Wagner PJ, Jester D, LeClair B *et al.* Taking the edge off – why patients choose St John's wort. *The Journal of Family Practice* 1999; **48**: 615–619.
12. Bore GM. Acute neuropathy after exposure to sun in a patient treated with St John's wort. *Lancet* 1998; **352**: 1121–1122.
13. Nierenburg AA, Burt T, Mathews J *et al.* Mania associated with St John's wort. *Biological Psychiatry* 1999; **46**: 1707–1708.
14. Ernst E. Second thoughts about safety of St John's wort. *Lancet* 1999; **354**: 2014–2015.
15. Johne A, Brockmoller J, Bauer S *et al.* Pharmacokinetic interaction of digoxin with a herbal extract from St John's wort (*Hypericum perforatum*). *Clinical Pharmacology and Therapeutics* 1999; **66**: 338–345.
16. Piscitelli SC, Burstein AH, Chaitt D *et al.* Indinavir concentrations and St John's wort. *Lancet* 2000; **355**: 547–548.
17. Reminder: St John's wort (*Hypericum perforatum*) interactions. *Current Problems in Pharmacovigilance* 2000; **26**: 6.
18. Lantz MS, Buchalter E, Giambanco V. St John's wort and antidepressant drug interactions in the elderly. *Journal of Geriatric Psychiatry and Neurology* 1999; **12**: 7–10.
19. Barnes J, Mills SY, Abbot NC *et al.* Different standards for reporting ADRs to herbal remedies and conventional OTC medicines: face-to-face interviews with 515 users of herbal remedies. *British Journal of Clinical Pharmacology* 1998; **45**: 496–500.

Further reading

Whiskey E, Werneke U, Taylor D. A systematic review and meta-analysis of *Hypericum perforatum* in depression: a comprehensive clinical review. *International Clinical Psychopharmacology* 2001; **16**: 239–252.

Drug interactions with antidepressants

Drugs can interact with each other in two different ways:

1. *Pharmacokinetic interactions* where one drug interferes with the Absorbtion, Distribution, Metabolism or Elimination of another drug. This may result in subtherapeutic effect or toxicity. The largest group of pharmacokinetic interactions involve drugs that inhibit or induce hepatic CYP450 enzymes (see the table opposite). Other enzyme systems include FMO[1] and UGT[2]. While both of these enzyme systems are involved in the metabolism of psychotropic drugs, the potential for drugs to inhibit or induce these enzyme systems is poorly studied.

2. *Pharmacodynamic interactions* where the effects of one drug are altered by another drug via physiological mechanisms such as direct competition at receptor sites (e.g. dopamine agonists with dopamine blockers negate any therapeutic effect), augmentation of the same neurotransmitter pathway (e.g. fluoxetine with tramadol can lead to serotonin syndrome) or affecting physiological functioning of an organ/organ system in different ways (e.g. two different antiarrythmic drugs). Most of these interactions can be easily predicted by a sound knowledge of pharmacology. A list can be found at the back of the *BNF*.

Pharmacodynamic interactions

Tricyclic antidepressants[8,9]:

- Are H_1 blockers (sedative). This can be exacerbated by other sedative drugs or alcohol. Beware respiratory depression.

- Are anticholinergic (dry mouth, blurred vision, constipation). This can be exacerbated by other anticholinergic drugs such as antihistamines or antipsychotics. Beware cognitive impairment and GI obstruction.

- Are adrenergic α_1-blockers (postural hypotension). This can be exacerbated by other drugs that block α_1-receptors and by antihypertensive drugs in general. Adrenaline, in combination with α_1-blockers can lead to hypertension.

- Are arrhythmogenic. Caution is required with other drugs that can alter cardiac conduction directly (e.g. antiarrhythmics or phenothiazines) or indirectly through a potential to cause electrolyte disturbance (e.g. diuretics).

- Lower the seizure threshold. Caution is required with other pro-convulsive drugs (e.g. antipsychotics) and particularly if the patient is being treated for epilepsy (higher doses of anticonvulsants may be required).

- May be serotonergic (e.g. amitriptyline, clomipramine). There is the potential for these drugs to interact with other serotonergic drugs (e.g. tramadol, SSRIs, selegiline) to cause serotonin syndrome.

Table	Pharmacokinetic interactions[3–7]		
p4501A2	**p4502C**	**p4502D6**	**p4503A**
Genetic polymorphism	5–10% of caucasians lack	3–5% of caucasians lack	60% P450 content
Induced by:	*Induced by:*	*Induced by:*	*Induced by:*
cigarette smoke	phenytoin	carbamazepine	carbamazepine
charcoal cooking	rifampicin	phenytoin	phenytoin
carbamazepine			prednisolone
omeprazole			rifampicin
phenobarbitone			
phenytoin			
Inhibited by:	*Inhibited by:*	*Inhibited by:*	*Inhibited by:*
cimetidine	cimetidine	chlorpromazine	erythromycin
ciprofloxacin	fluoxetine	citalopram	fluoxetine
erythromycin	fluvoxamine	fluoxetine	fluvoxamine
fluvoxamine	sertraline	fluphenazine	ketoconazole
paroxetine		haloperidol	nefazodone
		paroxetine	paroxetine
		sertraline	sertraline
		tricyclics	tricyclics
Metabolises:	*Metabolises:*	*Metabolises:*	*Metabolises:*
clozapine	diazepam	clozapine	benzodiazepines
haloperidol	omeprazole	codeine	calcium blockers
mirtazapine	phenytoin	donepezil	carbamazepine
olanzapine	tolbutamide	haloperidol	cimetidine
theophylline	tricyclics	methadone	clozapine
tricyclics	warfarin	phenothiazines	codeine
warfarin		risperidone	donepezil
		TCA secondary amines	erythromycin
		tramadol	galantamine
		trazodone	mirtazapine
		venlafaxine	risperidone
			steroids
			terfenadine
			tricyclics
			valproate
			venlafaxine
			Z-hypnotics

SSRIs[10,11]:

- Increase serotonergic neurotransmission. The main concern is serotonin syndrome (see page 143).

MAOIs[12]:

- Prevent the destruction of monoamine neurotransmitters. Sympathomimetic and dopaminergic drugs can lead to monoamine overload and hypertensive crisis. Pethidine and fermented foods can have the same effect.

- Can interact with serotonergic drugs to cause serotonin syndrome.

Avoid/minimise problems by:

1. Avoiding antidepressant polypharmacy.

2. Avoiding the co-prescription of other drugs with a similar pharmacology but not marketed as antidepressants (e.g. bupropion, sibutramine).

3. Knowing your pharmacology (most interactions can be easily predicted).

References

1. Cashman JR. Human Flavin Containing Mono-oxygenase: substrate specificity and role in drug metabolism. *Current Drug Metabolism* 2000; **1**: 181–191.
2. Anderson GD. A mechanistic approach to antiepileptic drug interactions. *Annals of Pharmacotherapy* 1998; **32**: 554–563.
3. Lin JH, Lu AYH. Inhibition and induction of cytochrome P450 and the clinical implications. *Clinical Pharmacokinetics* 1998; **35**: 361–390.
4. Mitchell PB. Drug interactions of clinical significance with selective serotonin reuptake inhibitors. *Drug Safety* 1997; **17**: 390–406.
5. Richelson E. Pharmacokinetic interactions of antidepressants. *Journal of Clinical Psychiatry* 1998; **59**(Suppl. 10): 22–26.
6. Greenblatt DJ, von Moltke LL, Harmatz JS *et al.* Drug interactions with newer antidepressants: role of human cytochromes P450. *Journal of Clinical Psychiatry* 1998; **59**(Suppl. 15): 19–27.
7. Taylor D. Pharmacokinetic interactions involving clozapine. *British Journal of Psychiatry* 1997; **171**: 109–112.
8. *British National Formulary.* Appendix 1 pp.618–658. Edition 43. London: British Medical Association and Royal Pharmaceutical Society of Great Britain, 2002.
9. Watsky EJ, Salzman C. Psychotropic drug interactions. *Hospital & Community Psychiatry* 1991; **42**: 247–256.
10. Mitchell PB. Drug interactions of clinical significance with serotonin reuptake inhibitors. *Drug Safety* 1997; **17**: 390–406.
11. Edwards JG, Anderson I. Systematic review and guide to selection of serotonin reuptake inhibitors. *Drugs* 1999; **57**: 507–533.
12. Livingstone MG, Livingstone HM. Monoamine oxidase inhibitors: an update on drug interactions. *Drug Safety* **14**: 219–227.

Table	Antidepressants: relative adverse effects – a rough guide			
Drug	Sedation	Hypotension	Anticholinergic effects	Forms available
Tricyclics				
Amitriptyline	+++	+++	+++	tabs/caps, liq, inj
Clomipramine	++	+++	++	tabs/caps, liq, inj
Desipramine	+	++	+	tabs
Dothiepin	+++	+++	++	tabs, caps
Doxepin	+++	++	++	caps
Imipramine	++	+++	+++	tabs, liq
Lofepramine	+	+	+	tabs
Nortriptyline	+	++	+	tabs
Trimipramine	+++	+++	++	tabs, caps
Other antidepressants				
Mianserin	++	–	–	tabs
Mirtazapine	+++	–	+	tabs
Nefazodone	++	–	–	tabs
Reboxetine	+	–	+	tabs
Trazodone	+++	++	–	caps, liq
Venlafaxine	+/–	–	+	tabs
Selective serotonin reuptake inhibitors (SSRIs)				
Citalopram	+/–	–	–	tabs
Fluoxetine	–	–	–	caps, liq
Fluvoxamine	+	–	–	tabs
Paroxetine	+	–	+	tabs, liq
Sertraline	–	–	–	tabs
Monoamine oxidase inhibitors (MAOIs)				
Isocarboxazid	+	++	++	tabs
Phenelzine	+	+	+	tabs
Tranylcypromine	–	+	+	tabs
Reversible inhibitor of monoamine oxidase A (RIMA)				
Moclobemide	–	–	–	tabs

KEY: +++ High incidence/severity
　　　++ Moderate
　　　+ Low
　　　– Very low/none

Anxiety spectrum disorders

Anxiety is a normal emotion that is experienced by everyone at some time. Symptoms can be psychological, physical, or a mixture of both. Intervention is required when symptoms become disabling.

There are several disorders within the overall spectrum of anxiety disorders, each with its own characteristic symptoms. These are outlined briefly in the table below. Anxiety disorders can occur on their own, be part of other psychiatric disorders (particularly depression), be a consequence of physical illness such as thyrotoxicosis or be drug-induced (e.g. by caffeine)[1]. Co-morbidity with other psychiatric disorders is very common.

Anxiety spectrum disorders tend to be chronic and treatment is often only partially successful.

Benzodiazepines

Benzodiazepines provide rapid symptomatic relief from acute anxiety states. All guidelines and consensus statements recommend that this group of drugs should only be used to treat anxiety that is severe, disabling, or subjecting the individual to extreme distress. Due to their potential to cause physical dependence and withdrawal symptoms, these drugs should be used at the lowest effective dose for the shortest period of time (max. 4 weeks), while medium/long-term treatment strategies are put in place. For the majority of patients these recommendations are sensible and should be adhered to. A very small number of patients with severely disabling anxiety may benefit from long-term treatment with a benzodiazepine and these patients should not be denied treatment[2].

SSRI dose and duration of treatment

When used to treat generalised anxiety disorder (**GAD**), SSRIs should initially be prescribed at half the normal starting dose for the treatment of depression and the dose titrated upwards into the normal antidepressant dosage range as tolerated (initial worsening of anxiety may be seen when treatment is started[3-6]). Response is usually seen within 6 weeks. The optimal duration of treatment has not been determined but should be at least 6 months. Effective treatment of GAD may prevent the development of major depression[7].

When used to treat **panic disorder**, the same starting dose and dosage titration as in GAD should be used. Doses of clomipramine[8], citalopram[9] and sertraline[10] towards the bottom of the antidepressant range give the best balance between efficacy and side-effects, whereas higher doses of paroxetine (40 mg and above) may be required[11]. Higher doses may be effective when standard doses have failed. Onset of action may take 6 weeks. The optimal duration of treatment is unknown, but should be at least 8 months[12,13], with some authors recommending up to 18 months[14]. Less than 50% are likely to remain well after medication is withdrawn[14].

Lower starting doses are also required in post-traumatic stress disorder (**PTSD**), with high doses (e.g. fluoxetine 60 mg) often being required for full effect. Response is usually seen within 8 weeks[15], but can take up to 12 weeks[14]. Treatment should be continued for at least 6 months (relapse rate of 5% on active drug at this point vs 26% of those switched to placebo after acute treatment[16]) and probably longer[17].

Although the doses of SSRIs licensed for the treatment of obsessive compulsive disorder (**OCD**) are higher than those licensed for the treatment of depression (e.g. fluoxetine 60 mg, paroxetine 40–60 mg), lower (standard antidepressant) doses may be effective, particularly for maintenance treatment[18,19]. Initial response is usually slower than in depression (can take 10–12 weeks). The relapse rate in those who continue treatment for 2 years is half that of those of stop treatment after initial response (25–40% vs 80%)[20,21].

Standard antidepressant starting doses are well tolerated in **social phobia**[22,23] and upward dosage titration may benefit some patients but is not always required. Response is usually seen within 8 weeks and treatment should be continued for at least a year and probably longer[24.]

SSRIs should not be stopped abruptly as patients with anxiety spectrum disorders are particularly sensitive to discontinuation symptoms (see page 148). The dose should be titrated down as tolerated over several weeks to months.

Psychological approaches

There is good evidence to support the efficacy of some psychological interventions in anxiety spectrum disorders. Examples include exposure therapy in OCD and social phobia. Initial drug therapy may be required to help the patient become more receptive to psychological input and some studies suggest that optimal outcome is achieved by combining psychological and drug therapies[1].

A discussion of the evidence base for psychological interventions is outside the scope of these guidelines. Further information can be found at www.doh.gov.uk[25] There are often long waiting lists for psychological therapies and some specialist interventions may not be available at all in some areas. The table on the following pages does not list psychological interventions as first-line treatments for these reasons, although it is recognised that for many patients their use as a first-line treatment would be appropriate.

References

1. Fineberg N, Drummond LM. Anxiety disorders: drug treatment or behavioural cognitive psychotherapy. *CNS Drugs* 1995; **3**: 448–466.
2. Royal College of Psychiatrists. Benzodiazepines: risks, benefits or dependence, a re-evaluation. Council Report CR 57. London: Royal College of Psychiatrists, 1997.
3. Scott A, Davidson A, Palmer K. Antidepressant drugs in the treatment of anxiety disorders. *Advances in Psychiatric Treatment* 2001; **7**: 275–282.
4. Rocca P, Fonzo V, Scotta M *et al*. Paroxetine efficacy in the treatment of generalised anxiety disorder. *Acta Psychiatrica Scandinavica* 1997; **95**: 444–450.
5. Davidson JR. Pharmacotherapy of generalised anxiety disorder. *Journal of Clinical Psychiatry* 2001; **62**: 46–50.
6. Ballenger JC, Davidson JRT, Lecrubier Y *et al*. Consensus statement on generalised anxiety disorder from the international consensus group on depression and anxiety. *Journal of Clinical Psychiatry* 2001; **62**(Suppl. 11): 53–58.
7. Goodwin RD, Gorman JM. Psychopharmacologic treatment of generalised anxiety disorder and the risk of major depression. *American Journal of Psychiatry* 2002; **159**: 1935–1937.
8. Caillard V, Rouillon F, Viel JF *et al*. Comparative effects of low and high doses of clomipramine and placebo in panic disorder: a double-blind controlled study. *Acta Psychiatrica Scandinavica* 1999; **99**: 51–58.
9. Wade AG, Lepola U, Koponen HJ *et al*. The effect of citalopram in panic disorder. *British Journal of Psychiatry* 1997; **170**: 549–553.
10. Londborg PD, Wolkov R, Smith WT *et al*. Sertraline in the treatment of panic disorder: a multi-site, double-blind, placebo-controlled, fixed dose investigation. *British Journal of Psychiatry* 1998; **173**: 54–68.
11. Ballanger JC, Wheadon DE, Steiner M *et al*. Double blind, fixed dose, placebo controlled study of paroxetine in the treatment of panic disorder. *American Journal of Psychiatry* 1998; **155**: 36–42.
12. Ridels K, Schweizer E. Panic disorder: Long term pharmacotherapy and discontinuation. *Journal of Clinical Psychopharmacology* 1998; **18**(Suppl. 2): 12–18.
13. Michelson D, Pollack M, Lydiard B *et al*. Continuing treatment of panic disorder after acute response: randomised, placebo-controlled trial with fluoxetine. *British Journal of Psychiatry* 1999; **174**: 213–218.
14. American Psychiatric Association. Practice Guideline for the Treatment of Panic disorder. *American Journal of Psychiatry* 1998; (Suppl.11).

(*cont.* on p. 162)

Table

	Generalised anxiety disorder[3–6,26–29]	*Obsessive compulsive disorder*[18–21,30–35]
Clinical presentation	• Irrational worries • Motor tension • Hypervigilance • Somatic symptoms (e.g. hyperventilation, tachycardia and sweating)	• Obsessional thinking (e.g. constantly thinking that the door has been left unlocked) • Compulsive behaviour (e.g. constantly going back to check)
Emergency management	Benzodiazepines (normally for short-term use only: max. 2–4 weeks, but see note overleaf & ref 2)	Not usually appropriate
First line drug treatment Treatment of anxiety may prevent the subsequent development of depression[7]	• SSRIs (although may initially exacerbate symptoms. A lower starting is often required) • Venlafaxine • Some TCAs (e.g. imipramine, clomipramine)	• SSRIs • Clomipramine
Other treatments (less well tolerated or weaker evidence base)	• Buspirone (has a delayed onset of action) • Hydroxyzine • β-blockers (useful for somatic symptoms, particularly tachycardia)	• Antipsychotics (evidence for quetiapine and risperidone as antidepressant augmentation, but not haloperidol) • Buspirone • Clomipramine (iv pulse loading) • Clonazepam (benzodiazepines in general are mainly useful in reducing associated anxiety)
Non-drug treatments See *www.doh.org.uk*	• Reassurance • Anxiety management, including relaxation training. • CBT	• Exposure therapy • Behavioural therapy • CBT • Combined drug and psychologicaltherapy may be the most effective option

Panic disorder[8–14,36,37,38–42]	Post-traumatic stress disorder[15–17,43,44]	Social phobia[22–24]
• Sudden unpredictable episodes of severe anxiety • Shortness of breath • Fear of suffocation/dying • Urgent desire to flee	• History of a traumatic life event (as perceived by the sufferer) • Emotional numbness or detachment • Intrusive flashbacks or vivid dreams • Disabling fear of re-exposure, causing avoidance of perceived similar situations	• Extreme fear of social situations (e.g. eating in public or public speaking) • Fear of humiliation or embarrassment • Avoidant behaviour (e.g. never eating in restaurants) • Anxious anticipation (e.g. feeling sick on entering a restaurant)
Benzodiazepines *(have a rapid effect, although panic symptoms return quickly if the drug is withdrawn).*	Not usually appropriate	Benzodiazepines (have a rapid effect and may be useful on a PRN basis)
• SSRIs (therapeutic effect can be delayed and patients can experience an initial exacerbation of panic symptoms) • Some TCAs (e.g. imipramine, clomipramine) • Reboxetine	• SSRIs • Serotonergic TCAs	• SSRIs • MAOIs
• MAOIs • Valproate • Inositol	• MAOIs • Valproate • Carbamazepine • Clonidine	• Moclobemide • Clonazepam • Propranolol (performance anxiety only) • Buspirone (adjunct to SSRIs only)
• CBT • Anxiety management, including relaxation, training • Combined drug and psychological therapy may be more effective	• Debriefing should be available if desired • Counselling • Anxiety management • CBT, especially for avoidance behaviours or intrusive images	• CBT • Exposure therapy (combined drug and exposure therapy may be more effective)

15. Stein DJ, Zungu-Dinwayi N, van der Linden GHJ *et al.* Pharmacotherapy for posttraumatic stress disorder. Cochrane database of systematic reviews. Cochrane Library, Update Software, 2002.
16. Davidson J, Pearlstein T, Londborg P *et al.* Efficacy of sertraline in preventing relapse of posttraumatic stress disorder: results of a 28-week double-blind, placebo controlled study. *American Journal of Psychiatry* 2001; **158**: 1974–1981.
17. Martenyi F, Brown EB, Zhang H *et al.* Fluoxetine v placebo in prevention of relapse in post-traumatic stress disorder. *British Journal of Psychiatry* 2002; **181**: 315–320.
18. Ravizza L, Maina G, Bogetto F *et al.* Long term treatment of obsessive-compulsive disorder. *CNS Drugs* 1998; **10**: 247–255.
19. March JS. Treatment of obsessive compulsive disorder: the expert consensus guideline series. *Journal of Clinical Psychiatry* 1997; **58**(Suppl. 4).
20. Ravizza L, Barzega G, Bellino S *et al.* Drug treatment of obsessive compulsive disorder: long term trial with clomipramine and SSRIs. *Psychopharmacology Bulletin* 1996; **32**: 167–173.
21. Greist JH, Jefferson JW, Kobak KA *et al.* Efficacy and tolerability of serotonin transport inhibitors in OCD. *Archives of General Psychiatry* 1995; **52**: 53–60.
22. Liebowitz MR, Stein MB, Tancer M *et al.* A randomized, double-blind, fixed-dose comparison of paroxetine and placebo in the treatment of generalised social anxiety disorder. *Journal of Clinical Psychiatry* 2002; **63**: 66–74.
23. Blomhoff S, Haug TT, Hellstrom K *et al.* Randomised controlled general practice trial of sertraline, exposure therapy and combined treatment in generalised social phobias. *British Journal of Psychiatry* 2001; **179**: 23–30.
24. Hood SD, Nutt DJ. Psychopharmacological treatments: an overview. In: Crozier R, Alden LE (ed). *International handbook of social anxiety*. Oxford: John Wiley & Sons Ltd, 2001.
25. Treatment choice in psychological therapies and counselling. Evidence based clinical practice guideline. www.doh.org.uk.
26. Lader M. Treatment of anxiety. *BMJ* 1994; **309**: 321–324.
27. Allgulander C, Hackett D, Salinas E. Venlafaxine extended release (ER) in the treatment of generalised anxiety disorder. *British Journal of Psychiatry* 2001; **179**: 15–22.
28. Rickels K, Downing R, Schweizer E *et al.* Antidepressants for the treatment of generalised anxiety disorder: a placebo controlled comparison of imipramine, trazodone and diazepam. *Archives of General Psychiatry* 1993; **50**: 884–895.
29. Lader M, Scotto JC. A multicentre double-blind comparison of hydroxyzine, buspirone and placebo in patients with generalised anxiety disorder. *Psychopharmacology* 1998; **139**: 402–406.
30. Atmaca M, Kuloglu M, Tezcan E *et al.* Quetiapine augmentation in patients with treatment resistant obsessive-compulsive disorder: a single blind, placebo controlled study. *International Clinical Psychopharmacology* 2002; **17**: 115–119.
31. McDougle CJ, Epperson CN, Pelton GH *et al.* A double-blind placebo-controlled study of risperidone addition in serotonin reuptake inhibitor-refractory obsessive compulsive disorder. *Archives of General Psychiatry* 2000; **57**: 794–801.
32. McDougle CJ, Goodman WK, Leckman JF. Haloperidol addition in fluvoxamine-refractory obsessive-compulsive disorder. *Archives of General Psychiatry* 1994; **51**: 302–308.
33. Koran LM, Sallee FR, Pallanti S. Rapid benefit of intravenous pulse loading of clomipramine in obsessive-compulsive disorder. *American Journal of Psychiatry* 1997; **154**: 396–401.
34. Piccinelli M, Pini S, Bellantovonoc C *et al.* Efficacy of drug treatment in obsessive-compulsive disorder. A meta-analytic review. *British Journal of Psychiatry* 1995; **166**: 424–433.
35. Park LT, Jefferson JW, Greist JH. Obsessive-compulsive disorder: treatment options. *CNS Drugs* 1997; **7**: 187–202.
36. Johnson MR, Lydiard RB, Ballenger JC. Panic disorder: pathophysiology and drug treatment. *Drugs* 1995; **49**: 328–344.
37. Versiani M, Cassano G, Perugi G *et al.* Reboxetine, a selective norepinephrine reuptake inhibitor, is an effective and well-tolerated treatment for panic disorder. *Journal of Clinical Psychiatry* 2002; **63**: 31–37.
38. Bakker A, van Balkom AJLM, Spinhoven P *et al.* SSRIs V TCAs in the treatment of panic disorder: a meta-analysis. *Acta Psychiatrica Scandinavica* 2002; **106**: 163–167.
39. Wade A. Antidepressants in panic disorder. *International Clinical Psychopharmacology* 1999; **X**(Suppl. 14): 13–17.
40. Benjamin J, Levine J, Fox M *et al.* Double-blind, placebo controlled, crossover trial of inositol treatment for panic disorder. *American Journal of Psychiatry* 1995; **152**: 1084–1086.
41. Baetz M, Bowen RC. Efficacy of divalproex sodium in patients with panic disorder and mood instability who have not responded to conventional therapy. *Canadian Journal of Psychiatry* 1998; **43**: 73–77.
42. Otto MW, Tuby KS, Gould RA *et al.* An effect-size analysis of the relative efficacy and tolerability of serotonin selective reuptake inhibitors for panic disorder. *American Journal of Psychiatry* 2001; **158**: 1989–1992.
43. Connor KM, Sutherland SM, Tupler LA *et al.* Fluoxetine in post-traumatic stress disorder: randomised, double-blind study. *British Journal of Psychiatry* 1999; **175**: 17–22.
44. Davidson J. Drug therapy of post-traumatic stress disorder. *British Journal of Psychiatry* 1992; **160**: 309–314.

Further reading

Hood SD, Argyroupoulos SV, Nutt DJ. Agents in development for anxiety disorders: current status and future potential. *CNS Drugs* 2000; **13**: 421–431.

Benzodiazepines

Benzodiazepines are normally divided into two groups depending on their half-life and classified as being hypnotics (short half-life) or anxiolytics (long half-life). Although benzodiazepines have a place in the treatment of some forms of epilepsy and severe muscle spasm, and as premedicants in some surgical procedures, the vast majority of prescriptions are written for their hypnotic and anxiolytic effects. A detailed account of the pharmacology of benzodiazepines, with respect to their anxiolytic and hypnotic properties, has been published by Nutt & Malizia[1]. Benzodiazepines are also used for rapid tranquillisation (see page 236) and, as adjuncts, in the treatment of depression and schizophrenia.

Anxiolytic effect

Benzodiazepines reduce pathological anxiety, agitation and tension. Although useful in the emergency management of anxiety, benzodiazepines are addictive, and in the majority of patients, use should be restricted to no more than a month[2]. In contrast with the commonly held belief that benzodiazepines should be avoided in bereavement as they are thought to inhibit psychological adjustment, a recent RCT by Warner et al[3] found that benzodiazepines had no effect on the course of bereavement.

Repeat prescriptions should be avoided in those with major personality problems, whose difficulties are unlikely ever to resolve. Benzodiazepines should also be avoided, if possible, in those with a history of substance misuse.

Hypnotic effect

Benzodiazepines inhibit REM sleep and a rebound increase is seen when they are discontinued. There is a debate over the significance of this property[4].

Many people have unrealistic sleep expectations and hypnotics are effective drugs, at least in the short term. A high proportion of hospitalised patients is prescribed hypnotics[5]. Care should be taken to avoid using hypnotics regularly or for long periods of time[6]. Physical causes (e.g. pain, dyspnoea, etc.) or substance misuse (most commonly high caffeine consumption) should always be excluded before a hypnotic drug is prescribed. Be particularly careful to avoid prescribing hypnotics on discharge from hospital as iatrogenic dependence may be the result.

Use in depression

Benzodiazepines are not a treatment for major depressive illness. The National Service Framework for Mental Health[7] highlights this point by including a requirement that GPs audit the ratio of benzodiazepines to antidepressants prescribed in their practice. However, benzodiazepines may have a place (as adjuncts to antidepressants) in the initial management of depression. A Cochrane review of this topic[8] concluded that 'patients receiving short term augmentation of their antidepressant with a benzodiazepine were 37% less likely to drop out of treatment, 63% more likely to show a response at 1 week, 42% at 2 weeks and 38% at 4 weeks'. The authors reminded clinicians to be mindful of the duration of benzodiazepine treatment (to minimise the risk of dependence).

Use in psychosis

Benzodiazepines have been shown to be effective in treating the prodromal symptoms of psychotic relapse[9]. The efficacy of benzodiazepines in RT, in conjunction with the fact that a significant minority of patients fail to respond adequately to antipsychotics alone, can result in benzodiazepines being prescribed on a chronic basis[10]. The literature in this area is confusing. There is evidence that some treatment-resistant patients may benefit from a combination of antipsychotics and benzodiazepines, either by showing a very marked antipsychotic response or by allowing the use of lower dose antipsychotic regimens[11]. Alprazolam and clonazepam are possibly more effective than the other benzodiazepines in this regard[11].

Side-effects

Headaches, confusion, ataxia, dysarthria, blurred vision, gastro-intestinal disturbances, jaundice and paradoxical excitement are all possible side-effect s. A high incidence of reversible psychiatric side-effects, specifically loss of memory and depression led to the withdrawal of triazolam[12]. The use of benzodiazepines has been associated with a 50% increase in the risk of hip fracture in the elderly[13]. The risk is greatest in the first few days and after 1 month of continuous use. This would seem to be a class effect (the risk is not reduced by using short half-life drugs). Benzodiazepines can cause anterograde amnesia[14] and can adversely affect driving performance[15].

Respiratory depression is rare with oral therapy but is possible when the IV route is used. A specific benzodiazepine antagonist, flumazenil, is available. Flumazenil has a much shorter half-life than diazepam, making close observation of the patient essential for several hours after administration.

Intravenous injections can be painful and lead to thrombophlebitis, due to the low water solubility of benzodiazepines, and therefore it is necessary to use solvents in the preparation of injectable forms. Diazepam is available in emulsion form (Diazemuls) to overcome these problems.

Drug interactions

Benzodiazepines do not induce microsomal enzymes and so do not precipitate pharmacokinetic interactions with any other drugs. Most benzodiazepines are metabolised by CYP3A4, which is inhibited by erythromycin, several SSRIs and ketoconazole. It is theoretically possible that co-administration of these drugs will result in higher serum levels of benzodiazepines. Pharmacodynamic interactions (usually increased sedation) can occur.

References

1. Nutt DJ, Malizia AL. New insights into the role of the GABAa-benzodiazepine receptor in psychiatric disorder. *British Journal of Psychiatry* 2001; **179**: 390–396.
2. Committee on Safety of Medicines. Benzodiazepines, dependence and withdrawal symptoms. *Current Problems* 1988; **21**: 1–2.
3. Warner J, Metcalfe C, King M. Evaluating the use of benzodiazepines following recent bereavement. *British Journal of Psychiatry* 2001; **178**: 36–41.
4. Vogel GW, Buffenstein A, Minter K *et al.* Drug effects on REM sleep and on endogenous depression. *Neuroscience and Behavioural Reviews* 1990; **14**: 49–63.
5. Mahomed R, Paton C, Lee E. Prescribing hypnotics in a mental health Trust: what consultants say and what they do. *Pharmaceutical Journal* 2002; **268**: 657–659.
6. Royal College of Psychiatrists. *Benzodiazepines: risks, benefits or dependence: a re-evaluation.* Council Report CR59. London: Royal College of Psychiatrists, 1997.
7. Department of Health. *The National Service Framework for Mental Health.* London: DoH, 1999.
8. Furakawa TA, Streiner OL, Young LT. Antidepressant plus benzodiazepine for major depression (Cochrane review). The Cochrane Library Issue 2. Oxford: The Cochrane Collaboration. Update Software, 2001.

9. Carpenter WT, Buchanan RW, Kirkpatrick B *et al.* Diazepam treatment of early signs of exacerbation in schizophrenia. *American Journal of Psychiatry* 1999; **156**: 299–303.
10. Paton C, Banham S, Whitmore J. Benzodiazepines in schizophrenia: is there a trend towards long-term prescribing? *Psychiatric Bulletin* 2000; **24**: 113–115.
11. Wolkowitz OM, Pickar D. Benzodiazepines in the treatment of schizophrenia: a review and re-appraisal. *American Journal of Psychiatry* 19991; **148**: 714–726.
12. The sudden withdrawl of triazolam – reasons and consequences. *Drug & Therapeutics Bulletin* 1991; **29**: 89–90.
13. Wang PS, Bohn RL, Glynn RJ *et al.* Hazardous benzodiazepine regimens in the elderly: effects of half-life, dosage and duration on risk of hip fracture. *American Journal of Psychiatry* 2001; **158**: 892–898.
14. Verway B, Eling P, Wientjes H *et al.* Memory impairment in those who attempted suicide by benzodiazepine overdose. *Journal of Clinical Psychiatry* 2000; **61**: 456–459.
15. Barbone F, McMahon AD, Davey PG *et al.* Association of road-traffic accidents with benzodiazepine use. *Lancet* 1998; **352**: 1331–1336.

Further reading

Ashton H. Guidelines for the rational use of benzodiazepines. *Drugs* 1994; **48**: 25–40.
Summers J, Brown KW. Benzodiazepine prescribing in a psychiatric hospital. *Psychiatric Bulletin* 1998; **22**: 480–483.
Williams DDR, McBride A. Benzodiazepines: time for reassessment. *British Journal of Psychiatry* 1998; **173**: 361–362.

Insomnia

A patient complaining of insomnia may describe one or more of the following symptoms:

- Difficulty falling asleep.

- Frequent waking during the night.

- Early-morning wakening.

- Daytime sleepiness.

- A general loss of well-being through the individual's perception of a bad night's sleep.

Insomnia is a common complaint affecting approximately one-third of the UK population in any one year[2]. It is more common in women, in the elderly (some reports suggest 50% of those over 65 years) and in those with medical or psychiatric disorders[1]. Population studies in the UK have found that the prevalence of symptoms of underlying psychiatric illness, particularly depression and anxiety, increases with the severity and chronicity of insomnia[3]. Insomnia that lasts for a year or more is an established risk factor for the development of depression[4]. Chronic insomnia rarely remits spontaneously[5].

Before treating insomnia with drugs, consider:

- Is the underlying cause being treated (e.g. depression, mania, breathing difficulties, urinary frequency, pain, etc.)?

- Is substance misuse or diet a problem?

- Are other drugs being given at appropriate times (i.e. stimulating drugs in the morning, sedating drugs at night)?

- Are the patient's expectations of sleep realistic (sleep requirements decrease with age)?

- Have all sleep hygiene approaches (see table below) been tried[1]?

Table Sleep hygiene approaches
• Increase daily exercise (not in the evening)
• Reduce daytime napping
• Reduce caffeine or alcohol intake, especially before bedtime
• Only use the bed for sleeping
• Use anxiety management or relaxation techniques
• Develop a regular routine of rising and retiring at the same time each day

Table   Guidelines for prescribing hypnotics[6]

1. Use the lowest effective dose.

2. Use intermittent dosing (alternate nights or less) where possible.

3. Prescribe for short-term use (no more than 4 weeks) in the majority of cases.

4. Discontinue slowly.

5. Be alert for rebound insomnia/withdrawal symptoms.

6. Advise patients of the interaction with alcohol and other sedating drugs.

7. Avoid the use of hypnotics in patients with respiratory disease or severe hepatic impairment and in addiction-prone individuals.

Short-acting hypnotics are better for patients who have difficulty dropping off to sleep, but tolerance and dependence may develop more quickly[4]. Long-acting hypnotics are more suitable for patients with frequent or early-morning wakening. These drugs may be less likely to cause rebound insomnia and can have next-day anxiolytic action, but next-day sedation and maybe loss of co-ordination are more likely to occur[6].

The most widely prescribed hypnotics are the benzodiazepines. Non-benzodiazepine hypnotics such as zopiclone and zolpidem are becoming more widely used but may be just as likely as the benzodiazepines to cause dependence and neuropsychiatric reactions[7,8]. Zopiclone may impair driving performance more than benzodiazepines[9].

Table   Drugs used as hypnotics

Drug	Usual therapeutic dose (mg/day)		Time until onset (minutes)	Duration of action
	Adult	Elderly		
Diazepam	5–10		30–60	Long
Lormetazepam	0.5–1.5		30–60	Short
Oxazepam	15–30		20–50	Medium
Nitrazepam	5–10		20–50	Long
Temazepam*	10–20	Quarter to half the adult dose	30–60	Short
Zaleplon	10		30	Very short
Zopiclone	3.75–7.5		15–30	Short
Zolpidem	5–10		7–27	Short
Promethazine (not licensed)	25–50		Unclear, but maybe 1–2 hours	Long

* Temazepam is a popular drug of misuse. Some of the Controlled Drug regulations apply to its prescription, supply and administration. Nursing paperwork can be simplified considerably by avoiding the use of this drug.

Although it is commonly believed that tolerance always develops rapidly to the hypnotic effect of benzodiazepines[10] and zopiclone, there are only limited objective data to support this and the magnitude of the problem may have been over-estimated[5]. Long-term treatment with hypnotics may be beneficial in a very small number of patients. Case reports, case series and consensus statements support this approach[4,5,6,11]. As with all prescribing, the potential benefits and risks of hypnotic drugs have to be considered in the context of the clinical circumstances of each case.

References

1. Shapiro CM (ed). *ABC of Sleep Disorders*. London: BMJ Publishing Group, 1993.
2. Hajak G. A comparative assessment of the risks and benefits of zopiclone. *Drug Safety* 1999; **21**: 457–469.
3. Nutt DJ, Wilson S. Evaluation of severe insomnia in the general population –implications for the management of insomnia: the UK perspective. *Journal of Psychopharmacology* 1999; **13**(Suppl. 1): 33–34.
4. Moller HJ. Effectiveness and safety of benzodiazepines (Benzodiazepine dependence and withdrawal: myths and management). *Journal of Clinical Psychopharmacology* 1999; **19**(Suppl. 2): 25–115.
5. Nowell PD, Mazumdar S, Buysse DJ *et al*. Benzodiazepines and zolpiderm for chronic insomnia. *JAMA* 1997; **278**: 2170–2177.
6. Royal College of Psychiatrists. *Benzodiazepines: risks, benefits or dependence: a re-evaluation*. Council Report CR59. London: Royal College of Psychiatrists, 1997.
7. Sikdar S, Ruben SM. Zopiclone abuse among polydrug users. *Addiction* 1996; **91**: 285–286.
8. Genick CA, Ludolph AC. Chronic abuse of zolpiderm. *JAMA* 1994; **272**: 1721–1722.
9. Barbone F, McMahon AD, Davey PG *et al*. Association of road traffic accidents with benzodiazepine use. *Lancet* 1998; **352**: 1331–1336.
10. Lader M. Withdrawal reactions after stopping hypnotics in patients with insomnia. *CNS Drugs* 1998; **10**: 425–440.
11. Mahomed R, Paton C, Lee E. Prescribing hypnotics in a mental health trust: what consultant psychiatrists say and what they do. *Pharmaceutical Journal* 2002; **268**: 657–659.

chapter 5

Treatment of childhood mental disorders

Pharmacological treatment for children with psychiatric disorder should always be considered as just one component part of a package of psychological, social and educational interventions. Sometimes (even for some cases of drug-responsive conditions such as obsessive compulsive disorder or Tourette's disorder), a knowledge of the natural history of disorder and a suitable psychoeducational intervention can make drug therapy unnecessary.

Table Summary of child psychiatric disorders in which drug treatment is indicated

Disorder	Drugs used first-line	Drugs used second-line
Psychosis	Atypical antipsychotics (risperidone, olanzapine, amisulpride)	Typical antipsychotics (haloperidol, chlorpromazine), clozapine
Hyperkinetic disorder/ADHD	Stimulants (methylphenidate, dexamphetamine)	Atomoxetine, imipramine, clonidine
Obsessive compulsive disorder	SSRIs (sertraline, fluoxetine, paroxetine, fluvoxamine, citalopram)	Clomipramine
Tourette syndrome/ tic disorders	Risperidone, haloperidol, sulpiride, clonidine	Pimozide, SSRIs
Depression	SSRIs (sertraline, fluoxetine, paroxetine, citalopram)	TCAs (imipramine, amitriptyline, clomipramine), venlafaxine

For many of the psychological disorders of childhood (eating disorders, sleep disorders, anxiety disorders, enuresis), medication plays only a minor role because of the availability of effective psychological treatments. Increasingly, medication is being used to control certain symptoms rather than syndromal control (for example, stimulant use to control hyperactivity, impulsivity and inattention in children with autism).

Experimental studies in children are difficult both from an ethical point of view and in practical terms, and so much of the current knowledge of pharmacokinetics and pharmacodynamics has been extrapolated from adult studies. Caution is needed until appropriate efficacy and safety studies are carried out in children. For this reason, manufacturers' labelling will often say 'not recommended for children' and sometimes licences, even of valuable and well-studied drugs, do not extend to children. This is a problem for all paediatric prescribers, not only in mental health. As a result, the psychiatrist's duty to offer the most valuable treatments to patients will often entail the recommendation of medicines beyond the terms of their licence. This should always be discussed with the patient and parents. The commonly-held idea that drugs are more hazardous in young people is not necessarily true. For example, antipsychotic-induced akathisia seems to be less common in children and adolescents (while acute dystonias are probably more common).

Drug response varies with age, weight, sex, disease-state, absorption, distribution, metabolism and excretion. For many drugs, apparent bioavailability is lower in children owing to rapid metabolism and distribution in a relatively larger extracellular fluid space; on the other hand, many drugs will more readily cross the blood–brain barrier in children than in adults. Titration of dosage within an mg/kg range is therefore the rule, since strict adherence to a single dose will undertreat some children and overtreat others.

Hyperkinetic disorder and ADHD

Children who meet the ICD-10 criteria for hyperkinetic disorder (HD) should have a treatment plan that includes the reduction of hyperactive behaviour as one of the goals. This is not the only goal: it will also be important to detect and treat any coexisting disorders, to prevent the development of conduct disorder (or reduce it if it has developed), to promote academic and social learning, improve emotional adjustment and self-esteem and relieve family distress. A multi-modal treatment approach will usually be needed. Behaviour therapy on its own appears to have a low impact in HD, while stimulants induce significant improvements[1]. Stimulants should therefore be considered for children over 4 years of age after a child mental health evaluation has established the HD. Once the treatment is established, however, routine prescribing and monitoring can reasonably be carried out within primary care. Advice to family and school and behavioural management remain an integral part of management.

For children with lesser degrees of hyperactivity – i.e. those with a DSM-IV diagnosis of Attention Deficit/Hyperactivity (ADHD), falling short of the more severe condition of hyperkinetic disorder – underlying causes such as learning disabilities, hearing impairment, family stresses, attachment disruptions and emotional disorders, should be carefully sought. Specific management of the underlying cause is essential in those in whom they are detected. The majority of those with ADHD will also respond to medication but in mild cases educational intervention and psychological treatment would be sufficient.

Prescription of stimulants

Methylphenidate and dexamphetamine are the only stimulant drugs licensed in the UK for the treatment of hyperactivity. There is a large evidence base, with many controlled trials asserting their value as an effective therapy[2–4] with few hazards. Recently, the sustained-release preparation of methylphenidate (Concerta XL) has been licensed in the UK for use in children and adolescents with ADHD. This capsule delivers methylphenidate over 12 hours to mimic the thrice-daily dosing of methylphenidate[5]. This has the advantage of ease of administration, and decreases the embarrassment and stigmatisation of taking medication in school. Atomoxetine[6,7], a noradrenaline reuptake inhibitor has recently been licensed in several countries for use in ADHD in both children and adults. The use of non-licensed drugs, or polypharmacy, should be on the advice of a specialist. Both stimulants have broadly similar effects on children's behaviour: they reduce hyperactive behaviour, enhance several aspects of information processing and increase on-task attentiveness.

Initial medication should be as a trial. Placebo control is not routinely necessary but helps in problem cases. Medication should be discussed and explained with the child, parents and teachers before it is started. While medication is being started, the family will need quick and ready access to the prescriber to report progress and any adverse effects. Methylphenidate will usually be the first choice. If titration of methylphenidate (see below) does not produce a clinically satisfactory response, then dexamphetamine should be prescribed. Pemoline has been used in the past but is now withdrawn from the market because of toxicity and is available only on a named-patient basis in the UK.

The usual starting dose of methylphenidate is 5 mg (dexamphetamine 2.5 mg) twice daily, with the dose being adjusted in the light of response. It is generally accepted that a thrice-daily dosing schedule of methylphenidate is more effective. The dose may need to rise as high as 20 mg with breakfast, 20 mg in the late morning or early afternoon, and 10 mg in the late afternoon. Some children require a higher second dose because of short-term tolerance developing to the morning dose of methylphenidate. If a dose range higher than 50 mg/day is contemplated, then more intensive monitoring should be used and a specialist consulted. Psychological action has a peak in the first hour and the effect wanes rapidly, with little action after about 4 hours. Accordingly, most children will be losing the effect of a breakfast dose by midday. Subsequent doses may then have to be given at school. The practicality and ease of administration of single-dose long-acting stimulants has increased their use in clinical practice.

Monitoring

Psychological response should be monitored with rating scales of behaviours (e.g. Conners abbreviated scale) completed regularly and systematically in different settings (e.g. by parents and school). Re-evaluation at the clinic should be carried out when rating scales suggest a therapeutic response is being achieved, or if there is no response after a month of therapy. Physical monitoring should include the plotting of height and weight along standardised growth curves, and examination for the appearance of any tics. Adverse psychological effects such as lack of spontaneity, depression and excessive perseveration should be assessed specifically, with ratings, interview and observational methods. Questioning should elicit any difficulties in getting to sleep, appetite disturbance, stomach-aches, headaches and dizziness. Many of the adverse effects of stimulants are transient and decrease with time.

The long-term aim is to maintain medication until the child's maturation and learning of cognitive skills make medication unnecessary. It is increasingly being recognised that some of the children continue to have symptoms into adulthood and that treatment may be long term. Periodically, approximately annually, there should be a gradual withdrawal of medication over a period of 2 weeks to assess whether there is indeed a continuing need for medication. Drug holiday (e.g. during weekends and vacations from school) are not required routinely unless the child's growth has been affected by medication.

Non-stimulant drugs

If stimulants are ineffective despite careful dose titration, or if adverse effects make them inappropriate, or if there are relative contraindications (such as tics or mood disorders), then specialist clinical review may lead to the prescription of second-line therapies. **Atomoxetine**[6,7] may be used as a second-line treatment. **Tricyclic antidepressants** (unlicensed for ADHD) have been shown to be more effective than placebo in randomised blinded controlled trials[8]. The dose (approx. 1 mg imipramine/kg body weight) is less than that for treating depression and the onset is quicker, usually in the first 3 days of treatment. The serious hazards are for the cardiovascular system: there can be tachycardia and deterioration of the ECG even years after the start of the treatment. A few cases of sudden death, presumably due to cardiac arrhythmia, have been reported in children using desipramine. Repeated ECGs and blood estimations (monthly at the start of treatment, quarterly after 6 months) are needed with doses over 50 mg daily of imipramine. Female patients seem to reach higher blood levels with the same weight-adjusted dose than male patients, and also show more side-effects. The blood level is unpredictably increased if methylphenidate is given simultaneously, so the combination should be given, if at all, only with close monitoring of blood level and ECG. In adolescents self-injury and overdose are quite common, so special care is needed and a good relationship between physician, parents and child is required.

Clonidine (unlicensed) has some effect in reducing hyperactive behaviour, although little benefit on cognitive performance can be expected. It does not worsen tics, and may even improve them.

Low-dose risperidone[9] reduces hyperactivity through a different mechanism from the stimulants and may be effective when they fail; however, weight gain is a common hazard and should be regarded as a treatment of last resort. Evaluation of the long-term effects on the CNS, lipid profile and glycaemic control is lacking in this population. Promising drugs such as venlafaxine[10], bupropion (amfebutamone)[11] and moclobemide[12] are still under evaluation.

Stimulants in younger children and adults

In the UK methylphenidate is officially not recommended below the age of 6 years. Dexamphetamine is licensed down to the age of 3. Clinicians should diagnose and treat hyperkinetic disorders from the age of 4, but should do so with some caution, remembering the difficulties of diagnosis in this age group and the possibility that oppositional and non-compliant behaviour may be mislabelled as attention deficit.

Stimulants have been tried in adults presenting with ADHD and trial evidence gives support to their use[13]. They should only be considered when there is both a childhood history of ADHD (preferably supported by contemporary evidence such as school reports or parental recall) and the current presentation includes high levels of inattentiveness and impulsiveness. Nicotine may also be effective[14,15]. Antisocial behaviour or occupational failure may be complications of ADHD, but they are unlikely to be helped by stimulants if the core symptoms of inattentiveness and impulsiveness have disappeared.

Depression in children

Major depressive disorders in childhood should be seen as serious psychiatric conditions that may become chronic or relapsing illness. Treatment of depression includes effective resolution of the current episode and effective prophylaxis to prevent further episodes or to reduce their morbidity if they do occur. Medication should be used in conjunction with interventions designed to improve interpersonal, social and academic functioning. Cognitive behavioural therapy, interpersonal psychotherapy, counselling and other non-pharmacological approaches are all useful in this population.

The trial evidence is not conclusive[16], but suggests that SSRIs are effective in child and adolescent depression, and should generally be the first choice of drug. Commonly-used SSRIs include sertraline, fluoxetine and paroxetine, and there is accumulating experience with citalopram and fluvoxamine.

In contrast, tricyclic antidepressant drugs are probably relatively ineffective in children. Meta-analysis of the efficacy of tricyclics in the treatment of childhood depression has concluded that there is no evidence that they are more effective than placebo for the broad group of children with depression[17]. They may still be useful in individual cases that are otherwise unresponsive. There is preliminary but weak evidence for effectiveness of venlafaxine[18].

Atypical antidepressants have not been adequately evaluated in childhood and the use of all these classes of drug is essentially unguided by evidence and should be used, if at all, only with specialist monitoring.

Obsessive compulsive disorder

Clomipramine is the treatment best established by trials in children[19,20], with its serotonin reuptake inhibition apparently being an essential part of its efficacy. In practice, the SSRIs have now largely superseded clomipramine as the first line of drug treatment because of their greater safety. Medication treatment for childhood obsessive compulsive disorder (OCD) may need to be long term; remissions may be prolonged if medication is combined with cognitive behavioural therapy.

Anxiety disorders[21]

Controlled studies of TCAs for separation anxiety disorder, with or without school refusal, have produced conflicting results. Literature is starting to emerge about the use of SSRIs for children with anxiety disorders. Fluoxetine, sertraline and paroxetine may be beneficial in the treatment of anxiety disorders and selective mutism and should be considered as a second line of therapy if psychological approaches are ineffective alone. SSRIs should be initiated in small doses and gradually increased as behavioural activation can occur in children. Other drugs (including benzodiazepines, buspirone and clonidine) have been advocated but do not yet have sound support from trial evidence.

Autism and other pervasive developmental disorders

Medication plays only a small role in management, which should be based largely on psychoeducational approaches and family support. Medication should be focused on target behaviours (such as hyperactivity) rather than on the condition as a whole. Antipsychotic drugs are quite widely used in autistic spectrum disorder, in an attempt to reduce repetitive and aggressive behaviours. Risperidone[22] has recently emerged as being effective in managing aggression, hyperactivity and difficult behaviour in children with autism. Even though atypical antipsychotics are considered safer than typicals, adverse effects such as obesity (and consequent metabolic abnormalities) are sufficiently severe that long-term use should be an uncommon event, reserved for the most intractable problems, and only persisted with if there is good clinical evidence that such therapy is indeed of value in the individual case. SSRIs such as fluoxetine and sertraline have been used in autistic children and adults with encouraging improvements in repetitive and maladaptive behaviour in the short term. Preliminary evidence suggests that despite stimulants occasionally increasing obsessionality and stereotypies in this group, they help manage hyperactivity and inattention. There is some evidence that clonidine may improve hyperactivity, irritability and oppositional behaviour in children with autism.

Enuresis

Desmopressin (a synthetic analogue of antidiuretic hormone) is a reasonably effective and safe means of reducing the frequency of bedwetting at night, at least in the short term, and may be useful for enabling children to go on school trips or holidays from which they would otherwise be barred. Imipramine can also be useful for this purpose. However, the value of both is very small and temporary by comparison with the safe, cheap and permanently effective therapy of the enuresis alarm.

Schizophrenia

Schizophrenia is rare in children but incidence increases rapidly in adolescence. Early onset schizophrenia is generally considered to be a variant of the adult form of schizophrenia. Outcome is particularly poor[23]: family histories are often heavily loaded for schizophrenia and various forms of cognitive impairment are particularly common. A multidisciplinary approach to treatment is needed and should include the family, teachers, social workers, pharmacist, paediatrician and GP. Antipsychotics are an essential component of the therapy. Acute dystonic reactions, hyperprolactinaemia and weight gain are particularly prominent adverse reactions in young people. The first choice of drug treatment is controversial[24]; we recommend an atypical antipsychotic such as risperidone, amisulpride or olanzapine, combined with sedation if required for the control of the acute stage. In general, the algorithm for adults applies for young people too. Limited trial evidence suggests that clozapine is indeed effective in this group[25], and this is in some contrast to the rather poor outcome with other antipsychotics. The responsible psychiatrist may therefore consider an earlier recourse to clozapine, especially when (as is often the case) severe negative symptoms are persistent. Many young people with schizophrenia enter specialist residential schools or homes; it is then particularly easy for psychiatric oversight to be lost, so the adolescent psychiatric team should review actively and assertively.

Bipolar disorder

There is considerable controversy surrounding the diagnosis of bipolar disorder in children, not least because of difficulties associated with distinguishing between mania and hyperactivity disorders[26]. Mood stabilisers are occasionally used in children, but the evidence base is particularly limited. Lithium[26] and valproate[27], among other drugs, may be effective. Note that anticonvulsants appear to be relatively more toxic in children than in adults[28].

Table Summary of recommendations – prescribing in children

Psychotropic group	Recommended dosage ranges in children & adolescents
Drugs for treatment of hyperkinetic disorder and ADHD	Methylphenidate 0.2–0.7 mg/kg for each dose; approx. 3 doses daily Dexamphetamine 0.1–0.4 mg/kg for each dose; approx. 3 doses daily Concerta XL 18 – 54 mg/day, single dose Tricyclics (e.g. imipramine 1–2 mg/kg/day, clonidine 3–4 µg/kg/day)
Antipsychotics in schizophrenia	Amisulpride 100–400 mg/day Risperidone 2–4 mg/day Olanzapine 2.5–15 mg/day Quetiapine 100–400 mg/day Clozapine: start with 12.5 mg/day and increase up to a max. of 500 mg daily
Antipsychotics for aggression and hyperactivity	Risperidone 0.25–2.0 mg daily Amisulpride 50–300 mg daily Haloperidol* 0.02–0.08 mg/kg/day
Antidepressants	Fluoxetine 10–20 mg/day Paroxetine 10–40 mg/day Sertraline 25–100 mg/day Citalopram 10–20 mg/day
Drugs for treatment of nocturnal enuresis	Desmopressin 20–40 µg nocte intranasally Imipramine 0.5–1.0 mg/kg
Bipolar disorder/mania	Lithium 30 mg/kg/day (has short half-life in children) Valproate 500–2000 mg/day Carbamazepine 100–600 mg/day

*Note: Dystonia very common in children; consider making procyclidine available to family.

References

1. The MTA Cooperative Group. A 14-month randomized clinical trial of treatment strategies for attention-deficit/hyperactivity disorder. *Archives of General Psychiatry* 1999; 56: 1073–1086.
2. Klein RG, Abikoff H, Klass E *et al*. Clinical efficacy of methylphenidate in conduct disorder with and without attention deficit hyperactivity disorder. *Archives of General Psychiatry* 1997; 54: 1073–1180.
3. Donnelly M, Rapoport JL, Potter WZ. Fenfluramine and dextroamphetamine treatment of childhood hyperactivity. *Archives of General Psychiatry* 1989; 46: 205–212.
4. Varley CK. Effects of methylphenidate in adolescents with attention deficit disorder. *Journal of the American Academy of Child Psychiatry* 1983; 22: 351–354.
5. Pelham WE, Gnagy EM, Burrows-Maclean L *et al*. Once-a-day concerta methylphenidate versus three-times-daily methylphenidate in laboratory and natural settings. *Pediatrics* 2001; 107: 1–15.

6. Michelson D, Allen AJ, Busner J *et al*. Once-daily atomoxetine treatment for children and adolescents with attention deficit hyperactivity disorder: a randomized, placebo-controlled study. *American Journal of Psychiatry* 2002; **159**: 1896–1901.
7. Kratochvil CJ, Heiligenstein JH, Dittmann R *et al*. Atomoxetine and methylphenidate treatment in children with ADHD: a prospective, randomized, open-label trial. *Journal of the American Academy of Child & Adolescent Psychiatry* 2002; **41**: 776–784.
8. Hazell P. Tricyclic antidepressants in children: is there a rationale for use? *CNS Drugs* 1996; **5**: 233–239.
9. Findling RL, Grcevich SJ, Lopez I *et al*. Antipsychotic medications in children and adolescents. *Journal of Clinical Psychiatry* 1996; **57**(Suppl. 9): 19–23.
10. Olvera RL, Pliszka SR, Luh J *et al*. An open trial of venlafaxine in the treatment of attention-deficit/hyperactivity disorder in children and adolescents. *Journal of Child & Adolescent Psychopharmacology* 1996; **6**: 241–250.
11. Conners CK, Casat CD, Gualtieri C *et al*. Bupropion hydrochloride in attention deficit disorder with hyperactivity. *Journal of the American Academy of Child and Adolescent Psychiatry* 1996; **35**: 1314–1321.
12. Trott GE, Friese HJ, Menzel M *et al*. Use of moclobemide in children with attention deficit/hyperactivity disorder. *Psychopharmacology* 1992; **106**: 134–136.
13. Spencer T, Wilens T, Biederman J *et al*. A double blind crossover comparison of methylphenidate and placebo in adults with childhood onset attention deficit hyperactivity disorder. *Archives of General Psychiatry* 1995; **52**: 434–443.
14. Levin ED, Conners CK, Sparrow ET *et al*. Nicotine effects on adults with attention-deficit/hyperactivity disorder. *Psychopharmacology* 1996; **123**: 55–63.
15. Levin ED, Conners CK, Silva D *et al*. Transdermal nicotine effects on attention. *Psychopharmacology* 1998; **140**: 135–141.
16. Findling RL, Reed MD, Blumer JL. Pharmacological treatment of depression in children and adolescents. *Paediatric Drugs* 1999; Jul-Sep 1: 161–182.
17. Hazell P, O'Connell D, Heathcote D *et al*. Efficacy of tricyclic drugs in treating child and adolescent depression: a meta-analysis. *BMJ* 1995; **310**: 897–901.
18. Mandoki MW, Tapia MR, Tapia MA *et al*. Venlafaxine in the treatment of children and adolescents with major depression. *Psychopharmacology Bulletin* 1997; **33**: 149–154.
19. Campbell M, Cueva JE. Psychopharmacology in child and adolescent psychiatry: a review of the past seven years. Part II. *Journal of the American Academy of Child and Adolescent Psychiatry* 1995; **34**: 1262–1272.
20. Kaplan CA, Hussain S. Use of drugs in child and adolescent psychiatry. *British Journal of Psychiatry* 1995; **166**: 291–298.
21. Labellarte MJ, Ginsburg GS, Walkup JT *et al*. The treatment of anxiety disorders in children and adolescents. *Biological Psychiatry* 1999; **46**: 1567–1578.
22. Findling RL, Maxwell K, Wiznitzer M. An open clinical trial of risperidone monotherapy in young children with autistic disorder. *Psychopharmacology Bulletin* 1997; **33**: 155–159.
23. Schulz SC, Findling RL, Friedman L *et al*. Treatment and outcomes in adolescents with schizophrenia. *Journal of Clinical Psychiatry* 1998; **59**(Suppl. 1): 50–54.
24. Remschmidt H, Schulz E, Herpertz-Dahlmann B. Schizophrenic psychoses in childhood and adolescence: a guide to diagnosis and drug choice. *CNS Drugs* 1996; **6**: 100–112.
25. Kumra S, Frazier JA, Jacobsen LK *et al*. Childhood-onset schizophrenia: a double-blind clozapine-haloperidol comparison. *Archives of General Psychiatry* 1996; **53**: 1090–1097.
26. Silva RR, Matzner F, Diaz J *et al*. Bipolar disorder in children and adolescents: a guide to diagnosis and treatment. *CNS Drugs* 1996; **12**: 437–450.
27. Dineen Wagner K, Weller EB, Carlson GA *et al*. An open-label trial of divalproex in children and adolescents with bipolar disorder. *Journal of the American Academy of Child and Adolescent Psychiatry* 2002; **41**: 1224–1230.
28. Verrotti A, Trotta D, Salladini C *et al*. Anticonvulsant hypersensitivity syndrome in children: incidence, prevention and management. *CNS Drugs* 2002; **16**: 197–205.

Further reading

Martin A, Scahill L, Charney DS, Leckman J (ed). *Pediatric Psychopharmacology: Principles and practice*. Oxford: Oxford University Press, 2003.
Heyman I, Santosh PJ. Physical treatments. In: Rutter M, Taylor E (eds). *Child and Adolescent Psychiatry: Modern approaches* 4th edition. Oxford: Blackwell Scientific Publications, 2002.
Hill P, Taylor E. An auditable protocol for treating attention deficit/hyperactivity disorder. *Archives of Disease in Childhood* 2001; **84**: 404–409.
Santosh PJ, Taylor E. Stimulant drugs. *European Child & Adolescent Psychiatry* 2000; **9**(Suppl 1): 127–143.
Santosh PJ, Baird G. Psychopharmacotherapy in children and adults with intellectual disability. *Lancet* 1999; **354**: 233–242.

chapter 6

Neuropsychiatric conditions

Alcohol and substance misuse

Pharmacotherapy for alcohol withdrawal

- Alcohol withdrawal is associated with significant morbidity and mortality when improperly managed.
- All patients need general support; a proportion will need pharmacotherapy to modify the course of reversal of alcohol-induced neuro-adaptation.
- Benzodiazepines are recognised as the treatment of choice for alcohol withdrawal. They are cross-tolerant with alcohol and have anticonvulsant properties.
- Parenteral vitamin replacement is an important adjunctive treatment for the prophylaxis and/or treatment of Wernicke–Korsakoff syndrome and other vitamin-related neuropsychiatric conditions.
- The majority of patients can be detoxified in the community. However, inpatient detoxification is indicated where there is:
  - a history of delirium tremens or withdrawal seizures
  - a history of failed community detoxification
  - poor social support
  - cognitive impairment

The alcohol withdrawal syndrome

In alcohol-dependent drinkers, the central nervous system has adjusted to the constant presence of alcohol in the body. When the blood alcohol level (BAC) is suddenly lowered, the brain remains in a hyperactive and hyperexcited state, causing the withdrawal syndrome.

The alcohol withdrawal syndrome is not a uniform entity. It varies significantly in clinical manifestations and severity. Symptoms can range from mild insomnia to delirium tremens (DTs).

The first symptoms and signs occur within hours of the last drink and peak within 24–48 hours. They include restlessness, tremor, sweating, anxiety, nausea, vomiting, loss of appetite and insomnia. Tachycardia and systolic hypertension are also evident. Generalised seizures occur rarely, usually within 24 hours of cessation. In DTs there is confusion, disorientation, agitation, tachycardia and hypertension. Fever is common. Visual and auditory hallucinations and paranoid ideation are also seen.

In most patients symptoms of alcohol withdrawal are mild-to-moderate and disappear within 5–7 days after the last drink. In more severe cases (approx. 5% of cases), DTs may develop.

Risk factors for DTs and seizures
- Severe alcohol dependence
- Past experience of DTs
- Long-standing history of alcohol dependence with previous episodes of inpatient treatment
- Older age
- Concomitant acute illness
- Severe withdrawal symptoms when presenting for treatment

Alcohol withdrawal assessment

1. History (including history of previous episodes of alcohol withdrawal)
2. Physical examination
3. Time of most recent drink
4. Concomitant drug intake
5. Severity of withdrawal symptoms
6. Co-existing medical/psychiatric disorders
7. Laboratory investigations: BAC, FBC, U&E, LFTs, INR, urinary drug screen

Withdrawal scales can be helpful. They can be used as a baseline against which withdrawal severity can be measured over time. Use of these scales can minimise over- and under-dosing with benzodiazepines.

The Clinical Institute Withdrawal Assessment for Alcohol-Revised version (CIWA-Ar) is a 10-item scale that can be used to monitor the clinical course of alcohol withdrawal. (Items 1–9 are scored from 0–7 and item 10 from 0–4; maximum possible score of 67).

1. Nausea and vomiting
2. Tremor
3. Paroxysmal sweats
4. Anxiety
5. Agitation

6. Tactile disturbances
7. Auditory disturbances
8. Visual disturbances
9. Headache and fullness in head
10. Orientation and clouding of sensorium

Severity of alcohol withdrawal	CIWA-Ar score
Mild	<10
Moderate	10–20
Severe	20+

Use of chlordiazepoxide

Outpatient/community detoxification

Mild dependence usually requires very small doses of chlordiazepoxide or else may be managed without medication.

Moderate dependence requires a larger dose of chlordiazepoxide. A typical regime might be 10–20 mg qds, reducing gradually over 5 days. Note that 5–7 days' treatment is adequate *and longer treatment is rarely helpful or necessary.*

Example – moderate dependence

Day 1	20 mg qds
Day 2	15 mg qds
Day 3	10 mg qds
Day 4	5 mg qds
Day 5	5 mg bd

Severe dependence requires even larger doses of chlordiazepoxide and will often require specialist/in-patient treatment. Daily monitoring is advised for the first 2–3 days, especially for severe dependence (see below). This may require special arrangements over a weekend. Prescribing should not start if the patient is heavily intoxicated, and in such circumstances they should be advised to return in a sober state at an early opportunity.

Inpatient protocol
The approach advocated here is to prescribe chlordiazepoxide according to a flexible regimen over the first 24 hours, with dosage titrated against the rated severity of withdrawal symptoms. This is followed by a fixed 5-day reducing regimen, based upon the dosage requirement estimated during the first 24 hours.

Occasionally (e.g. in DTs) the flexible regime may need to be prolonged beyond the first 24 hours. However, rarely (if ever) is it necessary to resort to the use of other drugs, such as antipsychotics (associated with reduced seizure threshold) or intravenous diazepam (associated with risk of over-dose).

The intention of the flexible protocol for the first 24 hours is to titrate dosage of chlordiazepoxide against severity of alcohol withdrawal symptoms. It is necessary to avoid either under-treatment (associated with patient discomfort and a higher incidence of complications such as seizures or DTs), or over-treatment (associated with excessive sedation and risk of toxicity/interaction with alcohol consumed prior to admission).

In the inpatient setting it is possible to be more responsive, with constant monitoring of the severity of withdrawal symptoms, linked to the administered dose of chlordiazepoxide.

Prescribing in alcohol withdrawal

First 24 hours (day 1)
On admission, the patient should be assessed by a doctor and prescribed chlordiazepoxide. (Diazepam is used in some centres and may be used for those with a history of sensitivity to chlordiazepoxide although some metabolites are shared.) Three doses of chlordiazepoxide must be specified:

FIRST DOSE (STAT)
This is the first dose of chlordiazepoxide which will be administered by ward staff immediately following admission, as a fixed 'stat' dose. It should be estimated upon:

- Clinical signs and symptoms of withdrawal (see below);

- Breath alcohol concentration on admission and 1 hour later.

The dose prescribed should usually be within the range of 5–50 mg. However, if withdrawal symptoms on admission are mild, or if the breath alcohol is very high, or rising, the initial dose may be 0 mg (i.e. nothing). It is the relative fall in blood alcohol concentration that determines the need for medication not the absolute figure (hence the need to take 2 Alcometer readings at an interval soon after admission). Caution is needed if a patient shows a high Alcometer level.

INCREMENTAL DOSE (RANGE)
This is the range within which subsequent doses of chlordiazepoxide should be administered during the first 24 hours (see below). A dose of 5–40 mg will cover almost all circumstances.

MAXIMUM DOSE IN 24 HOURS

This is the maximum cumulative dose that may be given during the first 24 hours. It may be estimated according to clinical judgement, but **250 mg should really be adequate for most cases.** Doses above 250 mg should not be prescribed without prior discussion with a consultant or specialist registrar.

The cumulative chlordiazepoxide dose administered during the initial 24-hour period assessment is called the *baseline dose*, and this is used to calculate the subsequent reducing regime.

Days 2–5

After the initial 24-hour assessment period a standardised reducing regime is used. Chlordiazepoxide is given in divided doses, 4 times daily. The afternoon and evening doses can be proportionately higher in order to provide night sedation (but note that the effect of chlordiazepoxide and its metabolites is long-lived). The dose should be reduced each day by approximately 20% of the baseline dose, so that no chlordiazepoxide is given on day 6. **However, a longer regime may be required in the case of patients who have DTs or a history of DTs. This should be discussed with a specialist registrar or consultant, and the dose tailored according to clinical need.**

Note
Chlordiazepoxide should not routinely be prescribed on a PRN basis after the initial assessment is complete. Patients exhibiting significant further symptoms may have psychiatric (or other) complications and should be seen by the ward or duty doctor.

Observations and administration

After chlordiazepoxide has been prescribed as above, the first 'stat' dose is given immediately. Subsequent doses during the first 24 hours are administered with a frequency and dosage that depend upon the observations of alcohol withdrawal status rated by the ward staff.

OBSERVATIONS

Each set of observations consist of:
- applying an alcohol withdrawal scale (e.g. CIWA-Ar) and/or clinical observations
- taking BP
- taking pulse
- Alcometer (first and second observations only).

Observations should be recorded:
- during the admission procedure, immediately after the patient has arrived on the ward;
- throughout the first 24-hours, at a frequency depending upon:
  – severity of withdrawal
  – whether or not chlordiazepoxide has been administered
- twice daily from days 2–6.

If a patient is asleep (and this is not due to intoxication), they should not be woken up for observations. However, it should be recorded that they were asleep.

During the first 24 hours chlordiazepoxide should be administered when withdrawal symptoms are considered significant (usually a CIWA-Ar score >15). If a patient suffers hallucinations or agitation, an increased dose should be administered, according to clinical judgement.

179

Table Alcohol withdrawal treatment interventions

Severity	Supportive care	Medical care	Pharmacotherapy for neuro-adaptation reversal	Setting
Mild CIWA-Ar <10	Moderate-to-high level required	Little required	Little to none required – maybe symptomatic treatment only (e.g. paracetamol)	Home
Moderate CIWA-Ar 10–20	Moderate-to-high level required	Little required	Little to none required – maybe symptomatic treatment only	Home or community
Severe CIWA-Ar >20	High level required	Medical monitoring	Usually required – probably symptomatic and substitution treatment (e.g. chlordiazepoxide)	Community or hospital
Complicated CIWA-Ar >10 plus medical problems	High level required	Specialist medical care required	Substitution and symptomatic treatments probably required	Hospital

Example of a chlordiazepoxide regimen – severe dependence

		Total (mg)
Day 1 (first 24 hours)	40 mg qds + 40 mg PRN	200
Day 2	40 mg qds	160
Day 3	30 mg tds and 40 mg nocte (or 30 mg qds)	120–130
Day 4	30 mg bd and 20 mg bd (or 25 mg qds)	100
Day 5	20 mg qds	80
Day 6	20 mg bd and 10 mg bd	60
Day 7	10 mg qds	40
Day 8	10 mg tds or 10 mg bd and 5 mg bd	30
Day 9	10 mg bd (or 5 mg qds)	20
Day 10	10 mg nocte	10

Vitamin supplementation

Parenteral vitamin supplements should be prescribed prophylactically for *all* inpatient detoxifications. There is considerable doubt about the usefulness of oral replacement.

Parenteral vitamin supplements should only be administered where suitable resuscitation facilities are available. The intramuscular route is usually used. Intravenous administration should be by dilution in 50–100 ml normal saline and infused over 15–30 minutes. This allows immediate discontinuation should anaphylaxis occur. Anaphylaxis is extremely rare after IM administration and this is the preferred route in most centres.

The classical triad of ophthalmoplegia, ataxia and confusion is rarely present in Wernicke's encephalopathy, and the syndrome is much more common than is widely believed. A presumptive diagnosis of Wernicke's encephalopathy should therefore be made in any patient undergoing detoxification who experiences any of the following signs:

- Ataxia
- Ophthalmoplegia/nystagmus
- Hypothermia & hypotension
- Memory disturbance
- Confusion
- Coma/unconsciousness

Parenteral B-complex must be administered before glucose is administered in all patients presenting with altered mental status.

Prophylactic treatment for Wernicke's encephalopathy should be:

1 pair IM/IV ampoules high potency B-complex vitamins (Pabrinex) daily for 3–5 days. (*Or:* thiamine 200–300 mg IM daily, if Pabrinex unavailable)

Note: All patients should receive this regime as an absolute minimum.

Therapeutic treatment of Wernicke's encephalopathy should be:

At least 2 pairs IM/IV ampoules high potency B-complex vitamins daily for 2 days.
- If no response, then discontinue treatment.
- If signs/symptoms respond, continue 1 pair ampoules daily for 5 days or for as long as improvement continues.

For outpatient detoxification, the options available are:
- No vitamin supplementation (not recommended).
- Oral vitamin supplementation with Vitamin B Compound Strong, one tablet 3 times daily (but this is unlikely to be absorbed effectively and is therefore of little or no benefit to alcohol-dependent patients).
- Parenteral supplementation, as above, in a clinical setting where appropriate resuscitation facilities are available.

Seizure prophylaxis

There is no clear consensus on seizure prophylaxis. Most clinicians prefer to use diazepam for medically-assisted withdrawal in those with a previous history of seizures. Some units advocate carbamazepine loading in patients with untreated epilepsy; those with a history of more than 2 seizures during previous withdrawal episodes; or previous seizures despite adequate diazepam loading. Phenytoin does not prevent alcohol-withdrawal seizures and is therefore not indicated.

Those who have a seizure for the first time should be investigated to rule out an organic disease or structural lesion.

Liver disease

For individuals with impaired liver functioning, oxazepam (a short-acting benzodiazepine) may be preferred to chlordiazepoxide, in order to avoid excessive build up of metabolites and over-sedation.

Hallucinations

Mild perceptual disturbances usually respond to chlordiazepoxide. However, hallucinations should be treated with oral haloperidol. Haloperidol may also be given intramuscularly or (very rarely) intravenously if necessary (but BP should be monitored for hypotension). Caution is needed because haloperidol can reduce seizure threshold. Have parenteral procyclidine available in case of dystonic reactions.

Symptomatic pharmacotherapy

Dehydration:	Ensure adequate fluid intake in order to maintain hydration and electrolyte balance. Dehydration can lead to cardiac arrythmia and death.
Pain:	Paracetamol.
Nausea & vomiting:	Metoclopramide (Maxolon) 10 mg or prochlorperazine (Stemetil) 5 mg 4–6 hourly.
Diarrhoea:	Diphenoxylate and atropine (Lomotil). Loperamide (Imodium).
Hepatic encephalopathy:	Lactulose.

Further reading

Claassen CA, Adinoff B. Alcohol withdrawal syndrome: guidelines for management. *CNS Drugs* 1999; **12**: 279–291.
Duncan D, Taylor D. Chlormethiazole or chlordiazepoxide in alcohol detoxification. *Psychiatric Bulletin* 1996; **20**: 599–601.
Mayo-smith MF. Pharmacological management of alcohol withdrawal. *JAMA* 1997; **278**: 144–151.

Prescribing for opioid dependence

> *Note:* treatment of opioid dependence usually requires specialist intervention – generalists should always contact substance misuse services (where available) before attempting to treat opioid dependence.

Treatment aims

- To reduce or prevent withdrawal symptoms
- To reduce or eliminate non-prescribed drug use
- To stabilise drug intake and lifestyle
- To reduce drug-related harm (particularly injecting behaviour)
- To help maintain contact and provide an opportunity to work with the patient

Treatment
This will depend upon:

- what is available;
- patient's previous history of drug use and treatment;
- patient's current drug use and circumstances.

Evidence of opioid dependence
Patient's self-reporting of opioid dependence must be confirmed by positive urine results for opioids, and objective signs of withdrawal or general restlessness should be present before considering prescribing any substitute pharmacotherapy. Recent sites of injection may also be present.

Table Objective opioid withdrawal scales			
Symptoms	*Absent/normal*	*Mild-moderate*	*Severe*
Lactorrhoea	Absent	Eyes watery	Eyes streaming/wiping eyes
Rhinorrhoea	Absent	Sniffing	Profuse secretion (wiping nose)
Agitation	Absent	Fidgeting	Can't remain seated
Perspiration	Absent	Clammy skin	Beads of sweat
Piloerection	Absent	Barely palpable hairs standing up	Readily palpable, visible
Pulse rate (BPM)	<80	>80 but <100	>100
Vomiting	Absent	Absent	Present
Shivering	Absent	Absent	Present
Yawning /10 min	<3	3–5	6 or more
Dilated pupils	Normal <4 mm	Dilated 4–6 mm	Widely dilated >6 mm

Subjective opioid withdrawal symptoms can include: nausea; stomach cramps; muscular tension; muscle spasms/twitching; aches and pains; insomnia.

> *Note:* Untreated heroin withdrawal symptoms typically reach their peak 32–36 hours after the last dose and symptoms will have subsided substantially after 5 days. Untreated methadone withdrawal typically reaches its peak between 4–6 days and symptoms do not substantially subside for 10–12 days.[1]

Induction and stabilisation of substitute prescribing

It is usually preferable to use a longer-acting opioid agonist or partial agonist (e.g. methadone or buprenorphine respectively) in opiate dependence, as it is generally easier to maintain stability[1]. However, patients with a less severe opioid dependency (e.g. history of using codeine or dihydrocodeine-containing preparations only) may in some cases be better managed by maintaining/detoxifying them using that preparation or an equivalent.

Choosing between buprenorphine and methadone for substitute treatment

Current evidence has not identified particular groups of patients who routinely do better on buprenorphine or methadone. Hence the decision should be made after discussion with the patient and taking the following into consideration:

- Buprenorphine appears to have a milder withdrawal syndrome than methadone and therefore may be preferred for detoxification programs[2,3].

- Side-effects: differences in side-effect profiles (e.g. buprenorphine is often described as less sedating) may affect patient preference.

- Buprenorphine appears to provide greater 'blockade' effects than doses of methadone <60 mg[4–7]. This may be considered an advantage or disadvantage by patients. In particular, patients with chronic pain conditions that frequently require additional opioid analgesia may have difficulties being treated with buprenorphine.

- Women who are pregnant or planning a pregnancy should consider methadone treatment, as the safety of buprenorphine in pregnancy has not been demonstrated.

- Methadone clients unable to reduce to doses of methadone <60 mg without becoming 'unstable' cannot easily be transferred to buprenorphine.

- Patients with a history of diversion of medication may be better served with methadone treatment, which has the capacity for daily supervised administration. Sublingual buprenorphine tablets can be more easily diverted with the risk of injecting tablets.

Methadone

Methadone is a controlled drug with a high dependency potential and a low lethal dose. The initial 2 weeks of treatment with methadone are associated with a substantially increased risk of overdose mortality[1,8–11]. It is important that appropriate assessment, titration of doses and monitoring is performed during this period.

Prescribing should only commence if:

- opioid drugs are being taken on a regular basis (typically daily);

- there is convincing evidence of dependence (see above);

- consumption of methadone can be supervised, especially for the initial doses.

Supervised daily consumption is recommended for new prescriptions, for a minimum of 3 months, if possible[1]. Alternatively, instalment prescriptions for daily dispensing and collection should be used. Certainly no more than 1 week's supply should be dispensed at one time, except in very exceptional circumstances[1].

Methadone should be prescribed in the oral liquid formulation (mixture or linctus). Tablets are likely to be crushed and inappropriately injected and therefore should not be prescribed[1,12].

Important: All patients starting a methadone treatment programme must be informed of the risks of toxicity and overdose, and the necessity for safe storage[1,10,11,13].

DOSE

For patients who are *currently prescribed* methadone and if *all* the criteria listed below are met, then it is safe to prescribe the same dose:

- Dose confirmed by prescriber

- Last consumption confirmed (e.g. pharmacy contacted) and is within last 3 days

- Prescriber has stopped prescribing and current prescription is completed or cancelled to date

- Patient is comfortable on dose (no signs of intoxication/withdrawal)

- No other contraindications or cautions are present

Otherwise the following recommendations should be followed.

STARTING DOSE

Consideration must be given to the potential for opioid toxicity, taking into account:

- Tolerance to opioids can be affected by a number of factors and it obviously significantly influences an individual's risk of toxicity[14]. Tolerance should be assessed on the history of quantity, frequency and route of administration (be aware of the likelihood of over-reporting). A person's tolerance to methadone can be significantly reduced within three to four days of not using, caution must be exercised when re-instating their dose.

- Use of other drugs, particularly depressants (e.g. alcohol and benzodiazepines).

- Long half-life of methadone, as cumulative toxicity may develop.[15,16]

Inappropriate dosing can result in potentially fatal overdose, particularly in the first few days[8-11]. Deaths have occurred following the commencement of a daily dose of 40 mg methadone[1]. It is safer to keep to a low dose that can subsequently be increased at intervals if this dose later proves to be insufficient.

Note: Opioid withdrawal is *not* a life-threatening condition. Opioid toxicity is.

Direct conversion tables for opioids and methadone should be viewed cautiously, as there are a number of factors influencing the values at any given time. It is much safer to titrate the dose against presenting withdrawal symptoms.

The **initial total** daily dose for most cases will be in the range of 10–40 mg methadone, depending on the level of tolerance (low: 10–20 mg, moderate: 25–40 mg). Starting doses >30 mg should be prescribed with caution because of the risk of overdose. It is safer to use a starting dose of 10–20 mg and reassess the patient after a period of 2–4 hours. Further incremental doses of 5–10 mg can be given, depending on the severity of the withdrawal symptoms. *Note:* onset of action should be evident within half an hour, with peak plasma levels being achieved after approximately four hours of dosing.

Heavily dependent users with high tolerance may require larger doses. A starting dose, not exceeding 30 mg can be given, followed by a second dose after a minimum interval of 2–4 hours. The second dose can be up to 30 mg, depending on the persisting severity of withdrawal symptoms. High doses should only be prescribed by experienced medical practitioners.

Table Methadone dose after initial dose	
Severity of withdrawal after initial dose	*Additional dosage*
Mild	Nil
Moderate (muscle aches & pains, pupil dilation, nausea, yawning, clammy skin)	5–10 mg
Severe (vomiting, profuse sweating, piloerection, tachycardia, elevated BP)	20–30 mg

STABILISATION DOSE
- First week
  Outpatients should attend daily for the first few days to enable assessment by the prescriber and any dose titration against withdrawal symptoms. Dose increases should not exceed 5–10 mg a day and 30 mg a week above the initial starting dose. Note that steady state plasma levels are only achieved approximately five days after the last dose increase. Once the patient has been stabilised on an adequate dose, methadone should be prescribed as a single daily dose. It should not be prescribed on a PRN basis.

- Subsequent period
  Subsequent increases should not exceed 10 mg per week, up to a total daily dose of 60–120 mg. Stabilisation is usually achieved within six weeks but may take longer.

CAUTIONS
- **Intoxication.** Methadone should not be given to any patient showing signs of intoxication, especially due to alcohol or other depressant drugs (e.g. benzodiazepines)[14,17]. Risk of fatal overdose is greatly enhanced when methadone is taken concomitantly with alcohol and other respiratory depressant drugs. Concurrent alcohol and illicit drug consumption must be borne in mind when considering subsequent prescribing of methadone due to the increased risk of overdose associated with polysubstance misuse[8,11,17,18]

- **Severe hepatic/renal dysfunction.** Metabolism and elimination of methadone may be affected in which case the dose or dosing interval should be adjusted accordingly against clinical presentation. Because of extended plasma half-life, the interval between assessments during initial dosing may need to be extended.

OVERDOSE
In the event of methadone overdose, naloxone should be administered following BNF guidelines.

Dose: by intravenous injection, 0.8–2 mg repeated at intervals of 2–3 minutes to a max. 10 mg if respiratory function does not improve.

By subcutaneous or intramuscular injection: as intravenous injection but only if intravenous route not feasible (onset of action slower).

By continuous intravenous infusion, 2 mg diluted in 500 ml intravenous infusion solution at a rate adjusted according to response.

> ## Always Call Emergency Services

Pregnancy & breastfeeding
There is no evidence of an increase in congenital defect with methadone, however, the newborn may suffer withdrawal syndrome[19]. It is important to prevent the patient going into a withdrawal state, since this is dangerous for both mother and foetus. Specialist advice should be obtained before prescribing or detoxing, particularly with regards to management and treatment plan during pregnancy.

Methadone is considered compatible with breastfeeding, with no adverse effects to nursing infant when mother is consuming 20 mg/24 hours or less[19].

Analgesia for methadone-prescribed patients
Non-opioid analgesics should be used in preference (e.g. paracetamol, NSAIDs).

If opioid analgesia is indicated (e.g. codeine, dihydrocodeine, MST), then this should be titrated accordingly against pain relief, with the methadone dose remaining constant to alleviate withdrawal symptoms. Avoid titrating the methadone dose to provide analgesia.

Buprenorphine (Subutex®)

Buprenorphine is a synthetic opioid. It is a partial opioid agonist with low intrinsic activity and high affinity at μ opioid receptors. It is effective in treating opioid dependence because:

- it alleviates/prevents opioid withdrawal and craving;
- it reduces the effects of additional opioid use because of its high receptor affinity[4-6];
- it is long-acting allowing daily (or less) dosing. The duration of action is related to the buprenorphine dose administered: low doses (e.g. 2 mg) exert effects for up to 12 hours; higher doses (e.g. 16–32 mg) exert effects for as long as 48–72 hours.

STARTING DOSE
The same principles for methadone apply when starting treatment with buprenorphine. However, of particular interest with buprenorphine is the phenomenon of precipitated withdrawal. Patient education is an important factor in reducing the problems during induction.

INDUCTING HEROIN USERS
The first dose of buprenorphine should be administered when the patient is experiencing opioid withdrawal symptoms to reduce the risk of precipitated withdrawal. The initial dose recommendations are as follows:

Patient in withdrawal and no risk factors	8 mg buprenorphine
Patient not experiencing withdrawal and no risk factors	4 mg buprenorphine
Patient has concomitant risk factors (e.g. medical condition, polydrug misuse, low or uncertain severity of dependence)	2–4 mg buprenorphine

Transferring from methadone

Patients transferring from methadone are at risk of experiencing precipitated withdrawal symptoms that may continue at a milder level for 1–2 weeks. Factors affecting precipitated withdrawal are listed in the table below.

Table Factors affecting risk of precipitated withdrawal with buprenorphine

Factor	Discussion	Recommended strategy
Dose of methadone	More likely with doses of methadone above 30 mg. Generally – the higher the dose the more severe the precipitate withdrawal[20]	Attempt transfer from doses of methadone <40 mg. Transfer from >60 mg should not be attempted
Time between last methadone dose and first buprenorphine dose	Interval should be at least 24 hours. Increasing the interval reduces the incidence and severity of withdrawal[21,22]	Cease methadone and delay first dose until patient experiencing withdrawal from methadone
Dose of buprenorphine	Very low doses of buprenorphine (e.g. 2 mg) are generally inadequate to substitute for methadone. High first doses of buprenorphine (e.g. 8 mg) are more likely to precipitate withdrawal	First dose should generally be 4 mg; review patient 2–3 hours later
Patient expectancy	Patients not prepared for precipitated withdrawal are more likely to become distressed and confused by the effect	Inform patients in advance. Have contingency plan for severe symptoms
Use of other medications	Symptomatic medication (e.g. lofexidine) can be useful to relieve symptoms	Prescribe in accordance to management plan

Transferring from methadone dose <40 mg

Methadone should be ceased abruptly, and the first dose of buprenorphine given at least 24 hours after the last methadone dose. The following conversion rates are recommended:

Last methadone dose	Initial buprenorphine dose	Day 2 buprenorphine dose
20–40 mg	4 mg	6–8 mg
10–20 mg	4 mg	4–8 mg
1–10 mg	4 mg	4 mg

Transferring from methadone dose 40–60 mg

- The methadone dose should be reduced as far as possible without the patient becoming unstable or chaotic, and then abruptly stopped.

- The first buprenorphine dose should be delayed until the patient displays clear signs of withdrawal, generally 48–96 hours after the last dose of methadone. Symptomatic medication (lofexidine) may be useful to provide transitory relief.

- An initial dose of 4 mg should be given. The patient should then be reviewed 2–3 hours later.

- If withdrawal has been precipitated further symptomatic medication can be prescribed.

- If there has been no precipitation or worsening of withdrawal, an additional 2–4 mg of buprenorphine can be dispensed on the same day.

- The patient should be reviewed the following day at which point the dose should be increased to between 8–12 mg.

Transferring from methadone doses >60 mg

Such transfers should not be attempted in an outpatient setting. Consider referral to inpatient unit if required.

Transferring from other prescribed opioids

There is little experience in transferring patients from other prescribed opioids (e.g. codeine, dihydrocodeine, morphine). Basic principles suggest that transferring from opioids with short half-lives should be similar to inducting heroin users; whereas transferring from opioids with longer half-lives will be similar to transferring from methadone.

Stabilisation dose of buprenorphine

Outpatients should attend regularly for the first few days to enable assessment by the prescriber and any dose titration. Dose increases should be made in increments of 2–4 mg at a time, daily if necessary, up to a maximum daily dose of 32 mg. Effective maintenance doses are usually in the range of 12–24 mg daily[23] 24 and patients should generally be able to achieve maintenance levels within 1–2 weeks of starting buprenorphine.

LESS THAN DAILY DOSING

Buprenorphine is registered in the UK as a medication to be taken daily. International evidence and experience indicates that many clients can be comfortably maintained on one dose every 2–3 days[25–28]. This may be pertinent for patients in buprenorphine treatment who are considered unsuitable for take-away medication because of the risk of diversion. The following conversion rate is recommended:

2-day buprenorphine dose = 2 x daily dose of buprenorphine (to a max. 32 mg)
3-day buprenorphine dose = 3 x daily dose of buprenorphine (to a max. 32 mg)

Note: In the event of patients being unable to stabilise comfortably on buprenorphine (often those transferring from methadone), the option of transferring to methadone should be available. Methadone can be commenced 24 hours after the last buprenorphine dose. Doses should be titrated according to clinical response, being mindful of the residual 'blockade' effect of buprenorphine which may last for several days.

Cautions with buprenorphine

- **Liver function:** There is some evidence suggesting that high dose buprenorphine can cause changes in liver function in individuals with a history of liver disease[29]. Such patients should have LFTs measured before commencing with follow-up investigations conducted 6–12 weeks after commencing buprenorphine. More frequent testing should be considered in patients of particular concern e.g. severe liver disease or those at risk of injecting the tablets.
- **Intoxication:** Buprenorphine should not be given to any patient showing signs of intoxication, especially due to alcohol or other depressant drugs (e.g. benzodiazepines). Buprenorphine in combination with other sedative drugs can result in respiratory depression, sedation, coma and death. Concurrent alcohol and illicit drug consumption must be borne in mind when considering subsequent prescribing of buprenorphine due to the increased risk of overdose associated with polysubstance misuse.

Overdose with buprenorphine
Buprenorphine as a single drug in overdose is generally regarded as safer than methadone and heroin because it causes less respiratory depression. However, in combination with other respiratory depressant drugs the effects may be harder to manage. Very high doses of naloxone (e.g. 10–15 mg) are needed to reverse buprenorphine effects, hence ventilator support is often required in cases where buprenorphine is contributing to respiratory depression (e.g. in polydrug overdose).

Always Call Emergency Services

Pregnancy and breastfeeding
Currently there is insufficient evidence regarding the use of buprenorphine as an opioid substitute treatment during pregnancy or breastfeeding to be able to define its safety profile[19]. More evidence is available on the safety of methadone, which for that reason makes it the preferred choice. Further evaluation and consideration would have to be made for individual cases.

Analgesia for buprenorphine-prescribed patients
Non-opioid analgesics should be used in preference (e.g. paracetamol, NSAIDs).

Buprenorphine reduces or blocks the effect of full agonist opioids therefore complicating their use as analgesics in patients on buprenorphine. If adequate pain control cannot be achieved then it may be necessary to transfer the patient to a stable methadone dose so that an opioid analgesic can be effectively used for pain control (see note on analgesia for methadone prescribed patients).

Opiate detoxification and reduction regimes

COMMUNITY SETTING

- **Methadone**
  Following a period of stabilisation with methadone, a contract should be negotiated between the patient and prescriber to reduce the daily methadone dose by 5–10 mg weekly or fortnightly. However, this should be reviewed regularly and remain flexible to adjustments and changes in the patient's readiness for total abstinence. Factors such as an increase in heroin or other drug use, worsening of the patient's physical, psychological or social well-being, may warrant a temporary increase, stabilisation or slowing-down of the reduction rate.

- **Buprenorphine**
  The same principles for methadone apply when planning a buprenorphine detoxification regime. Dose reduction should be gradual to minimise withdrawal discomfort. Suggested reduction regime:

Daily buprenorphine dose	Reduction rate
Above 16 mg	4 mg every 1–2 weeks
8–16 mg	2–4 mg every 1–2 weeks
2–8 mg	2 mg per week or fortnight
Below 2 mg	Reduce by 0.4–0.8 mg per week

- **Lofexidine**
  Lofexidine is licensed for the management of symptoms of opioid withdrawal. It is non-opioid and therefore less liable to misuse and diversion. Its use in community detoxification is more likely to be successful for patients with an average daily heroin use of up to $\frac{1}{2}$ g (or 30 mg methadone equivalent), for non-polydrug users and for those with shorter drug and treatment histories, or for those at an end stage of methadone detoxification (patients taking not more than 20 mg daily).
  - *Precautions:* severe coronary insufficiency, recent MI, bradycardia, cerebrovascular disease, chronic renal failure, pregnancy and breastfeeding.
  - *Interactions:* alcohol and other CNS depressants – lofexidine may enhance the effects. Tricyclic antidepressants – concomitant use may reduce the efficacy of lofexidine.
  - *Side-effects:* drowsiness, dryness of mouth, throat and nose, hypotension, bradycardia and rebound hypertension on withdrawal.
  Before commencing treatment with lofexidine, baseline blood pressure should be measured and monitored over the first few days. If there is a significant drop in BP (systolic less than 90 mmHg or 30 mmHg below baseline), or pulse is below 55, lofexidine should be withheld. Treatment should be reviewed with the option to either continue at a reduced dose or discontinue.
  - *Dose:* Initially, 0.4–0.6 mg twice daily, increased as necessary, to control withdrawal symptoms, in steps of 0.2–0.4 mg daily, to a maximum total daily dose of 2.4mg . The total daily dose should be given in 2–4 divided doses, with one dose at bedtime to offset insomnia associated with opioid withdrawal. Treatment course should be 7–10 days, followed by a gradual withdrawal over 2–4 days.
  Low, reducing doses of methadone (e.g. 15 mg/10 mg/5 mg daily) may be given over the initial days of treatment with lofexidine as a cross-over period, to minimise withdrawal symptoms. This is only appropriate for patients currently taking methadone before detoxification.
  Additional short-term medication may be required for nausea, stomach cramps, diarrhoea and insomnia.

- **Methadone**
  Patients should have a starting dose assessment of methadone, over 48 hours following the same guidelines listed above. The dose may then be reduced following a linear regime over 10 days.
- **Buprenorphine**
  Buprenorphine can be used effectively for short-term inpatient detoxifications following the same principles as for methadone.
- **Lofexidine** *(see community detoxification regimes above for more information)*
  Higher doses of lofexidine (up to the maximum daily dose of 2.4 mg) may be given initially, particularly for patients with an average daily heroin use over $\frac{1}{2}$ g (or 30 mg methadone equivalent). This is provided there is an adequate monitoring of BP, pulse and adverse effects, and appropriate action can be taken in any such event. If there is a significant drop in BP or pulse, (systolic less than 90 mmHg or 30 mmHg below baseline, or pulse is below 55) lofexidine should be withheld until normal measurements are obtained and then re-introduced cautiously at a lower dose. In certain cases lofexidine may need to be discontinued and alternative detoxification treatment regimes considered.

  The total daily dose should be given in four divided doses over the first 2–3 days with the full treatment course continuing for 7–10 days. This should then be followed by a gradual withdrawal over 2–4 days.

  Additional short-term medication may be required for nausea, stomach cramps, diarrhoea and insomnia.

Relapse prevention – naltrexone

Evidence for the effectiveness of naltrexone as a treatment for relapse prevention in opioid misusers is inconclusive[30]. Combined use of naltrexone and psychosocial therapy has proved to be more effective than either therapy alone in improving post treatment outcomes[31]. Naltrexone should be available as a treatment option to those who can benefit, due to the importance of avoiding relapse.

INITIATING TREATMENT

Naltrexone has the propensity to cause a severe withdrawal reaction in patients who are either currently taking opioid drugs or who were previously taking opioid drugs and have not allowed a sufficient wash-out period prior to administering naltrexone.

The minimum recommended interval between stopping the opioid and starting naltrexone depends on the opioid used, duration of use and the amount taken as a last dose. Opioid agonists with long half-lives such as methadone and will require a wash-out period of up to 10 days, whereas shorter acting opioids such as heroin may only require up to 7 days.

Experience with buprenorphine indicates that a wash-out period of up to 7 days is sufficient (final buprenorphine dose >2 mg; duration of use >2 weeks) and in some cases naltrexone may be started within 2–3 days of a patient stopping (final buprenorphine dose <2 mg; duration of use <2 weeks).

A test dose of naloxone (0.2–0.8 mg), which has a much shorter half-life than naltrexone, may be given to the patient prior to starting naltrexone treatment. Any withdrawal symptoms precipitated will be of shorter duration than if precipitated by naltrexone.

Patients *must* be advised of the risk of withdrawal prior to giving the dose. It is worth thoroughly questioning the patient as to whether they have taken any opioid containing preparation unknowingly (e.g. over-the-counter analgesic).

> Patients must also be warned of the risk of acute opioid toxicity occurring in an attempt to overcome the blockade effect of naltrexone. Changes in the individual's opioid tolerance level are likely to be very significant particularly following a detoxification program and any period of abstinence.

Dose of naltrexone

An initial dose of 25 mg naltrexone should be administered after a suitable opioid free interval (and naloxone challenge if appropriate). The patient should be monitored for 4 hours after the first dose for symptoms of opioid withdrawal. Symptomatic medication for withdrawal (lofexidine) should be available for use on the first day of naltrexone dosing (withdrawal symptoms may last up to 4–8 hours). Once the patient has tolerated this low naltrexone dose, subsequent doses can be increased to 50 mg daily as a maintenance dose.

References

1. Department of Health, The Scottish Office Department of Health, Welsh Office, Department of Health and Social Services, Northern Ireland. Drug misuse and dependence – guidelines on clinical management, 1999.
2. Seifert J, Metzner C, Paetzold W *et al.* Detoxification of opiate addicts with multiple drug abuse: a comparison of buprenorphine vs. methadone. *Pharmacopsychiatry* 2002; **35**: 159–164.
3. Jasinski DR, Pevnick JS, Griffiths JD. "Human pharmacology and abuse potential of the analgesic buprenorphine: a potential agent for treating narcotic addiction." *Archives of General Psychiatry* 1978; **35**: 501–16.
4. Bickel WK, Stitze ML *et al.* Buprenorphine: dose-related blockade of opioid challenge effects in opioid dependent humans. *Journal of Pharmacology & Experimental Therapeutics* 1988; **247**: 47–53.
5. Walsh SL, Preston KL *et al.* Acute administration of buprenorphine in humans: partial agonist and blockade effects. *Journal of Pharmacology and Experimental Therapeutics* 1995; **274**: 361–372.
6. Comer SD, Collins ED, Fischman MW. Buprenorphine sublingual tablets: effects on IV heroin self administration by humans. *Psychopharmacology* 2001; **154**: 28–37
7. Donny EC, Walsh SL, Bigelow GE, Eissenberg T, Stitzer ML. High-dose methadone produces superior opioid blockade and comparable withdrawal suppression to lower doses in opioid-dependent humans. *Psychopharmacology* 2002; **161**: 202–212.
8. Harding-Pink D. Methadone: one person's maintenance dose is another's poison. *Lancet* 1993; **341**: 665–666.
9. Drummer O.H, Opeskin K, Syrjanen M, Cordner S. Methadone toxicity causing death in ten subjects starting on methadone maintenance program. *American Journal of Forensic Medicine and Pathology* 1992; **13**: 346–350.
10. Caplehorn J. Deaths in the first two weeks of maintenance treatment in NSW in 1994: identifying cases of iatrogenic methadone toxicity. *Drug and Alcohol Review* 1998; **17**: 9–17.
11. Zador D, Sunjic S. Deaths in methadone maintenance treatment in NSW, Australia 1990–1995. *Addiction* 2000; **95**: 77–84.
12. Task Force To Review Services for Drug Misusers: Report of an independent review of drug treatment services in England. London: DOH publication, 1996.
13. Hall W. Reducing the toll of opioid overdose deaths in Australia. *Drug and Alcohol Review* 1999; **18**: 213–220.
14. White J, Irvine R. Mechanisms of fatal opioid overdose. *Addiction* 1999; **94**: 961–972.
15. Wolff K, Rostami-Hodjegan A, Shires S *et al.* The pharmacokinetics of methadone in healthy subjects and opiate users. *British Journal of Clinical Pharmacology* 1997; **44**: 325–334.
16. Rostami-Hodjegan A, Wolff K, Hay A, Raistrick D, Calvert R, Tucker GT. Population pharmacokinetics in opiate users: characterisation of time dependent changes. *British Journal of Clinical Pharmacology* 1999; **47**: 974–986.
17. Farrell M, Neeleman J, Griffiths P, Strang J. Suicide and overdose among opiate addicts. Editorial. *Addiction* 1996; **91**: 321–324.
18. Neal J. Methadone, methadone treatment and non-fatal overdose. *Drug and Alcohol Dependence* 2000; **58**: 117–124.
19. Briggs GG, Freeman RK, Yaffe SJ (eds). *Drugs in Pregnancy and Lactation* 6th edition. Philadelphia (PA): Lippincott, Williams and Wilkins, 2002.
20. Walsh SL, June HL, Schuh KJ *et al.* Effects of buprenorphine and methadone in methadone-maintained subjects. *Psychopharmacology* 1995; **119**: 268–276.
21. Strain EC, Preston KL, Liebson IA, Bigelow GE. Acute effects of buprenorphine, andhydromorphone and naloxone in methadone maintained volunteers. *Journal of Pharmacology & Experimental Therapeutics* 1992; **261**: 985–993.
22. Strain EC, Preston KL, Liebson IA, Bigelow GE. Buprenorphine effects in methadone maintained volunteers: effects at 2 hours after methadone. *Journal of Pharmacology & Experimental Therapeutics* 1995; **272**: 628–638.
23. Ling W, Charuvastra C *et al.* Buprenorphine maintenance treatment of opiate dependence: a multicenter, randomized clinical trial. *Addiction* 1998; **93**: 475–486.
24. Mattick RP, Kimber J, Breen C, Davoli M. Buprenorphine maintenance versus placebo or methadone maintenance for opioid dependence. Cochrane Database Systematic Review 4. Oxford: 2002.
25. Amass L, Bickel WK *et al.* Alternate day dosing during buprenorphine treatment of opioid dependence. *Life Sciences* 1994; **54**: 1215–1228.
26. Amass Bickel WK *et al.* Alternate day buprenorphine dosing is preferred to daily dosing by opioid dependent humans. Psychopharmacology 1998; **136**: 217–225.
27. Johnson RE, Eissenberg T, Stitzer ML *et al.* Buprenorphine treatment of opioid dependence: clinical trial of daily versus alternate day dosing. *Drug and Alcohol Dependence* 1995; **40**: 27–35.
28. Eissenberg TR, Johnson RE *et al.* Controlled opioid withdrawal evaluation during 72-hr dose omission in buprenorphine maintained patients. *Drug and Alcohol Dependence* 1997; **45**: 81–91
29. Berson A, Gervais A, Cazals D *et al.* Hepatitis after intravenous buprenorphine misuse in heroin addicts. *Journal of Hepatology* 2001; **34**: 346–350.
30. Kirchmayer U, Davoli M, Verster A. Naltrexone maintenance treatment for opioid dependence (Cochrane Review). The Cochrane Library, Issue 1. Oxford: 2003.
31. Tucker T, Ritter A. Naltrexone in the treatment of heroin dependence: a comprehensive review. *Drug and Alcohol Review* 2000; **19**: 73–82.

Drugs of misuse – a summary

One in ten adults use illicit drugs in any one year[1], and a third of those with mental illness can be classified as having a 'dual diagnosis'[2]. It is therefore important to be aware of the main mental state changes associated with drugs of abuse. Urine-testing for illicit drugs is routine on many psychiatric wards. It is important to be aware of the duration of detection of drugs in urine and of other commonly used substances and drugs that can give a false positive result.

Drug	Physical signs/ symptoms of intoxication	Most common mental state changes[6]	Withdrawal symptoms
Amphetamine[3]	Tachycardia Increased blood pressure Anorexia	Visual/tactile/ olfactory auditory hallucinations Paranoia Decreased concentration Elation	Extreme fatigue Hunger Depression
Benzodiazepines	Sedation Dizziness Respiratory depression	Relaxation Visual hallucinations Disorientation Sleep disturbance	Seizures Psychosis Paraesthesias
Barbiturates	Headache, Hypotension Respiratory depression	Restlessness/ataxia Confusion/ excitement Drowsiness	Similar to alcohol: tremor, vomiting, seizures, delirium tremens
Cannabis[4,5]	Tachycardia Lack of co-ordination Red eyes	Elation, psychosis Perceptual distortions Disturbance of memory/judgement	Not proven. Non-specific symptoms have been reported[5]
Cocaine	Tachycardia/ tachypnoea Increased BP/headache Respiratory depression	Euphoria Paranoid psychosis Panic attacks/anxiety Insomnia/excitement	Profound lethargy Decreased consciousness
Heroin	Pinpoint pupils Clammy skin Respiratory depression	Drowsiness Euphoria Hallucinations	Nausea General aches & pains/gooseflesh. Runny nose/eyes Diarrhoea
Methadone	Respiratory depression Pulmonary oedema	As above	As above but milder & longer lasting

References

1. Ramsey M, Spiller J. *Drug misuse declared in 1996: latest results from the British crime survey.* London: Home Office, 1996.
2. Menenzes PR, Johnson S, Thornicroft G *et al.* Drug and alcohol problems among individuals with severe mental illness in south London. *British Journal of Psychiatry* 1996; **168**; 612–619.
3. Srisuraponont M, Kittiratanapaiboon P, Jarusuraisin N. Treatment for amphetamine dependence and abuse. Cochrane Database of Systematic Reviews. Oxford: Update Software, 2001.
4. Hall W, Solowij N. Long-term cannabis use and mental health. *British Journal of Psychiatry* 1997; **171**: 107–108.
5. Johns A. Psychiatric effects of cannabis. *British Journal of Psychiatry* 2001; **178**: 116–122.
6. Micromedex Healthcare, Volume 13. Thomson Ltd, USA, 2002.
7. Euromed Ltd see info@euromed.ltd.uk.
8. HM Prison Service. *Non-instrumental drug screen test cross-reactivity manual.* Drug Strategy Unit. Prison Service Headquarters, 2001.

Duration of withdrawal	Duration of detection in the urine[6, 7]	Other substances which give a positive result[6,8]
Peaks 7–34 hours Lasts max 5 days	Up to 72 hours	Cough & decongestant preparations, selegiline, large quantities of tryramine, tranylcypromine, chloroquine, ranitidine
Usually short lived but may last weeks to months	2–21 days: depending on half life of drug taken	Zopiclone (possible)
Depends on half-life – likely to be at least several days	24 hours–14 days: depending on half life	None known
Uncertain Probably less than 1 month[5]	Single use: 3 days Chronic heavy use: up to 4 weeks	Passive 'smoking' of cannabis
12–18 hours	2–3 days	Food/tea containing coco leaves
Peaks after 36–72 hours	Up to 48 hours	Food/tea containing poppy seed. Procaine. Any opiate analgesic Diphenoxylate, naltrexone
Peaks after 4–6 days Can last 3 weeks	Up to 7 days with chronic use	Imipramine Meperidine

Interactions between 'street drugs' and prescribed psychotropic drugs

There are some significant interactions between 'street drugs' and drugs that are prescribed for the treatment of mental illness. Information comes from case reports or theoretical assumptions, rarely from systematic investigation. A summary can be found in the table below but remember that the knowledge base is poor. Always be cautious.

In all patients who misuse street drugs:
- infection with hepatitis B and C is common. This may lead to a reduced ability to metabolise other drugs and increased sensitivity to side-effects.
- prescribed drugs may be used in the same way as illicit drugs (i.e erratically and not as intended). Large quantities of prescribed drugs should not be given to outpatients.

Acute behavioural disturbance

Acute intoxication with street drugs may result in behavioural disturbance. Non-drug management is preferable. If at all possible, a urine drug screen should be done to determine the drugs that have been taken, before prescribing any psychotropic. A physical examination should be done if possible (BP, TPR & ECG).

If intervention with a psychotropic is unavoidable, haloperidol 5 mg *or* olanzapine 10 mg po/IM are probably the safest options. Temperature, pulse, respiration and blood pressure *must* be monitored afterwards. Benzodiazepines are commonly misused with other street drugs and so standard doses may be ineffective in tolerant users. Interactions are also possible (see table opposite). Try to avoid.

References for table opposite

1. Johns A. Psychiatric effects of cannabis. *British Journal of Psychiatry* 2001; **178**: 116–122.
2. Ashton S. Pharmacology and effects of cannabis: a brief review. *British Journal of Psychiatry* 2001; **178**: 101–106
3. Zullino DF, Delessert D, Eap CB *et al.* Tobacco and cannabis smoking cessation can lead to intoxication with clozapine or olanzapine. *International Clinical Psychopharmacology* 2002; **17**: 141–143.
4. Benowitz NL, Jones RT. Effects of delta-9-tetrahydrocannabinol on drug distribution and metabolism. *Clinical Pharmacology and Therapeutics* 1977; **22**: 259–268.
5. Annex 14, Drug interactions: in Drug Misuse and Dependence – Guidelines on Clinical Management. Department of Health, HM Stationery Office, Norwich.
6. Wines JD, Weiss RD. Opiod withdrawal during risperidone treatment. *Journal of Clinical Psychopharmacology* 1999; **11**: 198–203.
7. Eap CB, Bertschy G, Powell K. Fluvoxamine and fluoxetine do not interact in the same way with the metabolism of the enantiomers of methadone. *Journal of Clinical Psychopharmacology* 1997; **17**: 113–117.
8. Ketter TA, Post RM, Worthington K. Principles of clinically important drug interactions with carbamazepine. Part 1. *Journal of Clinical Psychopharmacology* 1991; **11**: 198–203.
9. Miller BL, Mena I, Giombetti R *et al.* Neuropsychiatric effects of cocaine: SPECT measurements. In: Miller EB (ed). *Cocaine: Physiological and physiopathological effects.* New York: Haworth Press Inc, 1992.
10. Gowing LR, Henry-Edwards SM, Irvine RJ *et al.* The health effects of ecstasy: a literature review. *Drug and Alcohol Reviews* 2002; **21**: 53–63.
11. Newton TF, Ling W, Kalechstein AD *et al.* Risperidone pre-treatment reduces the euphoric effects of experimentally administered cocaine. *Psychiatric Research* 2001; **102**: 227–233.
12. Grabowski J, Rhoades H, Silverman P *et al.* Risperidone for the treatment of cocaine dependence: randomised double-blind trial. *Journal of Clinical Psychopharmacology* 2000; **20**: 305–310.
13. Balki SL. Antidepressants in the treatment of cocaine dependence. Cochrane Database of Systematic Reviews. Update Software. Oxford: 2001.

Further reading

Howard LA, Sellers EM, Tyndale RF. The role of pharmacogenetically-variable cytochrome P450 enzyme in drug abuse and dependence. *Pharmacogenomics* 2002; **3**: 185–199.

Ley A, Jeffery DP, McLaren S *et al.* Treatment programmes for people with both severe mental illness and substance misuse. Cochrane Database of Systematic Reviews. Oxford: Update Software, 2002.

Williams R, Cohen J. Substance use and misuse in psychiatric wards. *Psychiatric Bulletin* 2000; **24**: 43–46.

Table Interactions between 'street drugs' and psychotropics (for references, see opposite)

	Cannabis	Heroin/methadone[5]	Cocaine Amphetamines Ecstasy	Alcohol
General considerations	• Usually smoked in cigarettes (induces CYP1A2) • Can be sedative[1] • Dose related tachycardia[2]	• Can produce sedation/respiratory depression	• Stimulants (cocaine can be sedative in higher doses) • Arrhythmias possible • Cerebral/cardiac ischaemia with cocaine[9] • Hyperthermia/dehydration with Ecstasy[10]	• Sedative • Liver damage possible
Older antipsychotics	• Antipsychotics reduce the psychotropic effects of almost all drugs of abuse by blocking dopamine receptors (dopamine is the neurotransmitter responsible for 'reward') • Patients prescribed antipsychotics may increase their consumption of illicit substances to compensate • Patients who have taken ecstasy may be more prone to EPSEs • Cardiotoxic or very sedative antipsychotics are best avoided, at least initially. Sulpiride is a reasonable safe first choice			
Atypicals	• Risk of additive sedation • Cannabis can reduce serum levels of olanzapine and clozapine via induction of CYP1A2[3]	• Risk of additive sedation • Case report of methadone withdrawal being precipitated by risperidone[6]	• Risperidone may reduce the euphoric effects of cocaine[11], but does not reduce cocaine use[12]	• Increased risk of hypotension with olanzapine (and possibly other β-blockers)
Antidepressants	• Tachycardia has been reported (monitor pulse and take care with TCAs[4])	• Avoid very sedative antidepressants • Some SSRIs can increase methadone plasma levels[7] (citalopram is SSRI of choice)	• Avoid TCAs (arrhythmias) • MAOIs contraindicated (hypertension) • Various antidepressants have been used in 'crack' withdrawal and may lower the 'high' experienced with stimulants. They are ineffective for cocaine dependence[13]	• Avoid very sedative antidepressants • Avoid antidepressants that are toxic in OD • Impaired psychomotor skills (*not* SSRIs)
Anticholinergics	• Misuse is likely. Try to avoid if at all possible (by using an atypical if an antipsychotic is required) • Can cause hallucinations, elation and cognitive impairment			
Lithium	• Very toxic if taken erratically • Always consider the effects of dehydration (particularly problematic with alcohol or Ecstasy)			
Carbamazepine/valproate		• Carbamazepine decreases methadone levels[8] (danger if CBZ stopped suddenly)		• Monitor LFTs
Benzodiazepines (Always remember that benzodiazepines are liable to misuse)	• Monitor level of sedation	• Oversedation (and respiratory depression possible) • Concomitant use can lead to accidental overdose • Possible pharmacokinetic interaction (increased methadone levels)	• Oversedation (if high doses of cocaine have been taken) • Widely used after cocaine intoxication	• Oversedation (and respiratory depression) possible • Future misuse possible • Widely used in alcohol detoxification

Depression and psychosis in epilepsy

The prevalence of clinical depression in people with epilepsy varies from 9 to 22%[1,2] and depressive symptoms may occur in up to 60% of people with intractable epilepsy[3]. Suicide rates have been estimated to be 4–5 times that of the general population[1,2]. The prevalence of psychotic illness in people with epilepsy is at least 4%[4]. Peri-ictal depression or psychosis (that is, symptoms temporally related to seizure activity) should initially be treated by optimising anticonvulsant therapy[4]. Interictal depression or psychosis (symptoms occurring independently of seizures) are likely to require treatment with antidepressants or antipsychotics[2,4].

Use of antidepressants and antipsychotics in epilepsy

The majority of antipsychotics and antidepressants can reduce the seizure threshold[1,2,5,6] and the risk is dose-related. Treatment with an antidepressant or antipsychotic drug increases the risk of de novo seizures in non-epileptic subjects 10-fold[5]. There are few systematic studies of antipsychotics or antidepressants in people with epilepsy. Data are mainly derived from animal studies, clinical trials, case reports and CSM reports. The table below gives some general guidance. Treatment should be commenced at the lowest dose and this should be gradually increased until a therapeutic dose is achieved[2,6,7]. As a general rule, the more sedating a drug is, the more likely it is to induce seizures[6].

Electroconvulsive therapy (ECT) has anticonvulsive properties and is worth considering in the treatment of depression in patients with unstable epilepsy[1,2].

Depression and psychosis associated with anticonvulsant drugs

Anticonvulsant drugs have been associated with new-onset depression and psychosis[1]. If anticonvulsants have recently been changed, this should always be considered as a potential cause of a new/worsening depressive or psychotic illness. Lowering of folate levels by some anticonvulsants may also influence the expression of depression[1]. Folate levels should be checked.

Psychosis[8]

Product data sheets and case reports associate the following anticonvulsants with the onset of psychotic symptoms: carbamazepine, ethosuximide, tiagabine, topiramate, valproate and vigabactrin. Some of these reports may relate to the process of 'forced normalisation' where a diminished frequency of seizures allows psychotic symptoms to emerge.

Depression[8]

Product data sheets and case reports associate the following anticonvulsants with the onset of depressive symptoms: acetazolamide, barbiturates, carbamazepine, ethosuximide, gabapentin, phenytoin, piracetam, tiagabine, topiramate and vigabatrin.

Interactions

Pharmacokinetic interactions between anticonvulsants and antidepressants/antipsychotics are common. These interactions are primarily mediated through cytochrome P450 enzymes[1,2]. Fluoxetine and paroxetine are potent inhibitors of several hepatic CYP enzyme systems (CYP2D6, CYP3A4). Sertraline is a less potent inhibitor, but this effect is dose-related and higher doses of sertraline are commonly used. Citalopram is a weak inhibitor. Carbamazepine and phenytoin have a narrow therapeutic range and serum levels can be increased by enzyme inhibitors. This is particularly dangerous with phenytoin. Plasma levels should be monitored and dosage adjustment may be required.

Carbamazepine is an enzyme inducer (mainly CYP3A4) and can lower serum levels of some antipsychotic drugs[9]. Many other medicines can cause problems in people with epilepsy by raising or reducing the seizure threshold or interacting with anticonvulsant drugs. Check Appendix 1 of the *British National Formulary* or contact pharmacy for advice (see also page 201 for a summary).

Table Psychotropics in epilepsy

Antidepressant	Safety in epilepsy	Special considerations
Moclobemide[10]	Good choice	Not known to be proconvulsive
SSRIs[11] Trazodone[11] Nefazodone[12]	Good choice	Low proconvulsive effect[2,13], but SSRIs have many potential interactions with anticonvulsant drugs (see above). Seizure risk is dose-related. Citalopram may be the safest SSRI[14]
Mirtazapine/reboxetine/venlafaxine[15]	Care required	Very limited data and clinical experience Use with care
Amitriptyline Dothiepin[16] Clomipramine[17]	Avoid	Most epileptogenic Ideally, should be avoided completely
Lithium[2]	Care required	Low proconvulsive effect at therapeutic doses Marked proconvulsive activity in overdose
Antipsychotic		
Trifluoperazine/haloperidol[2,6,18,19]	Good choice	Low proconvulsive effect. Carbamazepine increases the metabolism of some antipsychotics and larger doses of antipsychotic may be required
Sulpiride	Good choice	Low proconvulsive effect (less clinical experience) No known interactions with anticonvulsants
Risperidone[15] Olanzapine[20,21] Quetiapine Amisulpride	Care required	Limited clinical experience Use with care
Chlorpromazine[4,22,23] Loxapine[24]	Avoid	Most epileptogenic of the older drugs Ideally best avoided completely
Clozapine[5,25,4]	Avoid	Very epileptogenic. Approximately 4–5% who receive more than 600 mg/day develop seizures Sodium valproate is the anticonvulsant of choice as it has a lower incidence of leukopenia than carbamazepine
Zotepine[26]	Avoid	Has established dose-related proconvulsive effect Best avoided completely
Depot antipsychotics	Avoid	None of the depot preparations currently available is thought to be epileptogenic, however: • the kinetics of depots are complex (seizures may be delayed) • if seizures do occur, the offending drug may not be easily withdrawn Depots should be used with extreme care

Epilepsy and driving

People with epilepsy may not drive a car if they have had a seizure while awake in the previous year or, if seizures only occur during sleep, this has been an established pattern for at least 3 years. The consequences of inducing seizure with antidepressants or antipsychotics can therefore be significant. For further information see www.dvla.gov.uk.

References

1. Harden CL, Goldstein MA. Mood disorders in patients with epilepsy; Epidemiology and management. *CNS Drugs* 2002; **16**(Suppl. 5): 291–302.
2. Curran S, de Pauw K. Selecting an antidepressant for use in a patient with epilepsy; Safety considerations. *Drug Safety* 1998; **18**(Suppl. 2): 125–133.
3. Lambert MV, Robertson MM. Depression in epilepsy: etiology, phenomenology and treatment. *Epilepsia* 1999; **40**(Suppl.10): 21–47.
4. Blumer D, Wakhu S, Montouris G *et al.* Treatment of the interictal psychosis. *Journal of Clinical Psychiatry* 2000; **61**(Suppl. 2): 110–122.
5. Pisani F, Oteri G, Costa C *et al.* Effects of psychotropic drugs on seizure threshold. *Drug Safety* 2002; **25**: 91–110.
6. Marks RC, Luchins DJ. Antipsychotic medications and seizures. *Psychiatric Medicine* 1991; **9**: 37–52
7. Donald L, Rosentein MD, Craig J *et al.* Seizures associated with antidepressants: a review. *Journal of Clinical Psychiatry* 1993; **54**(Suppl. 8): 289–299.
8. http://emc.vhn.net
9. Tihonen J, Vartiainen H, Hakola P. Carbamazepine induced changes in plasma levels of neuroleptics. *Pharmacopsychiatry* 1995; **28**: 26–28.
10. Schiwy W, Heath WR, Delini-Stula A. Therapeutic and side effect profile of a selective and reversible MAOI inhibitor: results of dose finding trials in depressed patients. *Journal of Neural Transmission* 1989; **28**: 33–44.
11. Weden OP, Oderda GM, Klein-Schwartz W *et al.* Relative toxicity of cyclic antidepressants. *Annals of Emergency Medicine* 1986; **15**: 797–804.
12. Dunner DL, Laird LK, Zakecka J *et al.* Six-year perspectives on the safety and tolerability of nefazodione. *Journal of Clinical Psychiatry* 2002; **63**: 32–41.
13. Duncan D, Taylor D. Which is the safest antidepressant to use in epilepsy? *Psychiatric Bulletin* 1995; **19**: 355–357.
14. Hovorka K, Herman E, Nemacova I *et al.* Treatment of interictal depression with citalopram in patients with epilepsy. *Epilepsy & Behaviour* 2000; **1**: 444–447.
15. Alldredge BK. Seizure risk associated with psychotropic drugs: clinical and pharmacokinetic considerations. *Neurology* 1999; **53**(Suppl. 2): 68–75.
16. Buckley NA, Dawson AH, Whyte IM *et al.* Greater toxicity in overdose of dothiepin than other tricyclic antidepressants. *Lancet* 1994; **343**: 159–162.
17. Stimmel GL, Dopheide JA. Psychotropic drug-induced reductions in seizure threshold: incidence and consequences. *CNS Drugs* 1996; **5**: 37–50.
18. Markowitz JC, Brown RP. Seizures with neuroleptics and antidepressants. *General Hospital Psychiatry* 1987; **9**: 135–141.
19. Darbk JK, Pasta DJ, Dabin L. Haloperidol dose and blood level variability: toxicity and interindividual and intraindividual variability in the nonresponder patient in the clinical practice setting. *Journal of Clinical Psychopharmacology* 1995; **15**: 334–340.
20. Beasley CM, Tollefson GD, Tran PV. Safety of olanzapine. *Journal of Clinical Psychiatry* 1997; **58**(Suppl. 10): 13–17.
21. Lee JW, Crismon ML, Dorson PG. Seizure associated with olanzapine. *Annals of Pharmacotherapy* 1999; **33**: 554–556.
22. Itil TM, Soldatos C. Epileptogenic side effects of psychotropic drugs. *JAMA* 1980; **244**: 1460–1463.
23. Logothetis J. Spontaneous epileptic seizures and EEG changes in the course of phenothiazine therapy. *Neurology* 1967; **17**: 869–877.
24. Peterson CD. Seizures induced by acute loxapine overdose. *American Journal of Psychiatry* 1981; **138**: 1089–1091.
25. Toth P, Frankenberg FR. Clozapine and seizures: a review. *Canadian Journal of Psychiatry* 1994; **39**: 236–238.
26. Tscuchiya H, Kawahara R, Tanaka Y *et al.* Generalised seizure during treatment of schizophrenia with zotepine. *Yonago Acta Medica* 1986; **29**: 103–171.

Further reading

Centorrino F, Price BH, Tuttle MMS *et al.*. EEG abnormalities during treatment with typical and atypical antipsychotics. *American Journal of Psychiatry* 2002; **159**: 109–115.

Schmitz B. Antidepressant drugs: indications and guidelines for use in epilepsy. *Epilepsia* 2002; **43**(Suppl. 2): 14–18.

Van der Feltz-Cornelis CM. Treatment of interictal psychiatric disorder in epilepsy. I. Affective and anxiety disorders. *Acta Neuropsychiatrica* 2002; **14**: 39–43.

Van der Feltz-Cornelis CM. Treatment of interictal psychiatric disorder in epilepsy. II. Chronic psychosis. *Acta Neuropsychiatrica* 2002; **14**: 44–48.

Van der Feltz-Cornelis CM. Treatment of interictal psychiatric disorder in epilepsy. III. Personality disorder, aggression and mental retardation. *Acta Neuropsychiatrica* 2002; **14**: 49–54.

Drug interactions between antiepileptic drugs and other psychotropic drugs

Antiepileptic drug	Increases level of	Decreases level of	Level increased by	Level decreased by
Carbamazepine	Phenytoin	Clonazepam Clobazam Ethosuximide Primidone Valproic acid Lamotrigine Tiagabine Topiramate Phenytoin Haloperidol Clozapine Olanzapine Risperidone Quetiapine Zotepine TCAs ?Sertraline ?Citalopram Bupropion Donepezil Methylphenidate Thyroxine Methadone Benzodiazepines	Valproic acid and primidone increase levels of 10,11 epoxide metabolite of carbamazepine Fluoxetine Fluvoxamine Nefazodone	Phenobarbitone Phenytoin
Phenytoin	Carbamazepine Phenobarbitone Valrpoate	Carbamazepine Valproate Phenobarbitone Lamotrigine Tiagabine Topiramate Benzodiazepines Haloperidol Clozapine Quetiapine TCAs Paroxetine Methadone Donepezil Bupropion	Carbamazepine Phenobarbitone Valproate Topiramate Phenothiazines ?Zotepine Fluoxetine Fluvoxamine Trazodone TCAs Sertraline Diazepam Benzodiazepines Disulfiram Methylphenidate Alcohol (acute)	Vigabatrin Carbamazepine Phenobarbitone Valproate Alcohol (chronic) *cont.*

Antiepileptic drug	Increases level of	Decreases level of	Level increased by	Level decreased by
Lamotrigine	None known	None known	Valproate Sertraline	Phenytoin Carbamazepine Oxcarbazepine Phenobarbitone Primidone
Valproate	Phenobarbitone Primidone Free phenytoin TCAs Benzodiazepines	Total phenytoin Topiramate 10 monohydroxy metabolite of oxcarbazepine	Lamotrigine Oxcarbazepine Topiramate ?Fluoxetine	Phenytoin Phenobarbitone Carbamazepine ?Fluoxetine
Gabapentin	None known	None known	None known	None known
Levetiracetam	?Phenytoin	None known	None known	None known
Vigabatrin	Carbamazepine	Phenytoin ?Phenobarbitone	None known	None known
Oxcarbazepine	10,11 epoxide metabolite of carbamazepine phenobarbitone phenytoin	Carbamazepine Lamotrigine		Phenobarbitone Carbamazepine Phenytoin Valproate
Phenobarbitone	Phenytoin	Carbamazepine Clonazepam Lamotrigine Tiagabine Valproate Ethosuximide Phenytoin Haloperidol ?Chlorpromazine Clozapine Quetiapine zotepine Mianserin TCAs Nefazodone Paroxetine ?Donepezil Bupropion Benzodiazepines Methadone	Valproate Oxcarbazepine Phenytoin Alcohol (acute)	Vigabatrin Alcohol (chronic)
Tiagabine	None known	Valproate	?Nefazodone ?Fluoxetine ?Valproate	Phenytoin Phenobarbitone Carbamazepine Primidone

cont.

202

Antiepileptic drug	Increases level of	Decreases level of	Level increased by	Level decreased by
Topiramate	Phenytoin	?Valproate	?Valproate	Phenytoin Carbamazepine Phenobarbitone
Ethosuximide	?Phenytoin ?Valproate	None known	Valproate	Carbamazepine Phenobarbitone Phenytoin
Tiagabine	?Valproate	Valproate	?Nefazodone ?Fluoxetine	Phenytoin Phenobarbitone Carbamazepine Primidone

Further reading

Schmitz B. Antidepressant drugs: indications and guidelines for use in epilepsy. *Epilepsia* 2002; 43(Suppl. 2): 14–18.
British Medical Association and Royal Pharmaceutical Society (2003). *British National Formulary*, Issue 45, Appendix 1.
Patsalos PN, Fröscher W, Pisani F *et al.* The importance of drug interactions in epilepsy therapy. *Epilepsia* 2002; 43: 365–385.

chapter 7

Use of psychotropics in special patient groups

Drug choice in pregnancy

A 'normal' outcome to pregnancy can never be guaranteed. The spontaneous abortion rate in confirmed early pregnancy is 10–20% and the risk of spontaneous major malformation is 2–3% (approx. 1 in 40 pregnancies)[1]. Drugs account for a very small proportion of abnormalities (approximately 5%). Potential risks of drugs include major malformation (first trimester exposure), neonatal toxicity (third trimester exposure) and long-term neurobehavioural effects. The safety of psychotropics in pregnancy cannot be clearly established because robust, prospective trials are obviously unethical. Individual decisions on psychotropic use in pregnancy are therefore dependent upon an imperfect retrospective database and an assessment of the risks and benefits associated with withdrawal or continuation of drug treatment. The patient's view of risks and benefits will have paramount importance. This section provides a brief summary of knowledge to date.

General principles of prescribing in pregnancy

- Only treat when absolutely necessary (potential benefit outweighs potential harm).
- Ensure that the prospective parents are as fully involved as possible in all discussions.
- Always consider the risk of relapse when discontinuing psychotropics – relapse may ultimately be more harmful to the mother and child than continued, effective drug therapy.
- Try to avoid all drugs in the first trimester when major organs are being formed.
- Use an established drug at the lowest effective dose.
- Avoid polypharmacy whenever possible.
- Be prepared to adjust doses as pregnancy progresses and drug handling is altered. Plasma level monitoring is helpful, where available.
- Ensure adequate foetal screening during pregnancy.
- Be aware of potential problems with individual drugs around the time of delivery.
- Monitor the neonate for withdrawal effects after birth.
- Document all decisions.

Risk of psychosis during pregnancy and postpartum[2–5]

- The risk of peri-natal psychosis is 0.1–0.25% in the general population, but may be as high as 50% in women with a history of psychosis.
- During the month after childbirth there is an increase in the relative risk of psychosis that may be up to 20-fold.
- The risk of post-partum psychosis in patients with a history of post-partum psychosis is 30–50%.

The risks of not treating psychosis include:

- Harm to the mother through poor self-care, lack of obstetric care, poor judgement or impulsive acts.
- Harm to the foetus or neonate (ranging from neglect to infanticide).
- The mental health of the mother influences foetal well-being, obstetric outcome and child development.

Treatment with antipsychotics

It has long been established that people with schizophrenia are more likely to have minor physical anomalies than the general population[6]. Some of these anomalies may be apparent at birth, while others are more subtle and may not be obvious until later in life. This background risk complicates the assessment of antipsychotic drug risk.

Older, conventional antipsychotics are generally considered to have minimal risk of teratogenicity, although data are less than convincing, as might be expected[7,8]. It remains uncertain as to whether conventional antipsychotics are entirely without risk to the foetus or to later development. However, this uncertainty and the wide use of these drugs over several decades suggest that any risk is small – an assumption borne out by most studies[9].

Data relating to atypical antipsychotics are now appearing. The use of clozapine appears to present no increased risk of malformation, although gestational diabetes and neonatal seizures may be more likely to occur[10]. Similarly, limited data suggest that olanzapine is not associated with teratogenicity, but may increase the risk of gestational diabetes[7,10,11]. Still more limited data tentatively suggest that neither risperidone[12] nor quetiapine[13] are teratogenic in humans.

These data do not allow an assessment of relative risks associated with different agents and certainly do not confirm absolutely the safety of any particular drug. Older, conventional drugs may still be preferred in pregnancy but, considering data now available on some atypical drugs, it may not be appropriate always to switch to these drugs, should continued treatment be necessary. As with other drugs, decisions must be based on the latest available information and an individualised assessment of probable risks and benefits.

Recommendations – psychosis in pregnancy

- Patients with a history of psychosis who are maintained on antipsychotic medication should be advised to discuss a planned pregnancy as early as possible.
- Such patients, particularly if they have suffered repeated relapses, are best maintained on antipsychotics during and after pregnancy. This may minimise foetal exposure by avoiding the need for higher doses should relapse occur.
- There is most experience with chlorpromazine (constipation and sedation can be a problem), trifluoperazine, olanzapine and clozapine (gestational diabetes may be a problem with both atypicals). If the patient is established on another antipsychotic, always obtain the most up-to-date advice. Experience with other drugs is growing and a change in treatment may not be necessary or wise.
- Some authorities recommend discontinuation of antipsychotics 5–10 days before anticipated delivery to minimise the chances of neonatal EPSEs. This may, however, put mother and infant at risk and needs to be considered carefully. Antipsychotic discontinuation symptoms can occur in the neonate (e.g. crying, agitation, increased suckling).

Risk of depression during pregnancy and postpartum[4,14,15]

- Approximately 10% of pregnant women will develop a depressive illness and a further 16% a self-limiting depressive reaction.
- There is a significant increase in new psychiatric episodes in the first 3 months after delivery. At least 80% are mood disorders, primarily depression.
- Women who have had a previous episode of depressive illness (postpartum or not) are at higher risk of further episodes post-partum.
- The risk is highest in women with bipolar illness.

The risks of not treating depression include:
- Harm to the mother through poor self-care, lack of obstetric care or self-harm.
- Harm to the foetus or neonate (ranging from neglect to infanticide).
- The mental health of the mother influences foetal well being, obstetric outcome and child development.

Treatment with antidepressants

Tricyclic antidepressants have been widely used throughout pregnancy without apparent detriment to the foetus[8,16] and are agents of choice in pregnancy. Some authorities recommend the use of nortriptyline and desipramine (not available in UK) because these drugs are less anticholinergic and hypotensive than amitriptyline and imipramine (respectively, their tertiary amine parent molecules). Note that use of tricyclics in the third trimester is well known to produce neonatal withdrawal effects (agitation, irritability, seizures)[17]. In addition, little is known of the developmental effects of prenatal exposure to tricyclics, although one small study detected no adverse consequences[18].

SSRIs also appear not to be teratogenic, with most data supporting the safety of fluoxetine[16–18]. They have however been associated with both decreased gestational age (mean 1 week) and birth weight (mean 175 g)[19]. Third trimester exposure has been associated with reduced early APGAR scores[19]. Third trimester use of paroxetine may give rise to neonatal complications, presumably related to abrupt withdrawal[20]. Rather more scarce data suggest the absence of terotogenic potential with mocobemide[21], reboxetine[22] and venlafaxine (although neonatal withdrawal may occur)[23], but none of these drugs can be specifically recommended at the time of writing. Similarly, trazodone, bupropion (amfebutamone) and mirtazapine cannot be recommended because there are few, if any, data supporting their safety[8,16].

MAOIs should be avoided in pregnancy because of a suspected increased risk of congenital malformation and because of the risk of hypertensive crisis[24].

There is no evidence to suggest that ECT causes harm to either the mother or foetus during pregnancy[25].

Recommendations – depression in pregnancy

- Patients who are already receiving antidepressants and are at high risk of relapse are best maintained on antidepressants during and after pregnancy.
- Those who develop a depressive illness during pregnancy should be treated with antidepressant drugs if psychological management has failed or is not available.
- There is most experience with amitriptyline, imipramine (constipation & sedation can be a problem with both), and fluoxetine (increased chance of earlier delivery and reduced birthweight). If the patient is established on another antidepressant, always obtain the most up to date advice. Experience with other drugs is growing and a change in treatment may not be necessary, or wise.
- The neonate may experience a discontinuation symptoms such as agitation and irritability. The risk is assumed to be particularly high with short half life drugs such as paroxetine and venlafaxine.

Risks in patients with bipolar illness during pregnancy and postpartum

- There is no evidence to suggest that pregnancy increases the risk of relapse in patients with bipolar illness.
- The risk of relapse following delivery is hugely increased: up to 8 fold in the first month postpartum.

The risks of not treating depression include:
- Harm to the mother through poor self care, lack of obstetric care or self harm.
- Harm to the foetus or neonate (ranging from neglect to infanticide).
- The mental health of the mother influences foetal well being, obstetric outcome and child development.

Treatment with mood stabilisers

Lithium use during pregnancy has a well known association with the cardiac malformation Ebstein's anomoly[8] (relative risk 10–20 times more than control, but the absolute risk is low 1:1000)[27]. The period of maximum risk to the foetus is 2 to 6 weeks post conception[28]; before the majority of women will know that they are pregnant. Although the risk of major malformations in the infant has probably been overestimated, lithium should be avoided in pregnancy if possible. Slow discontinuation before conception is the preferred course of action[10] because abrupt discontinuation is suspected of worsening risk of relapse. The relapse rate post partum may be as high as 70% in women who discontinued lithium pre-conception[26]. If lithium is continued during pregnancy, then high-resolution ultrasound and echocardiography should be performed at 6 and 18 weeks of gestation. In the third trimester, the use of lithium may be problematic because of changing pharmacokinetics: an increasing dose of lithium is required to maintain the lithium level during pregnancy as total body water increases, but the requirements return abruptly to pre-pregnancy levels immediately after delivery. Neonatal goitre and cardiac arrythmias can occur.

Most data relating to carbamazepine and valproate come from studies in epilepsy; a condition associated with increased neonatal malformation. These data may not be precisely relevant to use in mental illness. Nonetheless, both carbamazepine and valproate have a clear causal link with an increased risk of a variety of foetal abnormalities, particularly spina bifida[8,16,29]. Both drugs should be avoided, if possible. Where continued use is deemed essential, low-dose monotherapy is strongly recommended. Ideally, all patients should take folic acid (5 mg daily) for at least a month before conception (this may reduce the risk of neonatal neural tube defects). Use of carbamazepine in the third trimester may necessitate the need for maternal vitamin K. There are too few data relating to lamotrigine to recommend its use.

Recommendations – bipolar disorder in pregnancy

- For women who have had a long period without relapse, the possibility of withdrawing treatment preconception and for at least the first trimester should be considered.
- The risk of relapse postpartum is very high.
- Women with severe illness or who are known to relapse quickly following discontinuation of a mood stabiliser may need to continue their medication.
- No mood stabiliser is clearly safe. Women prescribed lithium should undergo level 2 ultrasound of the foetus at 6 and 18 weeks gestation to screen for Ebsteins anomaly. Those prescribed valproate or carbamazepine should receive prophylactic folic acid to reduce the incidence of neural tube defects. Prophylactic vitamin K should be administered to the mother and neonate after delivery.
- Combinations of mood stabilisers should be avoided if possible.

Risks in patients with epilepsy during pregnancy and postpartum[30,31]

- There is an increased risk of maternal complications such as severe morning sickness, eclampsia, vaginal bleeding and premature labour. Women should get as much sleep and rest as possible and comply with medication (if prescribed) in order to minimise the risk of seizures.
- The risk of having a child with minor malformations may be increased regardless of treatment with antiepileptic drugs (AEDs).
- The risks of not treating epilepsy include:
  - If seizures are inadequately controlled there is an increased risk of accidents resulting in foetal injury. Postpartum, the mother may be less able to look after herself and her child.
  - The risk of seizures during delivery is 1–2%, potentially resulting in maternal and neonatal mortality.

Treatment with anticonvulsant drugs[32-35]

It is established that treatment with anticonvulsant drugs increases the risk of having a child with major congenital malformation to 2 to 3 fold that seen in the general population. Congential heart defects (1.8%) and facial clefts (1.7%) are the most common congenital malformations. Both carbamazepine and valproate are associated with a hugely increased incidence of spina bifida at 0.5–1% and 1–2% respectively. The risk of other neural tube defects is also increased. Higher doses (particularly doses of valproate exeeding 1,000 mg/day) and anticonvulsant polypharmacy are particularly problematic. Cognitive deficits have been reported in older children who have been exposed to valproate in utero. There are too few data about other anticonvulsants to evaluate their teratogenic risk.

Pharmacokinetics change during pregnancy. Dosage adjustment may be required to keep the patient seizure-free. Serum levels usually return to pre-pregnancy levels within a month of delivery. Doses may need to be reduced at this point.

Best practice guidelines recommend that a woman should receive the lowest possible dose of a single AED.

Recommendations – epilepsy in pregnancy

- For women who have had a long period seizure-free, the possibility of withdrawing treatment preconception and for at least the first trimester should be considered.

- No anticonvulsant is clearly safer. Women prescribed valproate or carbamazepine should receive prophylactic folic acid to reduce the risk of neural tube defects. Prophylactic vitamin K should be administered to the mother and neonate after delivery.

- Combinations of anticonvulsants should be avoided if possible.

- All women with epilepsy should have a full discussion with their neurologist to quantify the risks and benefits of continuing anticonvulsant drugs.

Sedatives

First trimester exposure to benzodiazepines appears to be associated with an increased risk of oral clefts in newborns, although there is debate about the magnitude of this risk[36]. Third trimester use is commonly associated with neonatal difficulties (floppy baby syndrome)[37]. Benzodiazepines are best avoided in pregnancy.

Promethazine has been used in hyperemesis gravidarum and appears not to be teratogenic, although data are limited.

Recommendations – psychotropics in pregnancy

Psychotropic group	Recommendations
Antidepressants	Nortriptyline Amitriptyline Imipramine Fluoxetine
Antipsychotics	**Conventional drugs** have been widely used, although safety is not fully established. Most experience with **chlorpromazine** and **trifluoperazine**. No evidence that **clozapine** and **olanzapine** have teratogenic potential but data are limited
Benzodiazepines	Best avoided
Mood stabilisers	Avoid unless risks and consequences of relapse outweigh known risk of teratogenesis. Women of child bearing potential taking carbamazepine or valproate should receive prophylactic folic acid
Sedatives	Promethazine widely used but supporting data scarce

References

1. McElhatton PR. General principles of drug use in pregnancy. *Pharmaceutical Journal* 2003; **270**: 232–234.
2. Oates M. Patients as patents: the risk to children. *British Journal of Psychiatry* 1997; **170**(Suppl. 32): 22–27.
3. Terp IM, Mortensen PB. Post-partum psychoses. *British Journal of Psychiatry* 1998; **172**: 521–526.
4. Stein G. Postpartum and related disorders. In: Stein G, Wilkinson G (eds). *Seminars in General Adult Psychiatry*. London: Royal College of Psychiatrists, 1998, pp. 903–953.
5. Spinelli M. A systematic investigation of 16 cases of neonaticide. *American Journal of Psychiatry* 2001; **158**: 811–813.
6. Ismail B, Cantor-Graae E, McNeil TF *et al*. Minor physical anomalies in schizophrenic patients and their siblings. *American Journal of Psychiatry* 1998; **155**: 1695–1702.
7. Patton SW, Misri S, Corral MR *et al*. Antipsychotic medication during pregnancy and lactation in women with schizophrenia: evaluating the risk. *Canadian Journal of Psychiatry* 2002; **47**: 959–965.
8. Cohen LS, Rosenbaum JF. Psychotropic drug use during pregnancy: weighing the risks. *Journal of Clinical Psychiatry* 1998; **59**(Suppl. 2): 18–28.
9. Trixler M, Tényi T. Antipsychotic use in pregnancy: what are the best treatment options? *Drug Safety* 1997; **16**: 403–410.
10. Ernst CL, Goldberg JF. The reproductive safety profile of mood stabilizers, atypical antipsychotics, and broad-spectrum psychotropics. *Journal of Clinical Psychiatry* 2002; **63**:(Suppl. 4): 42–55.
11. Zyprexa – use in pregnancy. Personal communication. Eli Lilly & Co. 2003.
12. Ratnayaka T, Libretto SE. No complications with risperidone treatment before and throughout pregnancy and during the nursing period. *Journal of Clinical Psychiatry* 2002; **63**: 76–77.
13. Tényi T, Trixler M, Keresztes Z. Quetiapine and pregnancy. *American Journal of Psychiatry* 2002; **159**: 674.
14. Simon GE, Cunningham ML, Davis RL. Outcome of prenatal antidepressant exposure. *American Journal of Psychiatry* 2002; **159**: 2055–2061.
15. Llewellyn AM, Stowe ZN, Nemeroff CB. Depression during pregnancy and the puerperium. *Journal of Clinical Psychiatry* 1997; **58**: 26–32.
16. Altshuler LL, Cohen L, Szuba MP. Pharmacologic management of psychiatric illness during pregnancy: dilemmas and guidelines. *American Journal of Psychiatry* 1996; **153**: 592–606.

17. Wisner KL, Gelenberg AJ, Leonard H *et al*. Pharmacologic treatment of depression during pregnancy. *JAMA* 1999; **282**: 1264–1268.
18. Nulman I, Rovet J, Stewart DE *et al*. Child development following exposure to tricyclic antidepressants or fluoxetine throughout fetal life: a prospective, controlled study. *American Journal of Psychiatry* 2002; **159**: 1889–1895.
19. Simon GE, Cunningham ML, Davis RL. Outcomes of prenatal antidepressant exposure. *American Journal of Psychiatry* 2002; **159**: 2055–2061.
20. Moldovan Costei A, Kozer E, Ho T *et al*. Perinatal outcome following third trimester exposure to paroxetine. *Archives of Paediatric & Adolescent Medicine* 2002; **156**: 1129–1132.
21. Rybakowski JK. Moclobemide in pregnancy. *Pharmacopsychiatry* 2001; **34**: 82–83.
22. Edronax®: Use in pregnancy, renally and hepatically impaired patients. Personal communication – Pharmacia Ltd. 2003.
23. Einarson A, Fatoye B, Sarkar M. Pregnancy outcome following gestational exposure to venlafaxine: a multicentre prospective controlled study. *American Journal of Psychiatry* 2001; **158**: 1728–1730.
24. Hendrick V, Altshuler L. Management of major depression during pregnancy. *American Journal of Psychiatry* 2002; **159**: 1667–1673.
25. Miller LJ. Use of electroconvulsive therapy during pregnancy. *Hospital & Community Psychiatry* 1994; **45**: 444–450.
26. Viguera AC, Nonacs R, Cohen LS *et al*. Risk of recurrence of bipolar disorder in pregnant and non-pregnant women after discontinuing lithium maintenance. *American Journal of Psychiatry* 2000; **157**: 179–184.
27. Cohen LS, Friedman JM, Jefferson JW *et al*. A re-evaluation of risk in utero exposure to lithium. *JAMA* 1994; **271**: 146–150.
28. Yonkers KA, Little BB, March D. Lithium during pregnancy. *CNS Drugs* 1998; **9**: 261–269.
29. Holmes LB, Harvey EA, Brent A *et al*. The teratogenicity of anticonvulsant drugs. *New England Journal of Medicine* 2001; **344**: 1132–1138.
30. Shorvon S. Antiepileptic drug therapy during pregnancy: the neurologist's perspective. *Journal of Medical Genetics* 2002; **39**: 248–250.
31. Cleland PG. Risk-benefit assessment of anticonvulsants in women of child-bearing potential. *Drug Safety* 1991; **6**: 70–81.
32. Dolk H, McElhatton P. Assessing epidemiological evidence for the teratogenic effects of anticonvulsant medication. *Journal of Medical Genetics* 2002; **39**: 243–244.
33. Holmes LB. The teratogenicity of anticonvulsant drugs: a progress report. *Journal of Medical Genetics* 2002; **39**: 245–247.
34. Citrin O, Shechtman S, Arnon J *et al*. Is carbamazepine teratogenic? A prospective controlled study of 210 pregnancies. *Neurology* 2001; **57**: 321–324.
35. Iqbal MM, Sohhan T, Mahmud SZ. The effects of lithium, valproic acid and carbamazepine during pregnancy and lactation. *Clinical Toxicology* 2001; **39**: 381–392.
36. Dolovich LR, Addis A, Vaillancourt JMR *et al*. Benzodiazepine use in pregnancy and major malformations or oral cleft: meta-analysis of cohort and case-control studies. *BMJ* 1998; **317**: 839–843.
37. McElhatton PR. A review of the effects of benzodiazepine use during pregnancy and lactation. *Reprod Toxicology* 1994; **8**: 461–475.

Further reading

Wisner KL, Zarin DA, Holmboe C *et al*.. Risk-benefit decision making for treatment of depression during pregnancy. *American Journal of Psychiatry* 2000; **157**: 1933–1940.
Einarson A, Selby P, Koren G. Abrupt discontinuation of psychotropic drugs during pregnancy: fear of teratogenic risk and impact of counselling. *Journal of Psychiatry & Neuroscience* 2001; **26**: 44–48.

Breast-feeding

There are no published controlled studies on the safety of psychotropic medication during breast-feeding. All the data available are in the form of case reports or case series. With the majority of data, only acute adverse effects (or absence of) are reported. Long-term safety cannot therefore be guaranteed for any of the psychotropics mentioned. The information presented must be interpreted with caution with respect to limited data from which it is derived and the need for such information to be regularly updated.

General principles of prescribing psychotropics in breast-feeding

- In each case, the benefits of breast-feeding to the mother and infant should be weighed against the risk of drug exposure in the infant.
- Premature infants and infants with renal, hepatic, cardiac or neurological impairment are at a greater risk from exposure to drugs.
- The infants should be monitored for any specific adverse effects of the drugs as well as for feeding patterns and growth and development

Wherever possible:
- continue the same medication given during pregnancy;
- use the lowest effective dose;
- avoid polypharmacy;
- avoid drugs with a long half-life;
- time the feeds to avoid peak drug levels in the milk.

Summary of recommendations (see full review below for details)

Drug group	Recommended drugs
Antidepressants	Paroxetine or sertraline
Antipsychotics	Sulpiride
Mood stabilisers	Avoid if possible
Sedatives	Lorazepam for anxiety; zolpidem for sleep

Antidepressants in breast-feeding

Drug	Comment
Tricyclic anti-depressants[1-5]	All TCAs are excreted in human breast milk. Infant serum levels range from undetectable to low. No adverse effects have been reported in infants exposed to amitriptyline, nortriptylline, clomipramine, imipramine, dothiepin (dosulepin) and desipramine. There are two case reports of doxepin exposure during breast-feeding leading to adverse effects in the infant. In one, an 8-week-old infant experienced respiratory depression, which resolved 24 hours after stopping nursing. In the other, poor suckling, muscle hypotonia and drowsiness were observed in a newborn, again resolving 24 hours after removing doxepin exposure. Data on TCAs not mentioned in this section were not available and their use can therefore not be recommended unless used during pregnancy. This group of antidepressants is the most widely studied in breast-feeding. On the whole, the maternal risk of not receiving treatment for depression appears to exceed the neonatal risks associated with exposure to TCAs.
Citalopram[1,6-10]	Citalopram is excreted in breast milk. Infant serum levels appear to be low or undetectable, although higher than reported with fluvoxamine, sertaline and paroxetine. Breast milk peak levels have been observed 3–9 hours after maternal dose. There is one case report of uneasy sleep in an infant exposed to citalopram while breast-feeding. This resolved on halving the mother's dose. No other adverse effects have been reported in exposed infants.
Fluvoxamine[1,11-16]	Fluvoxamine is excreted in breast milk. The levels detected in infants exposed to fluvoxamine while breast-feeding vary from undetectable to up to half the maternal dose. No adverse effects were noted in these infants. Peak drug levels in breast milk have been observed 4 hours after maternal dose.
Fluoxetine[1,17-20]	Of the SSRIs most data relate to fluoxetine. Fluoxetine is excreted into breast milk. Infant serum levels appear to be low, although higher than reported with paroxetine, fluvoxamine and sertraline, and close to those reported for citalopram. No adverse effects were noted in the majority of fluoxetine-exposed infants. However, in 2 infants adverse effects were noted; symptoms included excessive crying, decreased sleep, diarrhoea and vomiting in one and somnolence, decreased feeding, hypotonia, moaning, grunting and fever in the other. No developmental abnormalities were noted in 4 infants exposed to fluoxetine during breast-feeding.
Paroxetine[1,11,21-24]	Paroxetine is excreted in breast milk. Infant serum levels vary from low to undetectable. No adverse effects were noted in these infants.
Sertraline[1,11,25-28]	Sertraline is excreted in breast milk. Infant serum levels appear to be low. Peak drug levels in breast milk have been observed 8–9 hours after the maternal dose. No adverse effects were noted in these infants. Withdrawal symptoms (agitation, restlessness, insomnia and an enhanced startle reaction) developed in a breast-fed neonate, after abrupt withdrawal of maternal sertraline. The neonate was exposed to sertraline *in utero*.
Nefazodone[29,30]	From the 3 published case reports available, it appears that nefazodone is excreted into breast milk. Levels in the infant serum were low. However, one case reports drowsiness and poor feeding in an infant exposed to nefazodone in breast milk. These symptoms resolved over a 72-hour period after feeding ceased. Peak breast milk levels were seen 1–3 hours post-maternal dose.
Venlafaxine[1,31,32]	Venlafaxine is excreted in breast milk. In a study of 3 infants exposed to venlafaxine during breast-feeding, serum levels were found to be low. Although in this instance not directly compared, these levels appear to be higher than those seen with fluvoxamine, sertraline and paroxetine. No adverse effects were seen in these infants. Another small study of 6 women found levels to range from undetectable to low.
MAOIs	There are no published data available.
Moclobemide[33,34]	Moclobemide is excreted in breast milk. Infant serum levels appear to be low. No adverse effects were detected in these infants. Peak drug levels in breast milk were seen at 3 hours.

Antipsychotics in breast-feeding

Drug	Comment
Butyrophenones[1,2,35,36]	Haloperidol is excreted in breast milk. The extent appears variable. Normal development was noted in one infant. However, delayed development was noted in 3 infants exposed to a combination of haloperidol and chlorpromazine in breast milk. Data on butyrophenones not mentioned in this section were not available and their use can therefore not be recommended unless used during pregnancy.
Phenothiazines[1,2,35,36]	Most of the data relate to chlorpromazine. Chlopromazine is excreted into breast milk. There is a wide variation in the breast milk concentrations quoted. Similarly, infant serum levels vary greatly. Lethargy was reported in one infant whose mother was taking chlorpromazine while breast-feeding. In another case, however, an infant exposed to much higher levels showed no signs of lethargy. There is a report of delayed development in 3 infants exposed to a combination of chlorpromazine and haloperidol while breast-feeding. In the one case of perphenazine exposure and 2 cases of trifluoperazine exposure, no adverse effects were noted in the infants. Data on phenothiazines not mentioned in this section were not available and their use can therefore not be recommended unless used during pregnancy.
Thioxanthenes[1,37]	There is one case of infant exposure to flupenthixol and one to zuclopenthixol. The amount excreted in breast milk of both drugs is low. No adverse effects or developmental abnormalities were noted in the infant exposed to flupenthixol. The clinical status of the other infant was not reported.
Sulpiride[38–42]	There are a number of small studies in which sulpiride has been shown to improve lactation in nursing mothers. The amounts excreted into breast milk were low. No adverse effects were noted in the nursing infants.
Amisulpride	There are no published data available.
Aripiprazole	There are no published data available.
Clozapine[1,2,36]	Clozapine is excreted in breast milk. There are no data on infant exposure to clozapine during breast-feeding. Because of the risk of neutropenia and seizures, it is advisable to avoid breast-feeding while on clozapine until more data become available.
Olanzapine[1,43,44]	Olanzapine is excreted in breast milk. Estimates of 5 infant serum levels were low. There is one case of an infant developing jaundice and sedation on exposure to olanzapine during breast-feeding. This continued on cessation of breast-feeding. This infant was exposed to olanzapine *in utero* and had cardiomegaly.
Quetiapine	There are no published data available.
Risperidone[45,46]	Risperidone is excreted in breast milk. There are two case reports of infant exposure to risperidone. No developmental abnormalities were noted in either.
Sertindole	There are no published data available.
Ziprasidone	There are no published data available.

Mood stabilisers in breast-feeding

Drug	Comment
Carbamazepine[1,47–49]	Carbamazepine is excreted in breast milk. Infant serum levels range from 6% to 65% of maternal serum levels. Adverse effects have been reported in a number of infants exposed to carbamazepine during breast-feeding. These include one case of cholestatic hepatitis, and one of transient hepatic dysfunction with hyperbilirubinaemia and elevated GGT. The adverse effects in the first case resolved after discontinuation of breast-feeding and the second resolved despite continued feeding. Other adverse effects reported include seizure-like activity, drowsiness, irritability and high pitched crying in one infant whose mother was on multiple agents, hyperexcitability in 2 infants and poor feeding in another 3. In contrast, in a number of infants, no adverse effects were noted.
Gabapentin	There are no published data available.
Lamotrigine[49,50]	Lamotrigine is excreted in breast milk. Infant serum levels range between 25% and 50% of maternal serum levels. No adverse effects have been reported in exposed infants. However, because of the risk of life-threatening rashes, it is advisable to avoid lamotrigine while breast-feeding until more data on its effects become available.
Lithium[47,49]	Lithium is excreted in breast milk. Infant serum levels range from 5% to 200% of maternal serum concentrations. Adverse effects have been reported in infants exposed to lithium while breast-feeding. One infant developed cyanosis, lethargy, hypothermia, hypotonia and a heart murmur, all of which resolved within 3 days of stopping breast-feeding. The infant was exposed to lithium *in utero*. Non specific signs of toxicity have been reported in others. There are also reports of no adverse effects in some infants exposed to lithium while breast-feeding. Opinions on the use of lithium while breast-feeding vary from absolute contra-indication to mother's informed choice. Conditions which may alter the infant's electrolyte balance and state of hydration must be borne in mind. If used, the infant must be carefully monitored for signs of toxicity.
Valproate[1,47–51]	Valproate is excreted into breast milk. Infant serum levels vary from undetectable to 40% of maternal serum levels. Thrombocytopenia and anaemia were reported in a 3-month-old infant exposed to valproate *in utero* and while breast-feeding. This reversed on stopping breast-feeding.

Sedatives in breast-feeding

Drug	Comment
Benzo-diazepines[1,52–56]	Diazepam is excreted in breast milk. Infant serum levels vary from undetectable to nearly 14% of the maternal dose. In some infants, no adverse effects were noted. In others, reported adverse effects included sedation, lethargy and weight loss. Lorazepam, temazepam and clonazepam are excreted in breast milk in small amounts. Apart from one case report of persistent apnoea in one infant exposed to clonazepam in utero and during breast-feeding, no adverse effects were reported.
Zopiclone and zolpidem[1,52]	There are more data on zolpidem than zopiclone, although still limited. Both are excreted into breast milk in small amounts. No adverse effects were noted in exposed infants.

References

1. Burt VK, Suri R, Alshuler L *et al.* The use of psychotropic medications during breast-feeding. *American Journal of Psychiatry* 2001; **158**: 1001–1009.
2. Yoshida K, Smith B, Kumar R. Psychotropic drugs in mothers' milk: a comprehensive review of assay methods, pharmacokinetics and of safety of breast-feeding. *Journal of Psychopharmacology* 1999; **13**: 64–80.
3. Misri S, Kostaras X. Benefits and risks to mother and infant of drug treatment for postnatal depression. *Drug Safety* 2002; **25**: 903–911.
4. Yoshida K, Smith B, Craggs M *et al.* Investigation of pharmacokinetics and of possible adverse effects in infants exposed to tricyclic antidepressants in breast-milk. *Journal of Affective Disorders* 1997; **43**: 225–237.
5. Frey OR, Scheidt P, von Brenndorff AL. Adverse effects in a newborn infant breast-fed by a mother treated with doxepin. *Annals of Pharmacotherapy* 1999; **33**: 690–693.
6. Heikkinen T, Ekblad U, Kero P. Citalopram in pregnancy and lactation. *Clinical Pharmacology & Therapeutics* 2002; **72**: 184–191.
7. Jensen PN, Olesen OV, Bertelsen A *et al.* Citalopram and desmethylcitalopram concentrations in breast milk and in serum of mother and infant. *Therapeutic Drug Monitoring* 1997; **19**: 236–239.
8. Spigset O, Carleborg L, Öhman R *et al.* Excretion of citalopram in breast milk. *British Journal of Clinical Pharmacology* 1997; **44**: 295–298.
9. Rampono J, Kristensen JH, Hackett LP *et al.* Citalopram and demethylcitalopram in human milk; distribution, excretion and effects in breast fed infants. *British Journal of Clinical Pharmacology* 2000; **50**: 263–268.
10. Schmidt K, Olesen OV, Jensen PN. Citalopram and breast-feeding: serum concentration and side effects in the infant. *Biological Psychiatry* 2000; **47**: 164–165.
11. Hendrick V, Fukuchi A, Altshuler L *et al.* Use of sertraline, paroxetine and fluvoxamine by nursing women. *British Journal of Psychiatry* 2001; **179**: 163–166.
12. Piontek CM, Wisner KL, Perel JM *et al.* Serum fluvoxamine levels in breastfed infants. *Journal of Clinical Psychiatry* 2001; **62**: 111–113.
13. Yoshida K, Smith B, Channi Kumar R. Fluvoxamine in breast-milk and infant development. *British Journal of Clinical Pharmacology* 1997; **44**: 209–213.
14. Hägg S, Granberg K, Carleborg L. Excretion of fluvoxamine into breast milk. *British Journal of Clinical Pharmacology* 2000; **49**: 283–288.
15. Arnold LM, Suckow RF, Lichtenstein PK. Fluvoxamine concentrations in breast milk and in maternal and infant sera. *Journal of Clinical Psychopharmacology* 2000; **20**: 491–492.
16. Kristensen JH, Hackett P, Kohan R *et al.* The amount of fluvoxamine in milk is unlikely to be a cause of adverse effects in breastfed infants. *Journal of Human Lactation* 2002; **18**: 139–143.
17. Yoshida K, Smith B, Craggs M *et al.* Fluoxetine in breast-milk and developmental outcome of breast-fed infants. *British Journal of Psychiatry* 1998; **172**: 175–179.
18. Lester BM, Cucca J, Andreozzi L *et al.* Possible association between fluoxetine hydrochloride and colic in an infant. *Journal of American Academy of Child and Adolescent Psychiatry* 1993; **32**: 6.
19. Hendrick V, Stowe ZN, Altshuler LL *et al.* Fluoxetine and norfluoxetine concentrations in nursing infants and breast milk. *Biological Psychiatry* 2001; **50**: 775–782.
20. Hale TW, Shum S, Grossberg M. Fluoxetine toxicity in a breastfed infant. *Clinical Pediatrics* 2001; **40**: 681–684.
21. Begg EJ, Duffull SB, Saunders DA *et al.* Paroxetine in human milk. *British Journal of Clinical Pharmacology* 1999; **48**: 142–147.
22. Stowe ZN, Cohen LS, Hostetter A *et al.* Paroxetine in human breast milk and nursing infants. *American Journal of Psychiatry* 2000; **157**: 185–189.
23. Misri S, Kim J, Riggs KW *et al.* Paroxetine levels in postpartum depressed women, breast milk, and infant serum. *Journal of Clinical Psychiatry* 2000; **61**: 828–832.
24. Öhman R, Hägg S, Carleborg L *et al.* Excretion of paroxetine into breast milk. *Journal of Clinical Psychiatry* 1999; **60**: 519–523.
25. Stowe ZN, Hostetter AL, Owens MJ *et al.* The pharmacokinetics of sertraline excretion into human breast milk: determinants of infant serum concentrations. *Journal of Clinical Psychiatry* 2003; **64**: 73–80.
26. Stowe ZN, Owens MJ, Landry JC *et al.* Sertraline and desmethylsertraline in human breast milk and nursing infants. *American Journal of Psychiatry* 1997; **154**: 1255–1260.
27. Kristensen JH, Ilett KF, Dusci LJ *et al.* Distribution and excretion of sertraline and *N*-desmethylsertraline in human milk. *British Journal of Clinical Pharmacology* 1998; **45**: 453–457.
28. Kent LSW, Laidlaw JDD. Suspected congenital sertraline dependence. *British Journal of Psychiatry* 1995; **167**: 412–413.
29. Yapp P, Ilett KF, Kristensen JH *et al.* Drowsiness and poor feeding in a breast-fed infant: association with nefazodone and its metabolites. *Annals of Pharmacotherapy* 2000; **34**: 1269–1272.
30. Dodd S, Maguire KP, Burrows GD *et al.* Nefazodone in the breast milk of nursing mothers: a report of two patients. *J Clin Psychopharmacology* 2000; **20**: 717–718.
31. Ilett KF, Kristensen JH, Hackett LP *et al.* Distribution of venlafaxine and its O-desmethyl metabolite in human milk and their effects in breastfed infants. *British Journal of Clinical Pharmacology* 2002; **53**: 17–22.
32. Ilett KF, Hackett LP, Dusci LJ *et al.* Distribution and excretion of venlafaxine and O-desmethylvenlafaxine in human milk. *British Journal of Clinical Pharmacology* 1998; **45**: 459–462.

215

33. Pons G, Schoerlin MP, Tam YK. Moclobemide excretion in human breast milk. *British Journal of Clinical Pharmacology* 1990; **29**: 27–31.
34. Buist A, Dennerstein L, Maguire KP *et al.* Plasma and human milk concentrations of moclobemide in nursing mothers. *Human Psychopharmacology Clinical and Experimental* 1998; **13**: 579–582.
35. Yoshsida K, Kumar R. Breast feeding and psychotropic drugs. *International Review of Psychiatry* 1996; **8**: 117–124.
36. Patton SW, Misri S, Corral MR *et al.* Antipsychotic medication during pregnancy and lactation in women with schizophrenia: evaluating the risk. *Canadian Journal of Psychiatry* 2002; **47**: 959–965.
37. Matheson I, Skjeraasen J. Milk concentrations of flupenthixol, nortriptyline and zuclopenthixol and between-breast differences in two patients. *European Journal of Clinical Pharmacology* 1988; **35**: 217–220.
38. Ylikorkala O, Kauppila A, Kivinen S *et al.* Treatment of inadequate lactation with oral sulpiride and buccal oxytocin. *Obstetry & Gynecology* 1984; **63**: 57–60.
39. Aono T, Shioji T, Aki T *et al.* Augmentation of puerperal lactation by oral administration of sulpiride. *Journal of Clinical Endocrinology & Metabolism* 1979; **48**: 478–482.
40. Ylikorkala O, Kauppila A, Kivinen S *et al.* Sulpiride improves inadequate lactation. *BMJ* 1982; **285**: 249–251.
41. Aono T, Aki T, Koike K *et al.* (1982) Effect of sulpiride on poor puerperal lactation. *American Journal of Obstetrics and Gynecology* 143: 927–932.
42. Polatti F. Sulpiride isomers and milk secretion in puerperium *Clinical Experimental Obstetrics and Gynecology* 1982; **3**: 144–147.
43. Goldstein DJ, Corbin LA, Fung MC. Olanzapine-exposed pregnancies and lactation: early experience. *Journal of Clinical Psychopharmacology* 2000; **20**: 399–403.
44. Croke S, Buist A, Hackett LP *et al.* Olanzapine excretion in human breast milk: estimation of infant exposure. *International Journal of Neuropsychopharmacology* 2002; **5**: 243–247.
45. Ratnayake T, Libretto SE. No complications with risperidone treatment before and throughout pregnancy and during the nursing period. *Journal of Clinical Psychiatry* 2002; **63**: 76–77.
46. Hill RC, McIvor RJ, Wojnar–Horton RE *et al.* Risperidone distribution and excretion into human milk: case report and estimated infant exposure during breast–feeding. *Journal of Clinical Psychopharmacology* 2000; **20**: 285–286.
47. Chaudron LH, Jefferson JW. Mood stabilizers during breastfeeding: a review. *Journal of Clinical Psychiatry* 2000; **61**: 79–90.
48. Wisner KL, Perel JM. Serum levels of valproate and carbamazepine in breastfeeding mother–infant pairs. *Journal of Clinical Psychopharmacology* 1998; **18**: 167–169.
49. Ernst CL, Goldberg JF. The reproductive safety profile of mood stabilizers, atypical antipsychotics, and broad-spectrum psychotropics. *Journal of Clinical Psychiatry* 2002; **63**(Suppl. 4): 42–55.
50. Ohman I, Vitols S, Tomson T. Lamotrigine in pregnancy: pharmacokinetics during delivery, in the neonate, and during lactation. *Epilepsia* 2000; **41**: 709–713.
51. Piontek CM, Baab S, Peindl KS *et al.* Serum valproate levels in 6 breastfeeding mother–infant pairs. *Journal of Clinical Psychiatry* 2000; **61**: 170–172.
52. Spigset O, Hägg S. Excretion of psychotropic drugs into breast milk: pharmacokinetic overview and therapeutic implications. *CNS Drugs* 1998; Feb 9: 111–134.
53. Hägg S, Spigset O. Anticonvulsant use during lactation. *Drug Safety* 2000; **22**: 425–440.
54. Masud Iqbal M, Sobhan T, Ryals T. Effects of commonly used benzodiazepines on the fetus, the neonate, and the nursing infant. *Psychiatric Services* 2002; **53**: 39–49.
55. Buist A, Norman TR, Dennerstein L. Breastfeeding and the use of psychotropic medication: a review. *Journal of Affective Disorders* 1990; **19**: 197–206.
56. Fisher JB, Edgren BE, Mammel MC *et al.* Neonatal apnoea associated with maternal clonazepam therapy: a case report. *Journal of Obstetrics and Gynaecology* 1985; **66**: 345–355.

Renal impairment

- Using drugs in patients with renal impairment can be difficult. This is because some drugs are nephrotoxic and also because pharmacokinetics (absorption, distribution, metabolism, excretion) of drugs are altered in renal impairment.

- Essentially, **patients with renal impairment have a reduced capacity to excrete drugs** and their metabolites.

Prescribing in renal impairment – general principles

1. **Estimate the excretory capacity of the kidney** by calculating the glomerular filtration rate (GFR). GFR can also be directly measured by collection of urine over 24 hours.

> GFR in *adults* can be estimated by calculating the creatinine clearance (CrCl) using the Cockroft & Gault equation*:
>
> $$\text{CrCl (ml/min)} = \frac{F\,(140 - \text{age}) \times \text{ideal body weight (kg)}}{\text{Plasma creatinine (μmol/l)}}$$
>
> F = 1.23 (men) and 1.04 (women)
> For men, ideal body weight (kg) = 50 kg + 2.3 kg per inch over 5 foot
> For women, ideal body weight (kg) = 45.5 kg + 2.3 kg per inch over 5 foot
>
> * This equation is not accurate if plasma creatinine is unstable, in pregnant women or children or in diseases causing production of abnormal amounts of creatinine

2. Grade the severity of renal impairment as below:

Grade	GFR	Approx. serum creatinine
Mild	20–50 ml/min	150–300 μmol/l
Moderate	10–20 ml/min	300–700 μmol/l
Severe	<10 ml/min	>700 μmol/l

In severe renal impairment most patients require dialysis.

3. **Note that elderly patients are assumed to have mild renal impairment.** Their creatinine may not be raised because they have a smaller muscle mass.

4. **Avoid drugs that are nephrotoxic** (e.g. lithium) in moderate or severe renal failure.

5. **Choose a drug that is safer to use in renal impairment** (see tables below).

6. **Be cautious when using drugs that are extensively renally cleared** (e.g. sulpiride, amisulpride).

217

7. **Start at a low dose and increase slowly** because, in renal impairment, the half-life of a drug and the time for it to reach steady state are often prolonged. Plasma level monitoring may be useful for some drugs.

8. **Avoid long-acting drugs** (e.g. depot preparations). Their dose and frequency cannot be easily adjusted should renal function change.

9. **Prescribe as few drugs as possible.** Patients with renal failure take many medications requiring regular review. Interactions and side-effects can be avoided if fewer drugs are used.

10. **Monitor patient for adverse effects.** Patients with renal impairment are more likely to experience side-effects and these may take longer to develop than in healthy patients. Adverse effects such as sedation, confusion and postural hypotension can be more common.

11. **Be cautious when using drugs with anticholinergic effects,** since they may cause urinary retention.

12. There are **few clinical studies** of the use of psychotropic drugs in people with renal impairment. Advice about drug use in renal impairment is often based on knowledge of the drug's pharmacokinetics in healthy patients.

13. **The effect of renal replacement therapies on drugs is difficult to predict.** Dosing advice is available from tables and data on each drug's volume of distribution and protein-binding affinity. Seek specialist advice.

Table	Antipsychotics in renal impairment
Drug	**Comments**
Aripiprazole[1]	Less than 1% of unchanged aripiprazole renally excreted. Manufacturer states no dose adjustment required in renal failure, however, no published studies in patients with renal disease
Amisulpride[1-3]	Primarily renally excreted. Limited experience in renal disease, manufacturer states no data with doses >50 mg, but recommends following dosing: 50% of dose if CrCl 30–60 ml/min; 33% of dose if CrCl is 10–30 ml/min; no recommendations for CrCl <10 ml/min so best avoided in severe renal impairment
Chlorpromazine[1,2,4,5]	Less than 1% excreted unchanged in urine. Manufacturer advises caution in renal failure. Dosing: CrCl 10–50 ml/min, dose as in normal renal function; CrCl <10 ml/min, start with lower dose because of an increased risk of anticholinergic, sedative and hypotensive side-effects. Monitor carefully
Clozapine[2,6,7]	Only trace amounts of unchanged clozapine excreted in urine, however, there are case reports of interstitial nephritis and acute renal failure. Contraindicated by manufacturer in severe renal disease
Flupentixol oral[1,2]	Negligible renal excretion of unchanged flupenthixol. Preliminary data suggest dose adjustment may not be necessary in the presence of renal impairment. Manufacturer recommends caution in renal failure
Fluphenazine oral[2]	Little information available, manufacturer contraindicates in renal failure
Haloperidol[1,2,8,13]	No specific dose adjustment needed in renal impairment. Case report of haloperidol use in renal failure suggests starting at a low dose and increasing slowly
Olanzapine[1,2]	7% of olanzapine is excreted unchanged in urine. No dose adjustment needed in renal impairment, however, a single-dose study of olanzapine in severe renal impairment used 5 mg, so consider starting at this dose
Pimozide[1,2,4]	Less than 1% of pimozide is excreted unchanged in the urine, dose reductions not usually needed in renal impairment. Dosing: CrCl 10–50 ml/min, dose as in normal renal function; CrCl <10 ml/min start with 50% of normal dose. Manufacturer advises caution in renal dysfunction
Quetiapine[1,2,9]	Less than 5% of quetiapine excreted unchanged in the urine. Plasma clearance reduced by an average of 25% in patients with a CrCl <30 ml/min thus start at 25 mg/day and increase in daily increments of 25–50 mg to an effective dose
Risperidone[1,2,10]	Clearance of the active metabolite of risperidone is reduced by 50% in patients with renal disease. In renal impairment halve the starting and incremental doses. In CrCl <10 ml/min start at 0.5 mg bd and increase by 0.5 mg bd to 1.5 mg bd. If higher doses are needed, increase by 0.5 mg bd weekly
Sertindole[1,2,11]	Less than 1% of sertindole is excreted into urine. A single-dose study of sertindole found no dose adjustment needed in mild, moderate or severe renal impairment
Sulpiride[2,12]	Primarily renally excreted with 95% excreted in urine and faeces as unchanged sulpiride. Dosing regimen: CrCl 30–60 ml/min give 70% of normal dose; CrCl 10–30 ml/min give 50% of normal dose; CrCl < 10 ml/min give 30% of normal dose
Thioridazine[1,2,4,14]	<4% excreted unchanged in urine. Use doses as for normal renal function but use lower initial doses and increase gradually
Ziprasidone[1,15]	<1% is renally excreted unchanged. No dose adjustment needed for CrCl >10 ml/min but care needed when using the injection as it contains a renally-eliminated excipient (cyclodextrin sodium)
Zotepine[1,2]	<0.1% is excreted as unchanged zotepine in urine. Patients with renal dysfunction have higher plasma levels than healthy patients so start low, gradually titrate and reduce the maximum daily dose. The manufacturer suggests a starting dose 25 mg bd, gradually titrating to a max. 75 mg bd.

Table Antidepressants in renal impairment

Drug	Comments
Amitriptyline[1,2,4,13,16]	<10% excreted unchanged in urine, no dose adjustment needed in renal failure. Dose as in normal renal function but start at a low dose and increase slowly. Monitor patient for urinary retention, confusion, sedation, postural hypotension, as increased metabolite plasma levels may cause an increased incidence of side-effects
Citalopram[1,2,17,18]	<13% of citalopram is excreted unchanged in the urine. Single-dose studies in mild, moderate and severe renal impairment show no change in the pharmacokinetics of citalopram
Clomipramine[1,2,4]	<3% of unchanged clomipramine is excreted in the urine. Dosing: CrCl 20–50 ml/min, as normal renal function; CrCl <20 ml/min, effects unknown, start at a low dose and monitor effects
Dosulepin (dothiepin)[1,4,19]	56% of mainly active metabolites renally excreted. They have a long half-life (50 hours) and may accumulate, resulting in excessive sedation. Dosing: CrCl 20–50 ml/min, dose as for normal renal function; CrCl <20 ml/min, start with 25 mg **on**
Doxepin[1,2,4]	<1% excreted unchanged in urine. Dose as in normal renal function but monitor patient for urinary retention, confusion, sedation, postural hypotension, as increased plasma metabolite levels may cause an increased incidence of side-effects. Manufacturer advises caution
Fluvoxamine[1,2,13]	Little information on its use in renal impairment. Dose as for normal renal function but start on a low dose and monitor carefully
Fluoxetine[1,2,4,13,20,21]	2.5–5% of fluoxetine and 10% of the active metabolite norfluoxetine are excreted unchanged in the urine. Dose adjustments are not needed in renal impairment and failure, however, one source suggests alternate day dosing if CrCl <10 ml/min
Imipramine[1,2,13,16]	Approximately 6% of unchanged imipramine and active metabolite are excreted in the urine. Severe renal impairment does not affect the renal excretion of imipramine but inactive metabolites are raised, possibly resulting in an increased incidence of side-effects (see amitriptyline). No specific dose adjustment necessary in renal impairment
Lofepramine[1,2,22]	Most lofepramine is excreted in the urine along with some as the active metabolite desipramine. Desipramine has a long half-life (12–24 hours) and can accumulate so avoid in renal impairment. Manufacturer advises caution in impaired renal function
Mirtazapine[1,2]	Clearance reduced by 30% in patients with a CrCl of 11–39 ml/min and by 50% in patients with a CrCl <10 ml/min. Manufacturer advises careful dosing and regular monitoring. Mirtazapine's active metabolite is renally cleared
Moclobemide[1,2,23,24]	<1% of parent drug excreted unchanged in the urine. However, an active metabolite was found to be raised in patients with renal impairment but was not thought to affect dosing. Dose adjustments are not required in renal impairment
Nortriptyline[1,4,16,25]	If CrCl 10–50 ml/min, dose as in normal renal function; if CrCl <10 ml/min start at a low dose. Plasma level monitoring recommended at doses of >100 mg/day. Plasma concentrations of active metabolites are raised in renal impairment, possibly resulting in an increased incidence of side-effects (see amitriptyline). Worsening of CrCl in elderly patients has also been reported
Paroxetine[1,2,4,13,26,27]	Less than 2% of oral dose is excreted unchanged in the urine. Single-dose studies show increased plasma concentrations of paroxetine when CrCl <30 ml/min. Dosing advice differs. One source suggests starting at 10 mg/day if CrCl <30 ml/min and increasing dose according to response. Another suggests using 20 mg if CrCl 10–30 ml/min

Table Antidepressants in renal impairment (*cont.*)

Drug	Comments
Phenelzine[1,4]	Approximately 1% excreted unchanged in the urine. No dose adjustment required in renal failure
Reboxetine[1,2,28,29]	Approximately 9% of unchanged drug is excreted unchanged in the urine. Starting dose in patients with renal impairment is 2 mg bd. Half-life is prolonged as renal function decreases
Sertraline[1,2,4,13]	<0.2% of unchanged sertraline excreted in urine. Pharmacokinetics in renal impairment are unchanged but no published data on multiple dosing. Dosing is as in normal renal function
Trazodone[1,2,4,13,30]	<5% excreted unchanged in urine but care as approximately 70% of active metabolite also excreted. Dosing: CrCl 20–50 ml/min, dose as normal renal function; CrCl 10–20 ml/min, dose as normal renal function but start with small dose and increase gradually; CrCl <10 ml/min, avoid or use half the dose or half frequency
Trimipramine[13,16,31,32]	No dose reduction required in renal impairment, however, elevated urea and interstitial nephritis have been reported. As with all TCAs, monitor patient for urinary retention, confusion, sedation, and postural hypotension as patients with renal impairment are at increased risk of having these side-effects
Venlafaxine[1,2,13,33]	1–10% is excreted unchanged and 30% as the active metabolite. Decreased clearance and prolonged half-lives occur in renal impairment. Dosing: CrCl 30–50 ml/min, reduce dose by 25%; CrCl <30 ml/min reduce dose by 50%. Manufacturer's advice differs; CrCl >30 ml/min, dose as in normal renal function; CrCl 10–30 ml/min reduce dose by 50%; CrCl <10 ml/min, avoid use

Table Mood stabilisers in renal impairment

Drug	Comments
Carbamazepine[1,2,4,40–45]	2–3% of the dose is excreted unchanged in urine. Dose reduction not necessary in renal disease, although cases of renal failure, tubular necrosis and tubulointerstitial nephritis have been reported, as has renal impairment in children on carbamazepine for 2 years
Lithium[1,2,4,13,54]	Lithium is nephrotoxic and contraindicated in severe renal impairment; 95% is excreted unchanged in the urine. Long-term treatment may result in impaired renal function and both reversible and irreversible kidney damage. If lithium is used in renal impairment, toxicity is more likely. Dosing: CrCl 10–50 ml/min, avoid or reduce dose (50–75% of normal dose) and monitor levels; CrCl <10 ml/min, avoid
Lamotrigine[1,2,4,46–49]	<10% of lamotrigine is excreted unchanged in the urine. Single-dose studies in renal failure show pharmacokinetics are little affected, however, inactive metabolites can accumulate (effects unknown) and half-life can be prolonged. Renal failure and interstitial nephritis have also been reported. Dosing: CrCl <10–50 ml/min, use cautiously, start with a low dose and monitor closely
Valproate[1,2,4,40,50–53]	Approximately 2% excreted unchanged as valproate. Dose adjustment usually not required in renal impairment, however, free valproate levels may be increased (by 27% if CrCl <10 ml/min). Renal impairment, interstitial nephritis, Fanconi's syndrome, renal tubular acidosis and renal failure have been reported. Dose as in normal renal function, however, in severe impairment it may be necessary to alter doses according to free valproate levels

Table Anxiolytics and hypnotics in renal impairment

Drug	Comments
Buspirone[1,2,4,13]	<1% excreted unchanged, however, active metabolite is renally excreted. Dosing advice contradictory, however, suggest: CrCl 10–50 ml/min dose as normal; CrCl <10 ml/min avoid if possible due to accumulation of active metabolites or reduce dose by 25–50%
Chlormethiazole[1,2,4,34]	0.1–5% of unchanged drug excreted unchanged in urine. Dose as in normal renal function but monitor for excessive sedation. Manufacturer recommends caution in renal disease
Chlordiazepoxide[2,4,13]	<5% of unchanged drug excreted but chlordiazepoxide has a long-acting active metabolite that can accumulate. Dosing: CrCl 10–50 ml/min, dose as normal renal function; CrCl <10 ml/min, reduce dose by 50%. Monitor for excessive sedation
Clonazepam[1,2,4,13]	<5% of clonazepam excreted unchanged in urine. Dose adjustment not required in impaired renal function, however, in long-term administration, active metabolites may accumulate so lower doses may be needed. Monitor for excessive sedation
Diazepam[1,4,13,35]	Dosing: CrCl 20–50 ml/min, dose as in normal renal function; CrCl <20 ml/min, use small doses and titrate to response. Long-acting active metabolites accumulate in renal impairment, monitor patients for excessive sedation and encephalopathy. One case of interstitial nephritis in a patient with chronic renal failure has been reported
Lorazepam[1,2,4,36,37]	<5% excreted unchanged in urine, dose as in normal renal function but carefully according to response as some may need lower doses. Monitor for excessive sedation. Impaired elimination reported in 2 patients with severe renal impairment and also a report of propylene glycol (a vehicle) in lorazepam injection causing renal impairment
Oxazepam[1,4,13,38]	No dose adjustment needed except in severe renal impairment. Oxazepam may take longer to reach steady state in patients with renal impairment. Dosing: CrCl 10–50 ml/min, dose as in normal renal function; CrCl <10 ml/min, 10–20 mg tds or qds. Monitor for excessive sedation
Promethazine[1,2,13]	Dose reduction usually not necessary, however, promethazine has a long half-life so monitor for excessive sedative effects in patients with renal impairment. Manufacturer advises caution in renal impairment
Temazepam[1,2,4]	<2% excreted unchanged in urine. In renal impairment half-life prolonged and inactive metabolite can accumulate. Monitor for excessive sedative effects. Dosing: CrCl 20–50 ml/min, dose as normal renal function; CrCl 10–20 ml/min, start with small doses, max. 20 mg/day; CrCl <10 ml/min, start with small doses, max. 10 mg daily
Zaleplon[1,2]	In renal impairment inactive metabolites accumulate. No dose adjustment appears to be necessary in patients with a CrCl >20 ml/min. Zaleplon has not been studied in severe renal impairment so is probably best avoided in patients with a CrCl <20 ml/min
Zolpidem[1,2]	Clearance moderately reduced in renal impairment. No dose adjustment required in renal impairment, however, there are no published studies of zolpidem in severe renal impairment
Zopiclone[1,2,4,39]	<7% excreted unchanged in urine, manufacturer states no accumulation of zopiclone in renal impairment but suggests starting at 3.75 mg in those with CrCl <10 ml/min

222

Summary – psychotropics in renal impairment

Drug group	Recommended drugs
Antipsychotics	No agent clearly preferred to another, however: • avoid sulpiride and amisulpride • avoid highly anticholinergic agents because they may cause urinary retention • typical antipsychotic – suggest **haloperidol** 2–6 mg a day • atypical antipsychotic – suggest **olanzapine** 5 mg a day
Antidepressants	No agent clearly preferred to another, however: • **citalopram** and **sertraline** are suggested as reasonable choices
Mood stabilisers	No agent clearly preferred to another, however: • avoid lithium • suggest start one the following at a low dose and increase slowly, monitor for adverse effects: **valproate**, **carbamazepine** and **lamotrigine**
Anxiolytics and hypnotics	No agent clearly preferred to another, however: • excessive sedation more likely to occur in patients with renal impairment, monitor all patients carefully • **lorazepam** and **zopiclone** are suggested as reasonable choices

References

1. Drugdex® System, Micromedex Inc., Englewood, Colorado. Second quarter, 2003.
2. Electronic Medicines Compendium; www.emc.vhn.net/professional/
3. Noble S, Benfield P. Amisulpride. A review of its clinical potential in dysthymia. *CNS Drugs* 1999; **12**: 471–483
4. Moorhead J, Bunn R, Ashley C. *The Renal Drug Handbook*. Oxford: Radcliffe Medical Press, 1999.
5. Fabre J, De Freudenreich J, Duckert A *et al*. Influence of renal insufficiency on the excretion of chloroquine, phenobarbital, phenothiazines and methacycline. *Helvetica Medica Acta* 1966; **4**: 307–316.
6. Fraser D, Jibani M. An unexpected and serious complication of treatment with the atypical antipsychotic drug clozapine. *Clinical Nephrology* 2000; **43**: 78–80.
7. Elias TJ, Bannister KM, Clarkson AR *et al*. Clozapine induced acute interstitial nephritis. *Lancet* 1999; **354**: 11801–1811.
8. Lobeck F, Jethanandani V, Evans RL, Mirza MA. Haloperidol concentrations in an elderly patient with moderate chronic renal failure. *Journal of Geriatric Drug Therapy* 1986; **1**(2): 91–97.
9. Thyrum PT, Wong YWJ, Yeh C. Single-dose pharmacokinetics of quetiapine in subjects with renal or hepatic impairment. *Progress in Neuropsychopharmacology and Biological Psychiatry* 2000; **24**: 521–533.
10. Snoeck E, Van Peer A, Sack M *et al*. Influence of age, renal and liver impairment on the pharmacokinetics of risperidone in man. *Psychopharmacology* 1995; **122**: 223–229
11. Wong SL, Menacherry S, Mulford D *et al*. Pharmacokinetics of sertindole and dehydrosertindole in volunteers with normal or impaired renal function. *European Journal of Clinical Pharmacology* 1997; **52**: 223–227.
12. Bressolle F, Bres J, Mourad G. Pharmacokinetics of sulpiride after intravenous administration in patients with impaired renal function. *Clinical Pharmacokinetics* 1989; **17**: 367–373.
13. Aronoff GR Berns JS, Brier ME *et al*. *Drug Prescribing in Renal Failure – Dosing Guidelines for Adults*. Philadelphia (PA): American College of Physicians, 1998.
14. Sakalis G, Traficante LJ, Gershon S. Thioridazine metabolism and clinical response: A pilot study. *Current Therapeutic Research* 1977; **21**: 729–724.
15. Aweeka F, Jayesekara D, Horton M *et al*. The pharmacokinetics of ziprasidone in subjects with normal and impaired renal function. *British Journal of Clinical Pharmacology* 2000; **49**(S1): 27S–33S.
16. Lieberman JA *et al*. Tricyclic antidepressants and metabolite levels in chronic renal failure. *Clinical Pharmacology and Therapeutics* 1985; **37**: 301–307.
17. Spigset O, Hagg S, Stergmayr B *et al*. Citalopram pharmacokinetics in patients with chronic renal failure and the effect of haemodialysis. *European Journal of Clinical Pharmacology* 2000; **56**: 699–703
18. Joffe P, Larsen FS, Pedersen V *et al*. Single-dose pharmacokinetics of citalopram in patients with moderate renal insufficiency or hepatic cirrhosis compared with healthy subjects. *European Journal of Clinical Pharmacology* 1998; **54**: 237–242
19. Rees JA. Clinical interpretation of pharmacokinetic data on dothiepin hydrochloride (dosulepin, prothiaden). *Journal of International Medical Research* 1981; **9**: 98–102

20. Blumenfield M, Levy NB, Spinowitz B *et al.* Fluoxetine in depressed patients on dialysis. *International Journal of Psychiatry in Medicine* 1997; **27**: 71–80
21. Bergstrom RF, Beasley CM, Levy NB *et al.* The effects of renal and hepatic disease on the pharmacokinetics, renal tolerance and risk-benefit profile of fluoxetine. *International Clinical Psychopharmacology* 1993; **8**: 261–266
22. Lancaster SG, Gonzalez JP. Lofepramine. A review of its pharmacodynamic and pharmacokinetic properties and therapeutic efficacy in depressive illness. *Drugs* 1989; **37**: 123–140.
23. Schoerlin MP, Horber FF, Frey FJ *et al.* Disposition kinetics of moclobemide, a new MAO-A inhibitor, in subjects with impaired renal function. *Journal of Clinical Pharmacology* 1990; **30**: 272–274.
24. Stoeckel K, Pfefen JP, Mayersohn M *et al.* Absorption and disposition of moclobemide in patients with advanced age or reduced liver or kidney function. *Acta Psychiatrica Scandinavica* 1990; **360**(S): 94–97.
25. Pollock BG, Perel JM, Paradis CF *et al.* Metabolic and physiologic consequences of nortriptyline treatment in the elderly. *Psychopharmacology Bulletin* 1994; **30**: 145–150.
26. Doyle GD, Laher M, Kelly JG *et al.* The pharmacokinetics of paroxetine in renal impairment. *Acta Psychiatrica Scandinavica* 1989; **80**(S350): 89–90.
27. Kaye CM, Haddock RE, Langely PF *et al.* A review of the metabolism and pharmacokinetics of paroxetine in man. *Acta Psychiatrica Scandinavica* 1989; **80**(S350): 60–75.
28. Coulomb F, Ducret F, Laneury JP *et al.* Pharmacokinetics of single dose reboxetine in volunteers with renal insufficiency. *Journal of Clinical Pharmacology* 2000; **40**: 482–487.
29. Dostert P, Benedetti MS, Poggesi I. Review of the pharmacokinetics and metabolism of reboxetine, a selective noradrenaline reuptake inhibitor. *European Neuropsychopharmacology* 1997; 7(S1): S23–S35.
30. Catanese B, Dionisio A, Barillari G *et al.* A comparative study of trazodone serum concentrations in patients with normal or impaired renal function. *Bolletino di Chimica Farmaceutica* 1978; **117**: 424–427.
31. Simpson GM, Blair JH, Iqbal J *et al.* A preliminary study of trimipramine in chronic schizophrenia. *Current Therapeutics and Research* 1966; **99**: 248.
32. Leighton JD, Walker RJ, Lynn KL. Trimipramine induced acute renal failure (Letter). *New Zealand Medical Journal* 1986; **99**: 248.
33. Troy SM, Schultz RW, Parker VD *et al.* The effect of renal disease on the disposition of venlafaxine. *Clinical Pharmacology and Therapeutics* 1994; **56**: 14–21.
34. Pentikainen PJ, Neuvonen PJ, Jostell KG. Pharmacokinetics of chlormethiazole in healthy volunteers and patients with cirrhosis of the liver. *European Journal of Clinical Pharmacology* 1980; **17**: 275–284.
35. Sadjadi SA, McLaughlin K, Shah RM. Allergic interstitial nephritis due to diazepam. *Archives of Internal Medicine* 1987; **147**: 579.
36. Verbeeck RK, Tjandramaga TB, de Schepper PJ *et al.* Impaired elimination of lorazepam following subchronic administration in two patients with renal failure. *British Journal of Clinical Pharmacology* 1981; **12**: 749–751.
37. Reynolds HN, Teiken P, Regan ME *et al.* Hyperlactinemia, increased osmolar gap and renal dysfunction during continuous lorazepam infusion. *Critical Care Medicine* 2000; **28**: 1631–1634.
38. Murray TG, Chiang ST, Koepke HH *et al.* Renal disease, age and oxazepam kinetics. *Clinical Pharmacology and Therapeutics* 1981; **30**: 805–809.
39. Goa KL & Heel RC. Zopiclone. A review of its pharmacodynamic and pharmacokinetic properties and therapeutic efficacy as a hypnotic. *Drugs* 1986; **32**: 48–65.
40. Verrotti A, Greco R, Pascarella R *et al.* Renal tubular function in patients receiving anticonvulsant therapy: A long term study. *Epilepsia* 2000; **41**: 1432–1435.
41. Hogg RJ, Sawyer M, Hecox K *et al.* Carbamazepine-induced acute tubulointerstitial nephritis. *Journal of Pediatrics* 1981; **98**: 830–831.
42. Hegarty J, Picton M, Agarwal G *et al.* Carbamazepine-induced acute granulomatous interstitial nephritis. *Clinical Nephrology* 2002; **57**: 310–313.
43. Nicholls DP, Yasin M. Acute renal failure from carbamazepine (Letter). *British Medical Journal* 1972; **4**: 490.
44. Jubert P, Almirall J, Casanovas A *et al.* Carbamazepine-induced acute renal failure. *Nephron* 1994; **66**: 121
45. Imai H, Nakamoto Y, Hirokawa M *et al.* Carbamazepine-induced granulomatous necrotizing angiitis with acute renal failure. *Nephron* 1989; **51**: 405–408.
46. Fillasatre JP, Taburet AM, Failaire A *et al.* Pharmacokinetics of lamotrigine in patients with renal impairment – influence of hemodialysis. *Drugs Exp Clinical Research* 1993; **19**: 25–32.
47. Wootton R, Soul-Lawton J, Rolan PE *et al.* Comparison of the pharmacokinetics of lamotrigine in patients with chronic renal failure and healthy volunteers. *British Journal of Clinical Pharmacology* 1997; **43**: 23–27.
48. Schaub JEM, Williamson PJ, Barnes EW *et al.* Multisystem adverse reaction to lamotrigine. *Lancet* 1994; **344**: 481.
49. Fervenza FC, Kanakiriya S, Kunau RT *et al.* Acute granulomatous interstitial nephritis and colitis in anticonvulsant hypersensitivity syndrome associated with lamotrigine treatment. *American Journal of Kidney Diseases* 2000; **36**: 1034–1040.
50. Smith GC, Balfe JW & Kooh SW. Anticonvulsants as a cause of Fanconi syndrome. *Nephrol Dial Transplant* 1995; **10**: 543–545.
51. Fukuda Y, Watanabe H, Ohtomo Y *et al.* Immunologically mediated chronic tubulo-interstitial nephritis caused by valproate treatment. *Nephron* 1996; **72**: 328–329.
52. Zaki EL, Springate JE. Renal injury from valproic acid: case report and literature review. *Pediatric Neurology* 2002; **27**: 318–319.
53. Tanaka H, Onodera N, Ryosuke I et al. Distal type of renal tubular acidosis after anti-epileptic therapy in a girl with infantile spasms. *Clinical & Experimental Nephrology* 1999; **3**: 311–313.
54. Gitlin M. Lithium and the kidney, an updated review. *Drug Safety* 1999; **20**: 231–243.

Hepatic impairment

Patients with hepatic impairment may have:

- **Reduced capacity to metabolise** biological waste products, dietary proteins and foreign substances such as drugs. Clinical consequences include hepatic encephalopathy and increased dose-related side-effects from drugs.

- **Reduced ability to synthesise** plasma proteins and vitamin K-dependent clotting factors. Clinical consequences include hypoalbuminaemia, leading in extreme cases to ascites. Increased toxicity from highly protein bound drugs should be anticipated. There is also an increased risk of bleeding from GI irritant drugs.

- **Reduced hepatic blood flow.** Clinical consequences include oesophageal varices.

General principles

LFTs are a poor marker of hepatic metabolising capacity, as the hepatic reserve is large. There are few clinical studies relating to the use of psychotropic drugs in people with hepatic disease. The following principles should be adhered to:

1. Prescribe as **few drugs** as possible.

2. Use **lower starting doses**, particularly of drugs that are highly protein bound. TCAs, SSRIs (except citalopram), trazodone and antipsychotics may have increased free plasma levels, at least initially. This will not be reflected in measured (total) plasma levels. Use lower doses of drugs known to be subject to extensive first pass metabolism. Examples include TCAs and haloperidol.

3. Be **cautious with drugs that are extensively hepatically metabolised** (most psychotropic drugs). Lower doses may be required. Exceptions are sulpiride, amisulpride, lithium and gabapentin which all undergo no or minimal hepatic metabolism.

4. **Leave longer intervals between dosage increases.** Remember that the half-life of most drugs is prolonged in hepatic impairment, so it will take longer for plasma levels to reach steady state.

5. Always **monitor carefully for side effects**, which may be delayed.

6. **Avoid drugs that are very sedative** because of the risk of precipitating hepatic encephalopathy.

7. **Avoid drugs that are very constipating** because of the risk of precipitating hepatic encephalopathy.

8. **Avoid drugs that are known to be hepatotoxic** in their own right (eg MAOIs, chlorpromazine).

9. **Choose a low risk drug** (see tables below) and **monitor LFTs** weekly, at least initially. If LFTs deteriorate after a new drug is introduced, consider switching to another drug.

These rules should always be observed in severe liver disease (low albumin, increased clotting time, ascites, jaundice, encephalopathy, etc). Many patients with chronic liver disease are asymptomatic or have fluctuating clinical symptoms. The information above, and on the following pages, should be interpreted in the context of the patient's clinical presentation.

Table Antipsychotics in hepatic impairment

Drug	Comments
Amisulpride[1,2]	Predominantly renally excreted, so dosage reduction should not be necessary as long as renal function is normal BUT there are no clinical studies in people with hepatic impairment and little clinical experience. Caution required
Clozapine[1–5]	Very sedative and constipating. Contraindicated in active liver disease associated with nausea, anorexia or jaundice, progressive liver disease or hepatic failure. In less severe disease, start with 12.5 mg and increase slowly using plasma levels to gauge metabolising capacity and guide dosage adjustment Transient elevations in AST, ALT and GGT to over twice the normal range occur in over 10% of physically healthy people. Clozapine-induced hepatitis, jaundice, cholestasis and liver failure have been reported
Flupentixol/ zuclopenthixol[1,2,6,7]	Both are extensively hepatically metabolised. Small, transient elevations in transaminases have been reported in some patients treated with zuclopenthixol. No other literature reports of use or harm. Both drugs have been in use for many years. Depot preparations are best avoided as altered pharmacokinetics will make dosage adjustment difficult and side effects from dosage accumulation more likely
Haloperidol[1]	Drug of choice in clinical practice and no problems reported although UK SPC states 'caution in liver disease'
Olanzapine[1,2,8]	Although extensively hepatically metabolised, the pharmacokinetics of olanzapine seem to change little in severe hepatic impairment. It is sedative and anticholinergic (can cause constipation) so caution advised. Consider using plasma levels to guide dosage (aim for 20–40 µg/l). Dose related, transient, asymptomatic elevations in ALT & AST reported in physically healthy adults. People with liver disease may be at increased risk
Phenothiazines[1,2,9,10]	All cause sedation and constipation. Associated with cholestasis and some reports of fulminant hepatic cirrhosis. Best avoided completely in hepatic impairment. Chlorpromazine is particularly hepatotoxic
Quetiapine[1,2,11–13]	Extensively hepatically metabolised but short half-life. One single dose kinetic study suggests that no change in starting dose is required. Clearance reduced by a mean of 30% in hepatic impairment so small dosage adjustments may be required. Can cause sedation and constipation. Little clinical experience in hepatic impairment so caution recommended
Risperidone[1,2,14–16]	Highly protein bound. Manufacturers recommend a maximum dose of 4 mg in hepatic impairment. Transient, asymptomatic elevations in LFTs, cholestatic hepatitis and rare cases of hepatic failure have been reported. Clinical experience limited in hepatic impairment so caution recommended
Sulpiride[1,2,17,18]	Almost completely renally excreted with a low potential to cause sedation or constipation. Dosage reduction should not be required. Some clinical experience in hepatic impairment with few problems. Very old established drug. Isolated case reports of cholestatic jaundice and primary biliary cirrhosis

Table Antidepressants in hepatic impairment

Drug	Comments
Fluoxetine[1,2,19–23]	Extensively hepatically metabolised with a long half-life. Kinetic studies demonstrate accumulation in compensated cirrhosis. Although dosage reduction (of at least 50%) or alternate day dosing could be used, it would take many weeks to reach steady state serum levels, making fluoxetine complex to use. Asymptomatic increases in LFTs found in 0.5% of healthy adults. Rare cases of hepatitis reported
Other SSRIs[1,2,23–30]	All are hepatically metabolised and accumulate on chronic dosing. Dosage reduction may be required Raised LFTs and rare cases of hepatitis, including chronic active hepatitis have been reported with paroxetine. Sertraline and fluvoxamine have also been associated with hepatitis Citalopram has minimal effects on hepatic enzymes and may be the SSRI of choice although clinical experience is limited. Paroxetine is used by some specialised liver units with few apparent problems
Tricyclics[1,2,31]	All are hepatically metabolised, highly protein bound and will accumulate. They vary in their propensity to cause sedation and constipation. All are associated with raised LFTs and rare cases of hepatitis There is most clinical experience with imipramine. Sedative TCAs such as trimipramine, dothiepin (dosulepin) and amitriptyline are best avoided. Lofepramine is possibly the most hepatotoxic and should be avoided completely
Venlafaxine[1,2,32]	Dosage reduction of 50% advised in moderate hepatic impairment. Little clinical experience. Rare cases of hepatitis reported. Caution advised
MAOIs[1,2,33,34]	People with hepatic impairment reported to be more sensitive to the side-effects of MAOIs. MAOIs are also more hepatotoxic than other antidepressants, so best avoided completely
Moclobemide[1,2,35,36]	Clinical experience limited but probably safer than the irreversible MAOIs. 50% reduction in dose advised by manufacturers. Rare cases of hepatotoxicity reported. Caution advised
Reboxetine[1,2,37]	50% reduction in starting dose recommended. Clinical experience limited. Does not seem to be associated with hepatotoxicity. Caution advised
Mirtazapine[1,2]	Hepatically metabolised and sedative. 50% dose reduction recommended based on kinetic data, but clinical experience limited. Mild, asymptomatic increases in LFTs seen in healthy adults. Caution advised

Table Mood stabilisers in hepatic impairment

Drug	Comments
Carbamazepine[1,2,38–40]	Extensively hepatically metabolised and potent inducer of CYP450 enzymes. Contraindicated in acute liver disease. In chronic stable disease, caution advised. Reduce starting dose by 50%, and titrate up slowly using plasma levels to guide dosage. Stop if LFTs deteriorate Associated with hepatitis, cholangitis, cholestatic and hepatocellular jaundice and hepatic failure (rare). Adverse hepatic effects are most common in the first month of treatment
Lamotrigine[1,2,41]	Manufacturers recommend 50% reduction in initial dose, dose escalation and maintenance dose in moderate hepatic impairment and 75% in severe Lamotrigine induced rash (which can be serious) is associated with too rapid dosage titration. Extreme caution advised, particularly if co-prescribed with valproate. Elevated LFTs and hepatitis reported
Lithium[1,2,42,43]	Not metabolised so dosage reduction not required as long as renal function is normal. Use serum levels to guide dosage and monitor more frequently if ascites status changes (volume of distribution will change). One case of ascites and one of hyperbilirubinaemia reported over many decades of lithium use worldwide
Valproate[1,2,44–46]	Highly protein bound and hepatically metabolised. Dosage reduction with close monitoring of LFTs in moderate hepatic impairment. Use plasma levels (free levels if possible) to guide dosage. Caution advised. Contraindicated in severe and/or active hepatic impairment Associated with elevated LFTs and serious hepatotoxicity including fulminant hepatic failure. Mitochondrial disease may be a risk factor. Particularly hepatotoxic in children

Summary – psychotropics in hepatic impairment

Drug group	Recommended drugs
Antipsychotics	**Haloperidol**: low dose *or* **Sulpiride/amisulpride**: no dosage reduction required if renal function is normal
Antidepressants	**Imipramine**: start with 25 mg/day and titrate slowly (weekly at most) if required *or* **Paroxetine** or **citalopram**: start at 10 mg if severe hepatic impairment. Titrate slowly (if required) as above
Mood stablisers	**Lithium**: Use plasma levels to guide dosage. Care if ascites status changes
Sedatives	**Lorazepam, oxazepam, temazepam**: as short half-life with no active metabolites Use low doses with caution as sedative drugs can precipitate hepatic encephalopathy **Zopiclone**: 3.75 mg with care in moderate hepatic impairment

References

1. www.emc.vhn.net/professional/
2. micromedex.
3. Hummer M, Kurz M, Kurzthaler I et al. Hepatotoxicity of clozapine. Journal of Psychopharmacology 1997; **17**: 314–317.
4. Kellner CH. Toxic hepatitis by clozapine treatment. American Journal of Psychiatry 1993; **150**: 985–986.
5. Thatcher GW. Clozapine induced toxic hepatitis. American Journal of Psychiatry 1995; **152**: 296–297.
6. Amdisen A, Nielsen MS, Dencker SJ et al. Zuclopenthixol acetate in viscoleo. Acta Psychiatrica Scandinavica 1987; **75**: 99–107.
7. Wistedt B, Koskinen T, Thelander S et al. Zuclopenthixol decanoate and haloperidol decanoate in chronic schizophrenia: a double-blind multicentre study. Acta Psychiatrica Scandinavica 1991; **84**: 14–16.
8. Beasley CM, Tollefson GD, Tran PV. Safety of olanzapine. Journal of Clinical Psychiatry 1997; **58**(Suppl. 10): 13–17.
9. Regal R, Billi JE, Glazer HM. Phenothiazine-induced cholestatic jaundice. Clinical Pharmacy 1987; **6**: 787–794.
10. Zimmerman HJ & Lewis JH. Drug induced cholestasis. Medical Toxicology 1987; **2**: 112–160.
11. Thyrum PT, Wong YW, Yeh C. Single dose pharmacokinetics of quetiapine in subjects with renal or hepatic impairment. Progress in Neuropsychopharmacology and Biological Psychiatry 2000; **24**: 521–533.
12. Nemeroff CB, Kinkead B, Goldstein J. Quetiapine: preclinical studies, pharmacokinetics, drug interactions and dosing. Journal of Clinical Psychiatry 2002; **63**(Suppl. 13): 5–11.
13. Green B. Focus on quetiapine. Current Medical Research & Opinion 1999; **15**: 145–151.
14. Cordeiro Q, Elkis H. Pancreatitis and cholestatic hepatitis induced by risperidone. Journal of Clinical Psychopharmacology 2001; **21**: 529–530.
15. Phillips EJ, Liu BA, Knowles SR. Rapid onset of risperidone induced hepatotoxicity. Annals of Pharmacotherapy 1998; **32**: 843.
16. Whitworth AB. Liensberger D, Gleischhacker WW. Transient increase of liver enzymes induced by risperidone: two case reports. Journal of Clinical Psychopharmacology 1999; **19**: 475–476.
17. Melzer E, Knobel B. Severe cholestatic jaundice due to sulpiride. Israeli Journal of Medical Science 1987; **23**: 1259–1260.
18. Ohmoto K, Yamamoto S, Hirokawa M. Symptomatic primary biliary cirrhosis triggered by administration of sulpiride. American Journal of Gastroenterology 1999; **94**: 3660–3661.
19. Schenker S, Bergstrom RF, Wolen RL et al. Fluoxetine disposition and elimination in cirrhosis. Clinical Pharmacy & Therapeutics 1998; **44**: 353–359.
20. Cai Q, Benson MA, Talbot TJ et al. Acute hepatitis due to fluoxetine therapy. Mayo Clinic Proceedings 1999; **74**: 692–694.
21. Friedenberg FK, Rothstein KD. Hepatitis due to fluoxetine treatment. American Journal of Psychiatry 1996; **153**: 580.
22. Johnston DE, Wheeler DE. Chronic hepatitis related to use of fluoxetine. American Journal of Gastroenterology 1997; **92**: 1225–1226.
23. Hale AS. New antidepressants: use in high-risk patients. Journal of Clinical Psychiatry 1993; **54**(Suppl. 8): 61–70
24. Benbow SJ, Gill G. Paroxetine and hepatotoxicity. BMJ 1997; **314**: 1387.
25. Odeh M, Misselevech I, Boss JH et al. Severe hepatotoxicity with jaundice associated with paroxetine. American Journal of Gastroenterology 2001; **96**: 2494–2496.
26. Dunbar GC. An interim overview of the safety and tolerability of paroxetine. Acta Psychiatrica Scandinavica 1989; **80**(Suppl. 350): 135–137.
27. Kuhs H, Rudolf GAE. A double blind study of the comparative antidepressant effect of paroxetine and amitriptyline. Acta Psychiatrica Scandinavica 1989; **80**(Suppl. 350): 145–146.
28. DeBree H, Van der Schoot JB, Post LC. Fluvoxamine maleate: disposition in man. European Journal of Drug Metabolism & Pharmacokinetics 1983; **8**: 175–179.
29. Green BH. Fluvoxamine and hepatic function. British Journal of Psychiatry 1998; **153**: 130–131.
30. Milne RJ, Goa KL, Citalopram: a review of its pharmacodynamic and pharmacokinetic properties, and therapeutic potential in depressive illness. Drugs 1991; **41**: 450–477.
31. Committee on Safety of Medicines. Lofepramine (Gamanil) and abnormal blood tests of liver function. Current Problems 1988; **23**: 2.
32. Cardona X, Avila A, Castellanos P. Venlafaxine-associated hepatitis. Annals of Internal Medicine 2000; **132**: 417.
33. Gomez GE, Salmeron JM, Mas A. Phenelzine induced fulminant hepatic failure. Annals of Internal Medicine 1996; **124**: 692–693.
34. Bonkovsky HL, Blanchette PL, Schned AR. Severe liver injusry due to phenelzine with unique hepatic deposition of extracellular material. American Journal of Medicine 1986; **80**: 689–692.
35. Stoeckel K, Pfefen JP, Mayersohn M et al. Absorption and disposition of moclobemide in patients with advanced age or reduced liver or kidney function. Acta Psychiatrica Scandinavica 1990; **360**: 94–97.
36. Timmings P, Lamont D. Intrahepatic cholestasis associated with moclobemide leading to death. Lancet 1996; **347**: 762–763.
37. Tran A, Laneury JP, Duchene P et al. Pharmacokinetics of reboxetine in patients with hepatic impairment. Clinical Drug Investigations 2000; **9**: 473–477.
38. El-Serag HB, Johnston DE. Carbamazepine-associated severe bile duct injury. American Journal of Gastroenterology 1999; **92**: 526–527.
39. Forbes GM, Jeffrey GP, Shilkin KB et al. Carbamazepine hepatotoxicity: another cause of vanishing bile duct syndrome. Gastroenterology 1992; **102**: 1385–1388.
40. Morales-Diaz M, Pinilla-Roa E, Ruiz I. Suspected carbamazepine-induced hepatotoxicity. Pharmacotherapy 1999; **19**: 252–255.
41. Sauve G, Bresson-Hadni S, Prost P et al. Acute hepatitis after lamotrigine administration. Digestive Diseases and Sciences 2000; **45**: 1874–1877
42. Cohen LS, Cohen DE. Lithium-induced hyperbilirubinemia in an adolescent. Journal of Clinical Psychopharmacology 1991; **11**: 274–275.
43. Hazelwood RE. Ascites: a side effect of lithium? American Journal of Psychiatry 1981; **138**: 257.
44. Krahenbuhl S, Brandner S, Kleinle S et al. Mitochondrial diseases represent a risk factor for valproate-induced fulminant liver failure. Liver 2000; **20**: 346–348.
45. Klotz U, Rapp T, Muller WA et al. Disposition of valproate acid in patients with liver disease. European Journal of Clinical Pharmacology 1978; **13**: 550–560.
46. Pinkston R, Walker LA. Multiorgan system failure caused by valproic acid toxicity. American Journal of Emergency Medicine 1997; **15**: 504–506.

Prescribing in the elderly

General principles

The pharmacokinetics and pharmacodynamics of most drugs are altered to an important extent in the elderly. These changes in drug action must be taken into account if treatment is to be effective and adverse effects minimised. The elderly often have a number of concurrent illnesses and may require treatment with several drugs. This leads to a greater chance of problems arising because of drug interactions and to a higher rate of drug-induced problems in general[1]. It is reasonable to assume that all drugs are more likely to cause adverse effects in the elderly than in younger patients.

How drugs affect the ageing body (altered pharmacodynamics)

As we age, control over reflex actions such as blood pressure and temperature regulation is reduced. Receptors may become more sensitive. This results in an increased incidence and severity of side-effects. For example, drugs that decrease gut motility are more likely to cause constipation (e.g. TCAs and opioids) and drugs that affect blood pressure are more likely to cause falls (e.g. TCAs and diuretics). The elderly are more sensitive to the effects of benzodiazepines than younger adults. Therapeutic response can also be delayed; the elderly may take longer to respond to antidepressants than younger adults[2].

How the ageing body affects drug therapy (altered pharmacokinetics)[3]

ABSORPTION

Gut motility decreases with age, as does secretion of gastric acid. This leads to drugs being absorbed more slowly, resulting in a slower onset of action. The same *amount* of drug is absorbed as in a younger adult.

DISTRIBUTION

The elderly have more body fat, less body water and less albumin than younger adults. This leads to an increased volume of distribution and a longer duration of action for some fat-soluble drugs (e.g. diazepam), higher concentrations of some drugs at the site of action (e.g. digoxin) and a reduction in the amount of drug bound to albumin (increased amounts of active 'free drug', e.g. warfarin, phenytoin).

METABOLISM

The majority of drugs are hepatically metabolised. Liver size is reduced in the elderly, but in the absence of hepatic disease or significantly reduced hepatic blood flow, there is no significant reduction in metabolic capacity. The magnitude of pharmacokinetic interactions is unlikely to be altered but the pharmacodynamic consequences of these interactions may be amplified.

EXCRETION

Renal function declines with age: 35% of function is lost by the age of 65 years and 50% by the age of 80.

More is lost if there are concurrent medical problems such as heart disease, diabetes or hypertension. Measurement of serum creatinine or urea can be misleading in the elderly because muscle mass is reduced, so less creatinine is produced. Creatinine clearance is the only accurate measure of renal function in this age group. It is best to assume that all elderly patients have at most two-thirds of normal renal function.

Most drugs are eventually excreted by the kidney. A few do not undergo biotransformation first. Lithium and sulpiride are important examples. Drugs primarily excreted via the kidney will accumulate in the elderly, leading to toxicity and side-effects. Dosage reduction is likely to be required (see page 217 et seq. for full review of renal effects of psychotropics).

Drug interactions

Some drugs have a narrow therapeutic index (a small increase in dose can cause toxicity and a small reduction in dose can cause a loss of therapeutic action). The most commonly prescribed examples are: digoxin, warfarin, theophylline, phenytoin and lithium. Changes in the way these drugs are handled in the elderly and the greater chance of interaction with other drugs mean that toxicity and therapeutic failure are more likely. These drugs can be used safely but extra care must be taken and blood levels should be measured where possible.

Some drugs inhibit or induce hepatic metabolising enzymes. Important examples include the SSRIs, erythromycin and carbamazepine (see page 154 for further information). This may lead to the metabolism of another drug being altered. Many drug interactions occur through this mechanism. Details of individual interactions and their consequences can be found in Appendix 1 of the *British National Formulary*. Most can be predicted by a sound knowledge of pharmacology.

Reducing drug-related risk

Adherence to the following principles will reduce drug-related morbidity and mortality:

- Only use drugs when absolutely necessary.
- Avoid, if possible, drugs that block α_1 adrenoceptors, have anticholinergic side-effects, are very sedative, have a long half-life or are potent inhibitors of hepatic metabolising enzymes.
- Start with a low dose and increase slowly but do not undertreat. Some drugs still require the full adult dose.
- Try not to treat the side-effects of one drug with another drug. Find a better-tolerated alternative.
- Keep therapy simple, i.e. once daily administration whenever possible.

Administering medicines in foodstuffs[4,5]

Sometimes patients may refuse treatment with medicines, even when such treatment is thought to be in their best interests. Where the patient has a mental illness or has capacity, the mental health act should be used, but if the patient lacks capacity, this option may not be desirable. Medicines should never be administered covertly to elderly patients with dementia without a full discussion with the MDT and the patient's relatives. The outcome of this discussion should be clearly documented in the patient's clinical notes. Medicine should only ever be administered covertly if the clear and express purpose is to reduce suffering for the patient.

References

1. Royal College of Physicians. Medication for older people. Summary and recommendations of a report of a working party of the Royal College of Physicians. *Journal of the Royal College of Physicians of London* 1997; **3**: 254–257.
2. Paykel ES, Raman R, Cooper Z *et al.* Residual symptoms after partial remission: an important outcome in depression. *Psychological Medicine* 1995; **25**: 1171–1180.
3. Mayersohn M. Special pharmacokinetic considerations in the elderly. In: Evans WE, Schentag JJ, Jusko WJ (eds). *Applied Therapeutics: principles of therapeutic drug monitoring*. Spokane, WA: Applied Therapeutics Inc., 1986, pp. 229–293.
4. Treloar A, Philpot M, Beats B. Concealing medication in patients' food. *Lancet* 2001; **357**: 62–64.
5. Treloar A, Beck S, Paton C. Administering medicines to patients with dementia and other organic cognitive syndromes. *Advances in Psychiatric Treatment* 2001; **7**: 444–450.

Further reading

National Service Framework for Older People. London: Department of Health, 2001.

Alzheimer's disease

Acetylcholinesterase inhibitors

Four inhibitors of acetylcholinesterase are currently licensed in the UK for the treatment of Alzheimer's disease: tacrine, donepezil, rivastigmine, galantamine. Tacrine is very poorly tolerated and has been superseded by the other three drugs. Cholinesterase inhibitors differ in pharmacological action: donepezil and galantamine are selective inhibitors of acetylcholinesterase (AChE); rivastigmine affects both AChE and butyrylcholinesterase (BuChE); donepezil and rivastigmine are relatively selective for AChE in the brain; and galantamine also affects nicotinic receptors[1]. To date, these differences have not been shown to result in differences in efficacy or tolerability.

All three drugs seem to have broadly similar clinical effects, as measured using the Mini Mental State Examination (MMSE – a 30-point basic evaluation of cognitive function) and the Alzheimer's Disease Assessment Scale – cognitive sub-scale (ADAS-cog – a 70-point evaluation largely of cognitive dysfunction). Major trials of donepezil[2–4] suggest an advantage over placebo of 2.5–3.1 points on the ADAS-cog scale. For rivastigmine[5,6] the advantage is 2.6–4.9 points and for galantamine[7–9] 2.9–3.9. Estimates of the number needed to treat (NNT) (improvement of >4 points ADAS-cog) range from 4 to 12.

These results need to be interpreted with caution, especially as no head-to-head studies have been published. Alzheimer's disease is usually characterised by inexorable cognitive decline, which is generally well quantified by tests such as ADAS-cog and MMSE. The average rate of decline is 4–6 points on the ADAS-cog over 1 year, but the range is large. It is therefore difficult to accurately assess treatment effect in individual patients. The effect of anticholinesterases is, on average, to improve modestly cognitive function for several months (scores return to baseline after about 9–12 months)[4,8].

This average incorporates and to some extent conceals 3 groups of patients: 'non-responders', who continue to decline at the anticipated rate; 'non-decliners', who neither improve significantly nor decline; and 'improvers' who improve to a clinically relevant extent. This last group is usually defined as those who show a >4 point improvement on ADAS-cog. In trials of around 6 months, approximately 25–35% of those on anticholinesterases will be classified as 'improvers' compared with around 15–25% on placebo. Around 55–70% of patients treated with anticholinesterases will show no cognitive decline during a 5–6-month trial[6,8] – about 20% more patients in absolute terms than those on placebo. Note that, for the most part, results of trials so far conducted relate only to patients with mild-to-moderate Alzheimer's disease (those giving a score of 10–26 on MMSE).

Taking into account trial differences and all assessments made, available anticholinesterases can be said to have broadly similar efficacy against cognitive symptoms in clinical trials. Any minor differences observed may be accounted for by differences in trial design or patient characteristics. In the absence of any 'head-to-head' studies, the available drugs should be assumed to have equal efficacy. Overall, in a cohort of patients given anticholinesterases at optimal doses under clinical trial conditions, approximately one-third would be expected to improve over 6 months and around another third would be expected not to deteriorate. These observations appear to be broadly reflected in practice.

Other effects

Anticholinesterases may also affect non-cognitive aspects of Alzheimer's disease. For example, they seem to have useful psychotropic activity against neuropsychiatric symptoms[10–12]. These drugs may also lower care-giver burden[13] and improve patients' abilities with daily activities[14]. Differential effects for different drugs have yet to be demonstrated.

Tolerability

Drug tolerability may differ between anticholinesterases but, again, in the absence of direct comparisons, it is difficult to draw cogent conclusions. Overall tolerability can be broadly evaluated by reference to numbers withdrawing from clinical trials. Withdrawal rates in trials of donepezil[2,3], ranged from 4 to 16% (placebo 1–7%). With rivastigmine[5,6] rates ranged from 7 to 29% (placebo 7%) and with galantamine[7–9] from 7 to 23% (placebo 7–9%). (All figures relate to withdrawals specifically associated with adverse effects.)

Tolerability seems to be affected by speed of titration and, perhaps less clearly, by dose. Most adverse effects occurred in trials during titration and slower titration schedules are recommended in clinical use. This may mean that these drugs are equally well tolerated in practice.

Dosing

Different titration schedules do, to some extent, differentiate anticholinesterases. **Donepezil** is perhaps easiest to use, starting at 5 mg/day and increasing 'if necessary' (however this might be determined) to 10 mg after a month. **Rivastigmine** is taken twice daily, starting at 1.5 mg bd then increasing to 3 mg bd after 2 weeks or more and then to 4.5 mg bd after a further 2 weeks (max. 6 mg bd). With **galantamine**, the starting dose is 4 mg twice daily, increasing to 8 mg twice daily after 4 weeks and then to 12 mg bd, if necessary, 4 weeks later. Thus, both rivastigmine and galantamine need to be given twice daily and have prolonged titration schedules. These factors may be important to prescribers, patients and carers.

Interactions

Potential for interaction may also differentiate currently available cholinesterase inhibitors. Donepezil[15] and galantamine[16] are metabolised by cytochromes 2D6 and 3A4 and so drug levels may be altered by other drugs affecting the function of these enzymes. Also anticholinesterases themselves may interfere with the metabolism of other drugs, although this is perhaps a theoretical consideration. Rivastigmine has almost no potential for interaction since it is metabolised at the site of action and does not affect hepatic cytochromes. Overall, rivastigmine appears to be least likely to cause problematic drug interactions, a factor that may be important in an elderly population subject to polypharmacy.

Adverse effects

When adverse effects occur, they are largely predictable: excess cholinergic stimulation leads to nausea, vomiting, dizziness, insomnia and diarrhoea[17]. Urinary incontinence has also been reported[18]. There appear to be no important differences between drugs in respect to type or frequency of adverse events, although clinical trials do suggest relatively lower frequency of adverse events for donepezil. This may simply be a reflection of somewhat aggressive titration schedules used in trials of other drugs.

NICE recommendations[19]

Using a protocol like that suggested by NICE (overleaf) may mean that, of a cohort of patients referred for treatment, only three-quarters may be considered suitable for treatment and only one-third of these may continue treatment for a year or more[20]. In contrast, in the artificial environment of a clinical trial, nearly half of patients continued for 2 years or more[21].

Summary of NICE guidance on anticholinesterases

- Anticholinesterase drugs may be prescribed for those with Alzheimer's disease with a MMSE score of >12 points.
- Diagnosis must be made in a specialist clinic.
- Assessments of cognitive functioning and activities of daily living should be made before starting drug treatment.
- Only specialists should initiate treatment.
- Only those likely to comply with drug treatment should be considered.
- Further assessments should be made 2–4 months after starting treatment. If MMSE scores indicated no deterioration or improvement and there is evidence of global or functional improvement then treatment should continue.
- Those remaining on drug treatment should thereafter be assessed at 6-monthly intervals. Anticholinesterases should not normally be used in patients where MMSE scores fall before 12 points.

Memantine

Memantine is licensed in the UK for the treatment of moderately severe to severe Alzheimer's disease. It acts as an antagonist at N-methyl-D-aspartate (NMDA) receptors, an action which, in theory, may be neuroprotective and thus disease-modifying[22]. Memantine appears to be well tolerated[23] but clinical experience is limited. Trials in severe dementia[24] and vascular dementia[25] suggest an advantage over placebo of around 2 points on the ADAS-cog scale and NNTs (improvement) of 4–10. Improvement was also seen in other domains of functioning.

Memantine's place in therapy has yet to be established. It is effective, but the exact magnitude of its effect and its clinical importance have yet to be established. Combined treatment with anticholinesterases is possible, but is untested and currently not recommended.

Table Summary – anticholinesterases in Alzheimer's disease

Drug	Starting dose	Usual treatment dose	Adverse effects	Costs (1 month's treatment) at usual dose
Donepezil	5 mg daily	10 mg daily	Nausea Vomiting Insomnia Diarrhoea	£103
Rivastigmine	1.5 mg bd	6 mg bd	Nausea Vomiting Insomnia Diarrhoea	£67
Galantamine	4 mg bd	12 mg bd	Nausea Vomiting Insomnia Diarrhoea	£90
Memantine	5 mg daily	20 mg daily	Hallucinations Dizziness Confusion	£79

References

1. Weinstock M. Selectivity of cholinesterase inhibition: clinical implications for the treatment of Alzheimer's disease. *CNS Drugs* 1999; **12**: 307–323.
2. Rogers SL, Doody RS, Mohs RC *et al.* Donepezil improves cognition and global function in Alzheimer Disease: a 15-week, double-blind, placebo-controlled study. *Archives of Internal Medicine* 1998; **158**: 1021–1031.
3. Rogers SL, Farlow MR, Doody RS *et al.* A 24-week, double-blind, placebo-controlled trial of donepezil in patients with Alzheimer's disease. *Neurology* 1998; **50**: 136–145.
4. Rogers SL, Friedhoff LT. Long-term efficacy and safety of donepezil in the treatment of Alzheimer's disease: an interim analysis of the results of a US multicentre open label extension study. *European Neuropsychopharmacology* 1998; **8**: 67–75.
5. Corey-Bloom J, Anand R, Veach J. A randomized trial evaluating the efficacy and safety of ENA 713 (rivastigmine tartrate), a new acetylcholinesterase inhibitor, in patients with mild to moderately severe Alzheimer's disease. *International Journal of Geriatric Psychopharmacology* 1998; **1**: 55–65.
6. Rösler M, Anand R, Cicin-Sain A *et al.* Efficacy and safety of rivastigmine in patients with Alzheimer's disease: international randomised controlled trial. *BMJ* 1999; **318**: 633–640.
7. Tariot PN, Solomon PR, Morris JC *et al.* A 5-month, randomized, placebo-controlled trial of galantamine in AD. *Neurology* 2000; **54**: 2269–2276.
8. Raskind MA, Peskind ER, Wessel T *et al.* 6-month randomized, placebo-controlled trial with a 6-month extension. *Neurology* 2000; **54**: 2261–2268.
9. Wilcock GK, Lilienfeld S, Gaens E. Efficacy and safety of galantamine in patients with mild to moderate Alzheimer's disease: multicentre randomised controlled trial. *MBJ* 2000; **321**: 1445–1449.
10. Cummings JL, Askin-Edgar S. Evidence for psychotropic effects of acetylcholinesterase inhibitors. *CNS Drugs* 2000; **13**: 385–395.
11. Weiner MF, Martin-Cook K, Foster BM *et al.* Effects of donepezil on emotional/behavioral symptoms in Alzheimer's disease patients. *Journal of Clinical Psychiatry* 2000; **61**: 487–492.
12. Blesa R. Galantamine: therapeutic effects beyond cognition. *Dementia, Geriatric Cognitive Disorders* 2000; **11**(Suppl. 1): 28–34.
13. Gauthier S, Lussier I, and the TriAD™ Study Group. An open-label trial to assess the effectiveness of donepezil treatment on caregiver burden in Alzheimer's disease – an interim report. Poster presented at the Ninth Congress of the International Psychogeriatric Association, August 15–20, Vancouver, Canada, 1999.
14. Winblad B, Engedal K, Soininen H *et al.* Donepezil enhances global function, cognition and activities of daily living compared with placebo in a one-year, double-blind trial in patients with mild to moderate Alzheimer's disease. Poster presented at the Ninth Congress of the International Psychogeriatric Association, August 15–20, 1, Vancouver, Canada, 1999.
15. Dooley M, Lamb H. Donepezil. *Drugs and Aging* 2000; **16**: 199–226.
16. Scott LJ, Goa KL. Galantamine: a review of its use in Alzheimer's disease. *Drugs* 2000; **60**: 1095–1122.
17. Dunn NR, Pearce GL, Shakir SAW. Adverse effects associated with the use of donepezil in general practice in England. *Journal of Psychopharmacology* 2000; **14**: 406–408.
18. Hashimoto M, Imamura T, Tanimukai S *et al.* Urinary incontinence: an unrecognised adverse effect with donepezil. *Lancet* 2000; **356**: 568.
19. National Institute for Clinical Excellence. Guidance on the use of donepezil, rivastigmine and galantamine for the treatment of Alzheimer's disease. Technology Appraisal Guidance No. 19, 2001.
20. Matthews HP, Korbey J, Wilkinson DG *et al.* Donepezil in Alzheimer's disease: eighteen month results from Southampton Memory Clinic. *International Journal of Geriatric Psychiatry* 2000; **15**: 713–720.
21. Ieni JR, Perdomo CA, Pratt RD. Safety of donepezil in extended treatment of Alzheimer's disease. *European Neuropsychopharmacology* 1999; **9**(Suppl. 5): S328.
22. Danysz W, Parsons CG, Möbius J-J *et al.* Neuroprotective and symptomatological action of memantine relevant for Alzheimer's Disease – a unified glutamatergic hypothesis on the mechanism of action. *Neurotoxicity Research* 1999; **2**: 85–97.
23. Parsons CG, Danysz W, Quack G. Memantine is a clinically well tolerated *N*-methyl-D-aspartate (NMDA) receptor antagonist – a review of preclinical data. *Neuropharmacology* 1999; **38**: 735–767.
24. Winblad B, Poritis N. Memantine in severe dementia: results of the ⁹M-Nest study (benefit and efficacy in severely demented patients during treatment with memantine). *International Journal of Geriatric Psychiatry* 1999; **14**: 135–146.
25. Orgogozo J-M, Rigaud A-S, Stöffler A *et al.* Efficacy and safety of memantine in patients with mild to moderate vascular dementia: a randomized, placebo-controlled trial (MMM 300). *Stroke* 2002; **33**: 1834–1839.

Further reading

Areosa Sastre A, Sherriff F. Memantine for dementia. In: The Cochrane Library, Issue 1. Oxford: Update Software, 2003.
Reisberg B, Doody R, Stoffler A, Schmitt F, Ferris S. Mobius HJ for the Memantine Study Group. Memantine in moderate-to-severe Alzheimer's disease. *New England Journal of Medicine* 2003; **348**(14): 1333–1341.

Acutely disturbed or violent behaviour

Acute behavioural disturbance can occur in the context of psychiatric illness, physical illness, substance abuse or personality disorder. Psychotic symptoms are common and the patient may be aggressive towards others secondary to persecutory delusions or auditory, visual or tactile hallucinations.

The common clinical practice of rapid tranquillisation (RT) is used when appropriate psychological and behavioural approaches have failed to de-escalate acutely disturbed behaviour. It is, essentially, a treatment of last resort. RT is not underpinned by a strong evidence base. Patients who require RT are often too disturbed to give informed consent and therefore cannot participate in randomised controlled trials (RCTs). Recommendations are therefore based partly on research data, partly on theoretical considerations and partly on clinical experience.

There are few studies that directly compare antipsychotic drugs and none that directly compare benzodiazepines. A few RCTs compare benzodiazepines with antipsychotics. All reach the same conclusion; antipsychotics and benzodiazepines are broadly equally effective, although there is a suggestion in some studies that the onset of action of benzodiazepines is more rapid[1,2]. Some studies also address the efficacy of combinations over single drugs. The combination of lorazepam and haloperidol has been consistently found to be more effective than either drug alone[3-5], an advantage that may be generalisable to other combinations of antipsychotic and sedative drugs[3].

Plans for the management of individual patients should ideally be made in advance. The aim is to prevent disturbed behaviour and reduce risk of violence. Nursing interventions (de-escalation, time out), increased nursing levels, transfer of the patient to a psychiatric intensive care unit (PICU) or pharmacological management are all options that may be employed. Note that RT is often viewed as punitive by patients.

The aims of RT are threefold:

1. To reduce suffering for the patient: psychological or physical (through self-harm or accidents).
2. To reduce risk of harm to others by maintaining a safe environment.
3. To do no harm (by prescribing safe regimes and monitoring physical health).

In an emergency situation (NB: read attached notes carefully)

Step	Intervention		
1	De-escalation, time out, placement, etc., as appropriate		
2[a,b]	Offer **oral treatment**	**Haloperidol** 5 mg or **Olanzapine** 10 mg or **Risperidone**[6] 1–2 mg	with or without lorazepam 1–2 mg. Repeat every 45–60 minutes. Go to step 3 if three doses fail
3[b,c,e,f]	Consider **IM treatment**	**Haloperidol** 5 mg or **Olanzapine**[7] 5–10 mg or **Ziprasidone** 10–20 mg[8,h]	with or without lorazepam[d,g] 1–2 mg
		Repeat up to 3 times at 30 minute intervals, if insufficient effect	
		Promethazine[i] 50 mg IM is an alternative in benzodiazepine-tolerant patients	
4	Consider **IV treatment**	**Diazepam**[j,k,l] 10 mg over at least 5 minutes[9] Repeat after 5–10 minutes if insufficient effect (up to three times)	
5	**Seek expert advice.** Amylobarbitone[m] 250 mg IM or paraldehyde[n] 5–10 ml IM are options. Very very few episodes of RT should reach this point		

Notes

a Choice depends on current treatment. If the patient is established on antipsychotics, lorazepam may be used alone. If the patient uses street drugs or is already receiving benzodiazepines regularly, an antipsychotic may be used alone. For the majority of patients, the best response will be obtained with a combination of an antipsychotic and lorazepam.

b Ensure that parenteral anticholinergics are available. Procyclidine 5–10 mg IM or benzatropine 1–2 mg IM may be required to reverse acute dystonic reactions.

c Either an antipsychotic or benzodiazepine can be used alone as in (a), but for the majority of patients the best response will be obtained with a combination of an antipsychotic and lorazepam.

d Mix lorazepam 1:1 with water for injections before injecting. Some centres use 2–4 mg.

e From this point onwards, review the patient's legal status. The requirement for enforced IM medication in informal patients should prompt the use of the Mental Health Act.

f From this point onwards, consider consulting a senior colleague.

g Have flumazenil available to reverse the effects of lorazepam. (Monitor respiratory rate – give flumazenil if rate falls below 10/min).

h Ziprasidone is unlikely to be licensed in the UK, but is available in the USA and other countries.

i Promethazine has a slow onset of action but is often an effective sedative. Dilution is not required before IM injection. May be repeated up to a max. 100 mg/day. Wait 1–2 hours after injection to assess response.

j Use Diazemuls to avoid injection site reactions. IV therapy may be used instead of IM when a very rapid effect is required. IV therapy also ensures near immediate delivery of the drug to its site of action and effectively avoids the danger of inadvertent accumulation of slowly absorbed IM doses. Note also that IV doses can be repeated after only 5–10 minutes if no effect is observed.

k Have flumazenil available to reverse the effects of diazepam. (Monitor respiratory rate – give flumazenil if rate falls below 10/min).

l Caution in the very young and elderly and those with pre-existing brain damage or impulse control problems as disinhibition reactions are more likely[9].

m Amylobarbitone is a powerful respiratory depressant with no pharmacological antagonist. Have facilities for mechanical ventilation available.

n Paraldehyde is now used extremely rarely and is difficult to obtain. It should be used when all else has failed. In many cases, ECT may be more appropriate.

References

1. Salzman C, Soloman D, Miyawaki et al. Parenteral lorazepam versus parenteral haloperidol for the control of psychotic disruptive behaviour. Journal of Clinical Psychiatry 1991; 52: 177–180.
2. Foster S, Kessel J, Berman ME et al. Efficacy of lorazepam and haloperidol for rapid tranquillisation in a psychiatric emergency room setting. International Clinical Psychopharmacology 1997; 12: 175–179.
3. Garza-Trevino ES, Hollister LE, Overall JE et al. Efficacy of combinations of intramuscular antipsychotics and sedative-hypnotics for control of psychotic agitation. American Journal of Psychiatry 1989; 146: 1598–1601.
4. Guz I, Moraes R, Sartoretto JN et al. The therapeutic effects of lorazepam in psychotic patients treated with haloperidol: a double blind study. Current Therapeutic Research 1972; 14: 767–774.
5. Bieniek SA, Ownby RL, Penalver A et al. A double-blind study of lorazepam versus the combination of haloperidol and lorazepam in managing agitation. Pharmacotherapy 1998; 18: 57–62.
6. Currier GW, Simpson GM. Risperidone liquid concentrate and oral lorazepam versus intramuscular haloperidol and intramuscular lorazepam for treatment of psychotic agitation. Journal of Clinical Psychiatry 2001; 62: 153–157.
7. Wright P, Birkett M, David SR et al. Double-blind, placebo-controlled comparison of intramuscular olanzapine and intramuscular haloperidol in the treatment of acute agitation in schizophrenia. American Journal of Psychiatry 2001; 158: 1149–1151.
8. Brook S, Lucey JV, Gunn KP. Intramuscular ziprasidone compared with intramuscular haloperidol in the treatment of acute psychosis. Journal of Clinical Psychiatry 2000; 61: 933–944.
9. Paton C. Benzodiazepines and disinhibition: a review. Psychiatric Bulletin 2002; 26: 460–462.

Further reading

Pilowsky LS, Ring H, Shine PJ et al. (1992). Rapid tranquillisation. A survey of emergency prescribing in a general psychiatric hospital. British Journal of Psychiatry 160: 831–835.
Kerr IB, Taylor DM (1997). Acute disturbed or violent behaviour: principles of treatment. Journal of Psychopharmacology 11: 271–277.

Rapid tranquillisation – monitoring

After any parenteral drug administration monitor as follows:

Temperature

Pulse

Blood pressure

Respiratory Rate

Every 5–10 minutes for one hour, then half-hourly until patient is ambulatory.

If the patient is asleep or **unconscious**, the use of pulse oximetry to continuously measure oxygen saturation is desirable. A nurse should remain with the patient until they are ambulatory again.

ECG and haematological monitoring are also strongly recommended when parenteral antipsychotics are given, especially when higher doses are used[1,2]. Hypokalaemia, stress and agitation place the patient at risk of cardiac arrhythmias[3] (see page 75).

References

1. Appleby L, Thomas S, Ferrier N *et al.* Sudden unexplained death in psychiatric in-patients. *British Journal of Psychiatry* 2000; **176**: 405–406.
2. Yap YG, Camm J. Risk of torsades de pointes with non-cardiac drugs. *BMJ* 2000; **320**: 1158–1159.
3. Taylor DM. Antipsychotics and QT prolongation. *Acta Psychiatrica Scandinavica* 2003; **107**: 85–95.

Remedial measures in rapid tranquillisation

Problem	Remedial measures
Acute dystonia (including oculogyric crises)	Give **procyclidine** 5–10 mg IM or IV or **benzatropine** 1–2 mg IM
Reduced respiratory rate (<10/min) or oxygen saturation (<90%)	Give oxygen; raise legs; ensure patient is not lying face down. Give **flumazenil** if benzodiazepine-induced respiratory depression suspected (see protocol) If induced by any other sedative agent: **ventilate mechanically**.
Irregular or slow (<50/min) **pulse**	**Refer** to specialist medical care immediately.
Fall in blood pressure (>30 mmHg orthostatic drop or <50 mmHg diastolic)	**Lie patient flat**, tilt bed towards head. Monitor closely.
Increased temperature	**Withhold antipsychotics:** (risk of NMS and perhaps arrhythmias). Check creatinine kinase urgently.

Guidelines for the use of flumazenil

Indication for use	If, after the administration of lorazepam or diazepam, respiratory rate falls below 10/minute.
Contra-indications	Patients with epilepsy who have been receiving long-term benzodiazepines.
Caution	Dose should be carefully titrated in hepatic impairment.
Dose and route of administration	*Initial:* 200 mcg **intravenously** over 15 seconds – if required level of consciousness not achieved after 60 seconds then, *Subsequent dose:* 100 mcg over 10 seconds.
Time before dose can be repeated	60 seconds.
Maximum dose	1 mg in 24 hours (one initial dose and eight subsequent doses).
Side effects	Patients may become agitated, anxious or fearful on awakening. Seizures may occur in regular benzodiazepine users.
Management	Side effects usually subside.

Monitoring

● **What to monitor?**	Respiratory rate
● **How often?**	Continuously until respiratory rate returns to baseline level. Flumazenil has a short half life (much shorter that diazepam) and respiratory function may recover then deteriorate again.
	Note: If respiratory rate does not return to normal or patient is not alert after initial doses given then assume sedation due to some other cause.

Guidelines for the use of Clopixol Acuphase (zuclopenthixol acetate)

Acuphase should only be used after an acutely psychotic patient has required <u>repeated</u> injections of short-acting antipsychotic drugs such as haloperidol, olanzapine or ziprasidone, or sedative drugs such as lorazepam.

Acuphase should only be given when enough time has elapsed to assess the full response to previously injected drugs: allow 15 minutes after IV injections; 60 minutes after IM.

*Acuphase should **never** be administered:*
- In an attempt to 'hasten' the antipsychotic effect of other antipsychotic therapy
- For rapid tranquillisation
- At the same time as other parenteral antipsychotics or benzodiazepines
- At the same time as depot medication
- As a 'test dose' for zuclopenthixol decanoate depot
- To a patient who is physically resistive (risk of intravasation and oil embolus).

*Acuphase should **never** be used for, or in, the following:*
- Patients who accept oral medication
- Patients who are neuroleptic–naïve
- Patients who are sensitive to EPSE
- Patients who are unconscious
- Patients who are pregnant
- Those with hepatitis or renal impairment
- Those with cardiac disease

Onset and duration of action
Sedative effects usually begin to be seen 2 hours after injection and peak after 12 hours. The effects may last for up to 72 hours. Note: Acuphase has no place in rapid tranquillisation: *its action is not rapid.*

Dose
Acuphase should be given in a dose of 50–150 mg, up to a maximum of 400 mg over a two-week period. This maximum duration ensures that a treatment plan is put in place. It does not indicate that there are known harmful effects from more prolonged administration, although such use should be very exceptional. There is no such thing as a 'course of acuphase'. The patient should be assessed before each administration.

Injections should be spaced at least 24 hours apart.

Note: Zuclopenthixol acetate is widely misused as a sort of 'chemical straightjacket'. In reality, it is a potentially toxic preparation with very little published information to support its use[1]. It is perhaps best reserved for those few patients who have a prior history of good response to Acuphase.

Reference

1. Fenton M, Coutinho ESF, Campbell C. Zuclopenthixol acetate in the treatment of acute schizophrenia and similar serious mental illnesses (Cochrane Review). In: *The Cochrane Library*, Issue 4, 2002. Oxford: Update Software.

Chronic behavioural disturbance in learning disability

Behavioural disturbance is common in those with a learning disability. It is often very difficult to determine the aetiology. The following may be useful prompts:

1. Is there or could there be an underlying physical illness? (Look for and treat)
2. Could environmental factors be contributing? (Consider and alter if possible)
3. Is there an underlying psychiatric illness? (Consider and treat if applicable)

Then consider:

4. Does the patient have a history of mood disturbance? (Try an antidepressant/mood stabiliser)
5. Is the disturbance cyclical? (Try a mood stabiliser)
6. Is/might epilepsy be a contributing factor? (Try an anticonvulsant)
7. Is the patient aggressive? (Try carbamazepine or a β-blocker)
8. Are there any signs of adrenergic overactivity, such as tachycardia or tremor? (Try a β-blocker)
9. Is the patient impulsive? (Try an SSRI)
10. Is the patient self-injurious? (Try an antipsychotic, SSRI or naltrexone)
11. Could the behaviour be driven by psychosis? (Try an antipsychotic)

Reference

Tyrer P. The use of psychotropic drugs In: Russell O (ed). *The Psychiatry of Learning Disabilities*, ch. 14. London: Royal College of Psychiatrists, 1997.

Self-injurious behaviour in learning disabilities

Repetitive or stereotypical acts that produce self-inflicted injury (self-injurious behaviour (SIB))[1-3]:

- Occur in approximately 20% of adults with a learning disability, (up to 50% in those requiring institutional care).
- Most commonly take the form of head-banging, banging other body parts, biting, scratching, pinching, gouging, hair-pulling and pica.
- Occur more frequently in males, younger adults, those with impairments in hearing, vision, mobility and communication, and those with a diagnosis of autism and epilepsy. As the IQ falls, the prevalence of SIB (and multiple behaviours) increases.

SIB is a major cause of distress to carers and a major cause of institutional care.

Aetiology[4-7]

SIB is best understood as being caused by a combination of organic and environmental factors. Organic factors include rare genetic syndromes (such as Lesch–Nyhan or Smith–Magenis syndrome), developmental brain damage, neurological disorders (such as epilepsy), physical illness, psychiatric illness and communication problems. SIB may be linked to the menstrual cycle in some women. Environmental factors include lack of stimulation/overstimulation, lack of/too much affection, rejection/lack of attention and adverse life events.

Some factors may predispose to SIB (e.g. genetic syndromes), others precipitate SIB (e.g. depression, dysphoria) and others perpetuate it (e.g. secondary changes in neuroregulatory systems).

The prevalence of mental illness is increased in those with learning disabilities and non-specific and atypical presentations of mental illness increase in frequency as the IQ falls. Diagnosis often has to be made from observing behaviour rather than directly eliciting symptoms.

Non-drug treatments[8-10]

It is important to try to understand why the patient self-harms (e.g. self-stimulation, relief of dysphoria, attention, social escape through being removed from communal areas, material reward). Psychological/behavioural strategies for dealing with the behaviour can then be put in place. This should always be tried before resorting to drug treatment.

Successfully preventing one form of SIB may lead to the emergence of another form. Staff may perceive SIB to be due to different causes in the same patient and may react with fear, irritation, anger, disgust or despair. Interventions based on individual belief systems will lead to inconsistent care. Effective management and support of staff is essential.

Drug treatment options – SIB in learning disability

Drug	Rationale
Antipsychotics[11,12]	• Supersensitivity of dopamine neurones in nigrostriatal pathways may predispose to SIB. D_1 blockers (such as thioridazine) may be more effective than D_2 blockers. Atypical antipsychotics are poorly evaluated (may have less severe side-effects). There is most experience with risperidone. • Dopamine is involved in reward mechanisms (blocking dopamine blocks reward). • Low dose antipsychotics reduce stereotypies.
Opiate antagonists[4,7]	• SIB leads to the release of endogenous opiates (endorphins), which may lead to a rewarding mood state (positive re-inforcement). • Naltrexone (an opiate antagonist) may decrease SIB acutely but is less effective in the long term (?opiate mechanisms are important in the early stages, but SIB is perpetuated via dopamine reward mechanisms).
Anticonvulsants[12]	• The prevalence of epilepsy is high in moderate/severe learning disabilities. • Aggression (to others or self) can be related to seizure activity (pre-ictal, ictal or post-ictal). Note: vigabatrin and topiramate may cause behavioural problems. • Rapid cycling mood disorders and mixed affective states are more common in learning disabilities and may respond best to carbamazepine or valproate.
SSRIs[4,7] **Lithium**[12,13] **Buspirone**[14]	• Drugs that increase 5HT neurotransmission have been shown to reduce SIB in some patients. • These drugs may act by targeting the behaviour that precipitates SIB (e.g. fear, irritability, anxiety or depression). • Lithium is licensed for 'the control of aggressive behaviour or intentional self-harm.'
Others[7,12,15]	• Other drugs may be useful in some circumstances (e.g. propranolol – probably through reducing anxiety), methylphenidate (when ADHD has been diagnosed), cyproterone (when severely problematic sexual behaviour contributes)

Most data originate from case reports and small open trials, often of heterogeneous patient groups.

Lithium is the only drug licensed for the treatment of SIB.

Prescribing and monitoring[12,16–19]

There is concern that antipsychotic drugs are prescribed excessively and inappropriately in the learning disability population and may cause undue harm. It is unclear if this patient population is more prone to side effects. It is therefore important to document:

- The rationale for treatment (including some measure of baseline target behaviours), potential risk/benefit and consent in the patient's notes. If the patient is unable to understand the nature, purpose and side-effects of treatment, a relative or carer should be consulted.
- The impact of medication and any side-effects experienced should also be documented each time the patient is reviewed.
- Drug interactions should always be considered (both kinetic and dynamic) before prescribing, particularly when anticonvulsant drugs are involved.

References

1. Schroeder SR, Oster-Granite ML, Berkson G *et al*. Self-injurious behaviour: gene-brain-behaviour relationships. *Mental Retardation and Developmental Disability Research Review* 2001; 7: 3–12.
2. Saloviita T. The structure and correlates of self-injurious behaviour in an institutional setting. *Research in Developmental Disabilities* 2000; 21: 501–511.
3. Collacott R, Cooper SA, Branford D *et al*. Epidemiology of self-injurious behaviour in adults with learning disabilities. *British Journal of Psychiatry* 1998; 173: 428–432.
4. Mikhail AG, King BH. Self-injurious behaviour in mental retardation. *Current Opinions in Psychiatry* 2001; 14: 457–461.
5. Moss S, Emerson E, Kiernan C *et al*. Psychiatric symptoms in adults with learning disability and challenging behaviour. *British Journal of Psychiatry* 2000; 176: 452–456.
6. Deb S. Self-injurious behaviour as part of genetic syndromes. *British Journal of Psychiatry* 1998; 172: 385–388.
7. Clarke DJ. Psychopharmacology of severe self-injury associated with learning disabilities. *British Journal of Psychiatry* 1998; 172: 389–394.
8. Xeniditis K, Russell A, Murphy D. Management of people with challenging behaviour. *Advances in Psychiatric Treatment* 2001; 7: 109–116.
9. Halliday S, Mackrell K. Psychological interventions in self-injurious behaviour. *British Journal of Psychiatry* 1998; 172: 395–400.
10. Bromley J, Emerson E. Beliefs and emotional reactions of care staff working with people with challenging behaviour. *Journal of Intellectual Disability Research* 1995; 39: 341–352.
11. Branford D. Antipsychotic drugs in learning disabilities (mental handicap). *Pharmaceutical Journal* 1997; 258: 451–456.
12. Einfeld SL. Systematic management approach to pharmacotherapy for people with learning disabilities. *Advances in Psychiatric Practice* 2001; 7: 43–49.
13. Craft M, Ismail IA, Krishnamurti D *et al*. Lithium in the treatment of aggression in mentally handicapped patients: a double-blind trial. *British Journal of Psychiatry* 1987; 150: 685–689.
14. Ratey JJ, Sovner R, Mikkelsen E *et al*. Buspirone therapy for maladaptive behaviour and anxiety in developmentally disabled persons. *Journal of Clinical Psychiatry* 1989; 50: 382–384.
15. Aman MG, Marks RE, Turbott SH *et al*. Clinical effects of methylphenidate and thioridazine in intellectually subaverage children. *Journal of the American Academy of Child and Adolescent Psychiatry* 1991; 30: 246–256.
16. Deb S, Fraser W. The use of psychotropic medication in people with learning disability: towards rational prescribing. *Human Psychopharmacology* 1994; 9: 259–272.
17. Cooray SE, Tolmac J. Antipsychotic medications in learning disability. *Psychiatric Bulletin* 1988; 22: 601–604.
18. Miller HEJ, Foster SE. Psychotropic medication in learning disabilities: audit as an alternative to legislation. *Psychiatric Bulletin* 1997; 21: 286–289.
19. Ahmed Z, Fraser W, Kerr MP *et al*. Reducing antipsychotic medication in people with a learning disability. *British Journal of Psychiatry* 2000; 176: 42–46.

Further reading

Read S. Self-injury and violence in people with severe learning disabilities. *British Journal of Psychiatry* 1998; 172: 381384.
Santosh PJ, Baird G. Psychopharmacology in children and adults with intellectual disability. *Lancet* 1999; 354: 233–240.
Thompson C, Read A. Behavioural symptoms among people with severe and profound intellectual disabilities: a 26-year follow-up study. *British Journal of Psychiatry* 2002; 181: 67–71.

chapter 8

Miscellaneous conditions and substances

Nicotine

The most common method of consuming nicotine is by smoking cigarettes. One-third of the general population, 40–50% of those with depression and up to 90% of those with schizophrenia smoke[1]. Nicotine causes peripheral vasoconstriction, tachycardia and increased blood pressure[2]. Smokers are at increased risk of developing cardiovascular disease. As well as nicotine, cigarettes also contain tar (a complex mixture of organic molecules, many carcinogenic), a cause of cancers of the respiratory tract, chronic bronchitis and emphysema[3].

Nicotine is highly addictive. People with mental illness are 2–3 times more likely than the general population to develop and maintain a nicotine addiction[1]. Chronic smoking contributes to the increased morbidity and mortality from respiratory and cardiovascular disease that is seen in this patient group. Nicotine also has psychotropic effects. Smoking can affect the metabolism (and therefore the efficacy and toxicity) of drugs prescribed to treat psychiatric illness[4]. Nicotine use may be a gateway to experimenting with other psychoactive substances.

Psychotropic effects
Nicotine is highly lipid-soluble and rapidly enters the brain after inhalation. Nicotine receptors are found on dopaminergic cell bodies and stimulation of these receptors leads to dopamine release[1]. Dopamine release in the limbic system is associated with pleasure: dopamine is the brain's 'reward' neurotransmitter. Nicotine may be used by people with mental health problems as a form of 'self-medication' (e.g. to alleviate the negative symptoms of schizophrenia or antipsychotic-induced EPSEs or for its anxiolytic effect[5]). Drugs that increase the release of dopamine reduce the craving for nicotine. They may also worsen psychotic illness (see under smoking cessation below).
  Nicotine improves concentration and vigilance[1]. It also enhances the effects of glutamate, acetylcholine and serotonin[5].

Schizophrenia
Up to 90% of people with schizophrenia regularly smoke cigarettes[1]. Possible explanations include: smoking casues dopamine release leading to feelings of well-being and a reduction in negative symptoms[5], alleviation of some of the side effects of antipsychotics such as drowsiness and EPSEs[1],

as a means of structuring the day (a behavioural filler) or as a means of alleviating the deficit in auditory gaiting that is found in schizophrenia[6]. It has been suggested that people with schizophrenia find it particularly difficult to tolerate nicotine withdrawal symptoms[4].

Depression and anxiety

In 'normal' individuals a moderate consumption of nicotine is associated with pleasure and a decrease in anxiety and feelings of anger[7]. The mechanism of this anxiolytic effect is not understood. People who suffer from anxiety and/or depression are more likely to smoke and find it more difficult to stop[7]. This is compounded by the fact that nicotine withdrawal can precipitate or exacerbate depression in those with a history of the illness[7]. Patients with depression are at increased risk of cardiovascular disease. By directly causing tachycardia and hypertension[2], nicotine may, in theory, exacerbate this problem.

Movement disorders and Parkinson's disease

By increasing dopaminergic neurotransmission, nicotine provides a protective effect against both drug-induced EPSEs and idiopathic Parkinson's disease. Smokers are less likely to suffer from antipsychotic-induced movement disorders than non-smokers[1] and use anticholinergics less often[4]. Parkinson's disease occurs less frequently in smokers than in non-smokers and the onset of clinical symptoms is delayed[1].

Drug interactions

Polycyclic hydrocarbons in cigarette smoke are known to stimulate the hepatic microsomal enzyme system, particularly P4501A2[5], the enzyme responsible for the metabolism of many psychotropic drugs. Smoking can lower blood levels of some drugs by up to 50%[5]. This can affect both efficacy and side-effects and needs to be taken into account when making clinical decisions. The drugs most likely to be affected are: clozapine, fluphenazine, haloperidol, chlorpromazine, olanzapine, many tricyclic antidepressants, mirtazapine, fluvoxamine and propranolol.

Withdrawal symptoms[4]

Withdrawal symptoms occur within 12–14 hours of stopping smoking and include depressed mood, insomnia, anxiety, restlessness, irritability, difficulty concentrating and increased appetite. Nicotine withdrawal can be confused with depression, anxiety, sleep disorders and mania. It can also exacerbate the symptoms of schizophrenia.

Smoking cessation

People with mental health problems generally have low motivation to stop smoking and may find withdrawal intolerable[5]. Although the efficacy of nicotine replacement treatments in people with enduring mental illness has not been evaluated, the adverse effects of smoking on physical health are so great that patients should always be encouraged to stop. Nicotine replacement is available in the form of patches, microtabs, gum, lozenges and inhalers. Full details can be found in the *BNF*. Bupropion/amfebutamone (a noradreline and dopamine reuptake inhibitor) is also licensed for smoking cessation[8] and may be effective even in schizophrenia[9].

References

1. Goff DC, Henderson DC, Amico E. Cigarette smoking in schizophrenia: relationship to psychophathology and medication side-effects. *American Journal of Psychiatry* 1992; **149**: 1189–1194.
2. Benowitz NL, Hansson A, Jacob P. Cardiovascular effects of nasal and transdermal nicotine and cigarette smoking. *Hypertension* 2002; **39**: 1107–1112.
3. Anderson JE, Jorenby DE, Scott WJ *et al*. Treating tobacco use and dependence: an evidence based clinical practice guideline for tobacco cessation. *Chest* 2002; **121**: 932–941.
4. Douglas M, Ziedonis P, George TP. Schizophrenia and nicotine use: report of a pilot smoking cessation programme and review of neurobiological and clinical issues. *Schizophrenia Bulletin* 1997; **23**: 247–254.
5. Edward R, Lyon M. A review of the effects of nicotine and schizophrenia antipsychotic medication. *Psychiatric Services* 1999; **50**: 1346–1350.
6. McEvoy JP, Freudenreich O, Wilson HW. Smoking and therapeutic response to clozapine in patients with schizophrenia. *Biological Psychiatry* 1999; **46**: 125–129.
7. Alexander H, Glassman MD. Cigarette smoking: implications for psychiatric illness. *American Journal of Psychiatry* 1993; **150**: 546–552.
8. Electronic SPC. Zyban, 2002.
9. George TP, Vessicchio JC, Termine A *et al*. A placebo controlled trial of tupropion for smoking cessation in schizophrenia. *Biological Psychiatry* 2002; **52**: 53–61.

Further reading

De Leon J, Mahmood D, Canuso C *et al*. Schizophrenia and smoking: an epidemiological survey in a state hospital. *American Journal of Psychiatry* 1995; **152**: 453–455.
Desai HD, Seabolt J, Jann MW. Smoking in patients receiving psychotropic medications: a pharmacokinetic perspective. *CNS Drugs* 2001; **15**: 469–494.
Zevin S, Benowitz N. Drug interactions with tobacco smoking. *Clinical Pharmacokinetics* 1999; **36**: 425–438.

Caffeine

Caffeine is probably the most popular psychoactive substance in the world. Mean daily consumption in the UK is 350–620 mg[1]. A quarter of the general population and half of those with psychiatric illness regularly consume over 500 mg caffeine/day [2]. Caffeine has 'de novo' psychotropic effects and may also worsen existing psychiatric illness. It may also interact with psychotropic drugs.

Table	Caffeine content of drinks
Brewed coffee	100 mg/cup
Instant coffee	60 mg/cup
Tea	45 mg/cup
Soft drinks	25–50 mg/can

Chocolate also contains caffeine. Martindale lists over 600 medicines that contain caffeine[3]. Most are available without prescription and are marketed as analgesics or appetite suppressants.

Pharmacokinetics

Caffeine is rapidly absorbed after oral administration and has a half-life of 2.5–4.5 hours. It is metabolised by CYP1A2, a hepatic cytochrome enzyme that may exhibit genetic polymorphism. Metabolic pathways also become saturated at higher doses[4]. These factors may account for the large inter-individual differences that are seen in the ability to tolerate caffeine[5].

Psychotropic effects

Caffeine is associated with CNS stimulation and increased catecholamine release[6]. Low-to-moderate doses are associated with favourable subjective effects such as elation and peacefulness[2]. Doses of >600 mg/day invariably produce anxiety, insomnia, psychomotor agitation, excitement, rambling speech (and sometimes delirium and psychosis)[7]. In sensitive people, these effects are produced by much lower doses. At high doses, caffeine can inhibit benzodiazepine receptor binding[6,7]. Tolerance develops to the effects of caffeine and an established withdrawal syndrome exists (headache, depressed mood, anxiety, fatigue, irritability, nausea, dysphoria and craving)[9].

Caffeine intoxication (caffeinism)

DSM IV[8] defines caffeinism as the recent consumption of caffeine, usually in excess of 250 mg accompanied by 5 or more of: restlessness, nervousness, excitement, insomnia, flushed face, diuresis, GI disturbance, muscle twitching, rambling flow of thought and speech, tachycardia or cardiac arrhythmia, periods of inexhaustibility and psychomotor agitation: when these symptoms cause significant distress or impairment in social, occupational or other important areas of functioning *and* are not due to a general medical condition or better accounted for by another mental disorder (e.g. an anxiety disorder).

Schizophrenia

Patients with schizophrenia often consume large amounts of caffeine-containing drinks[1]. This may be to relieve dry mouth (as a side effect of antipsychotic drugs), for the stimulant effects of caffeine (to relieve dysphoria/sedation/negative symptoms) or simply because coffee/tea drinking structures the day or relieves boredom. Excessive caffeine consumption is of concern because caffeine increases the release of catecholamines and so may theoretically precipitate or worsen psychosis. Kruger[6] found that large doses of caffeine can worsen psychotic symptoms (in particular elation & conceptual disorganisation) and result in the prescription of larger doses of antipsychotic drugs. De Freitas & Schwartz[10] found that the removal of caffeine from the diets of chronically disturbed (challenging behaviour) patients, led to decreased levels of hostility, irritability and suspiciousness. These findings have not been replicated in less disturbed populations[11].

Caffeine can also interfere with the effectiveness of drug treatment. Clozapine serum levels can be raised by up to 60%[12], presumably through competetive inhibition of CYP1A2. Other drugs metabolised by this enzyme, such as olanzapine, imipramine and clomipramine, may be similarly affected. The potential effects of caffeine on the metabolism of other drugs, as well as the potential to induce a caffeine-withdrawal syndrome should always be considered before substituting caffeine-free drinks.

Mood disorders

Caffeine may elevate mood through increasing noradrenaline release[13]. The practice of self-medication with caffeine to improve mood is common in the general population. Depressed patients may be more sensitive to the anxiogenic effects of caffeine[14].

Caffeine can increase cortisol secretion (gives a false positive in the dexamethasone suppression test)[15], increase seizure length during ECT[16] and increase the clearance of lithium by promoting diuresis[17]. Caffeine toxicity can be precipitated by drugs that inhibit CYP1A2. Fluvoxamine is an important example.

Anxiety disorders

Caffeine increases vigilance, decreases reaction times, increases sleep latency and worsens subjective estimates of sleep quality; effects that may be more marked in poor metabolisers. It can also precipitate or worsen generalised anxiety and panic attacks[18]. These effects are so marked that caffeine intoxication should always be considered when patients complain of anxiety symptoms or insomnia. Symptoms may diminish considerably or even abate completely if caffeine is avoided[19]. High doses of caffeine can reduce the efficacy of benzodiazepines (by reducing receptor binding[6,7]).

References

1. Rihs M, Muller C, Bauman P. Caffeine consumption in hospitalised psychiatric patients. *European Archives of Psychiatry and Clinical Neuroscience* 1996; **246**: 83–92.
2. Clementz G, Dailey JW. Psychotropic effects of caffeine. *American Family Physician* 1988; **37**: 167–172.
3. Martindale, *The Extra Pharmacopoeia* 32nd edition. London: Pharmaceutical Press, 1999.
4. Kaplan GB, Greenblatt DJ, Ehrenberg BL *et al.* Dose-dependent pharmacokinetics and psychomotor effects of caffeine in humans. *Pharmacokinetics and Pharmacodynamics* 1997; **37**: 693–703.
5. Butler MA, Lang NP, Young JF *et al.* Determination of CYP1A2 and NAT2 phenotypes in human populations by analysis of caffeine urinary metabolites. *Pharmacogenetics* 1992; **2**: 1211–1214.
6. Kruger A. Chronic psychiatric patients use of caffeine: pharmacological effects and mechanisms. *Psychology Reports* 1996; **78**: 915–923.
7. Sawynok J. Pharmacological rationale for the clinical use of caffeine. *Drugs* 1995; **49**: 37–50.
8. American Psychiatric Association. *Diagnostic and Statistical Manual of Mental Disorders* 4th edition. Washington DC: American Psychiatric Association, 1994.
9. Silverman K, Evans SM, Strain EC *et al.* Withdrawal syndrome after the double-blind cessation of caffeine consumption. *New England Journal of Medicine* 1992; **327**: 1109–1114.
10. De Freitas B, Schwartz G. Effects of caffeine in chronic psychiatric patients. *American Journal of Psychiatry* 1979; **136**: 1337–1338.
11. Roczapski A, Paredes J, Kogan C *et al.* Effects of caffeine on behaviour of schizophrenic inpatients. *Schizophrenia Bulletin* 1989; **15**: 339–344.
12. Carrillo JA, Herraiz AG, Ramos SL *et al.* Effects of caffeine withdrawal from the diet on the metabolism of clozapine in schizophrenic patients. *Journal of Clinical Psychopharmacology* 1998; **18**: 311–316.

13. Achor MB, Extein I. Diet aids, mania and affective illness. *American Journal of Psychiatry* 1981; **138**: 392.
14. Lee MA, Flegel P, Greden JF. Anxiogenic effects of caffeine on panic and depressed patients. *American Journal of Psychiatry* 1988; **145**: 632–635.
15. Uhde TW, Bierer LM, Post RM. Caffeine-induced escape from dexamethasone suppression. *Archives of General Psychiatry* 1985; **42**: 737–738.
16. Cantu TG, Korek JS. Caffeine in electroconvulsive therapy. *DICP* 1991; **25**: 1079–1080.
17. Mester R, Toren P, Mizrachi I *et al.* Caffeine withdrawal increases lithium blood levels. *Biological Psychiatry* 1995; **37**: 348–350.
18. Bruce MS. The anxiogenic effects of caffeine. *Postgraduate Medicine* 1990; **66**(Suppl. 2): 518–524.
19. Bruce MS, Lader M. Caffeine abstention in the management of anxiety disorders. *Psychological Medicine* 1989; **19**: 211–214.

Further reading

Drugdex Drug Evaluation. *Caffeine.* Micromedex Healthcare Series Vol 109. Micromedex Inc. USA, 2002.
Paton C, Beer D. Caffeine: the forgotten variable. *International Journal of Psychiatry in Clinical Practice* 2002; **5**: 231–236.

Complementary therapies

A large proportion of the population currently use or have recently used complementary therapies (CTs)[1-4]. As health professionals are rarely consulted before purchase, a diagnosis is often not made and efficacy and side-effects are not monitored. The majority of those who use CTs are also taking conventional medicines[4] and many people use more than one CT simultaneously. Many do not tell their doctor[5]. The public associate natural products with safety and may be unwilling to report possible side-effects[6]. Herbal medicines, in particular, can be toxic as they contain pharmacologically-active substances. Many conventional drugs prescribed today were originally derived from plants. These include medicines as diverse as aspirin, digoxin and the vinca alkaloids used in cancer chemotherapy. Herbal medicines such as St John's wort, *Gingko biloba* and valerian are increasingly used as self-medication for psychiatric and neurodegenerative illnesses[2,3,7]. Few CTs have been subject to randomised controlled trials, so efficacy is largely unproven[2,8,9]. There is no systematic monitoring of side-effects caused by CTs, so safety is largely unknown. Some herbs are known to be very toxic[10-12].

Whatever the perceived 'evidence base' for the use of complementary therapies, the feelings of autonomy engendered by taking control of one's own illness and treatment can result in important psychological benefits irrespective of any direct therapeutic benefits of the CT[4,13,14]. There are many different complementary therapies, the most popular being homeopathy and herbal medicine with its branches of Bach's flower remedies, Chinese and Ayurvedic medicine. Non-drug therapies such as acupuncture and osteopathy are also popular. To master one can take years of study, therefore to ensure safe and effective treatment, referral to a qualified practitioner is recommended. The majority of doctors and pharmacists have no qualifications or specific training in CTs. The following table gives a brief introduction. Further reading is strongly recommended.

Table An introduction to complementary therapies

	Homeopathy[8,9,15,20]	Herbal medicine (phytotherapy)[15-17]	Aromatherapy[15]
Health beliefs	• Treatment is selected according to the individual characteristics of the patient (hair colour and personality are as important as symptoms) • Treatment stimulates the body to restore health (there is no scientifically plausible theory to support this claim) • Like is treated with like (e.g. substances that cause a fever, treat a fever) • The more diluted the preparation, the more potent it is thought to be • Very potent preparations are unlikely to contain even 1 molecule of active substance	• Treatment is selected according to the individual characteristics of the patient (as with homeopathy) • Herbs are believed to stimulate the elimination of toxins by increasing diuresis, defecation, bile flow and sweating • Attention to diet is important • The whole plant is used, not the specific active ingredient (this is believed to reduce side-effects) • Active ingredients vary with the source of the herb (standardisation is contrary to the philosophy of herbal medicine) • Herbalists believe that if the correct treatment is chosen, treatment will be completely free of side-effects	• Treatment is selected according to the individual characteristics of the patient (as with homeopathy and herbal medicine). • Illness is believed to be the result of imbalance in mental, emotional and physical processes, and aromatherapy is believed to promote balance • Purified oils are not used (the many natural constituents and believed to protect against adverse effects: similar to the beliefs held by herbalists) • There is no standard dose • Individual oils may be used for several unrelated indications
Used for	• A wide range of indications (except those outlined below) • May be taken with conventional treatments • Over 2,000 remedies and many dilutions are available	• Everything except as outlined below • May be taken with conventional treatments but many significant interactions are possible (some have been reported) • Advertised in the lay press for a wide range of indications	• Everything except as outlined below • May be used as an adjunct to conventional treatments • Usually administered by massage onto the skin which is known to relieve pain and tension, increase circulation and aid relaxation

	Homeopathy[8,9,15,20]	Herbal medicine (phytotherapy)[15,16,17]	Aromatherapy[15]
Not suitable for	• Infection • Organ failure • Vitamin/mineral/hormone deficiency	• Use in pregnancy and lactation (many herbs are abortifacient)[18] • Evening primrose oil should not be used in epilepsy[18]	• Use in pregnancy (jasmine, peppermint, rose and rosemary may stimulate uterine) contractions ● Rosemary should be avoided in epilepsy and hypertension
Side-effects & other information	• None known or anticipated • Inactivated by aromatherapy & strong smells (eg coffee, peppermint, toothpaste). • Inactivated by handling. • Healing follows the law of cure: symptoms disappear down the body in the reverse order to which they appeared, move from vital to less vital organs and ultimately appear as a rash (which is a sign of cure).	● Herbal remedies are occasionally adulterated (with conventional medicines such as steroids or toxic substances such as lead[19]) ● Many side-effects can be anticipated (e.g. kelp and thyrotoxicosis, St John's wort and serotonin syndrome) ● Overuse, adulteration, variation in plant constituents and misidentification of plants are common causes of toxicity. Some Chinese herbs are toxic[10–12]	● Skin sensitivity ● Significant systemic absorption can occur during massage ● Ingestion can cause liver/kidney toxicity ● All aromatherapy products should be stored in dark containers away from heat to avoid oxidation

References

1. Fisher P, Ward A. Complementary medicine in Europe. *BMJ* 2001; **309**: 107–111.
2. Barnes J, Anderson LA, Phillipson JD. *Herbal Medicines: A guide for health care professionals* 2nd edition. London: Pharmaceutical Press, 2002.
3. Kessler RC, Soukup J, Davis RB. The use of complementary and alternative therapies to treat anxiety and depression in the United States. *American Journal of Psychiatry* 2001; **158**: 289–294.
4. Astin JA. Why patients use alternative medicine: results of a national study. *JAMA* 1998; **279**:1548–1553.
5. Berry MI, Tinorva E. The use of traditional Chinese medicine in Liverpool. *Pharmaceutical Journal* 1993; **251**: 12.
6. Barnes J, Mills SY, Abbot NC *et al.* Different standards for reporting ADRs to herbal remedies and conventional OTC medicines: face-to-face interviews with 515 users of herbal remedies. *British Journal of Clinical Pharmacology* 1998; **45**: 496–500.
7. Pies R. Adverse neuropsychiatric reactions to herbal and over-the-counter 'antidepressants'. *Journal of Clinical Psychiatry* 2000; **61**: 815–820.
8. Kleijnen J, Knipschild P, Riet G. Clinical trials of homeopathy. *BMJ* 1991; 302: 316–323.
9. Reilly D, Taylor MA, Beattie NGM *et al.* Is evidence for homeopathy reproducible. *Lancet* 1994; **344**: 1601–1606.
10. Kava Kava and hepatotoxicity. *Current Problems in Pharmacovigilance* 2002; **28**: 6.
11. Renal failure associated with traditional Chinese medicines. *Current Problems in Pharmacovigilance* 1999; **15**: 18.
12. Hypoglycaemia following the use of Chinese herbal medicine xiaoke wan. *Current Problems in Pharmacovigilance* 2001; **27**: 8.
13. Downer SM, Cody MM, McClusky P *et al.* Pursuit and practice of complementary therapies by cancer patients receiving conventional treatment. *BMJ* 1994; **309**: 86–89.
14. The placebo effect: can we use it better? *BMJ* 1994; **309**: 67–70.
15. Fulder S. *The Handbook of Complementary Medicine* 2nd edition. London: Hodder & Stoughton, 1989.
16. Mills SY. *The Essential Book of Herbal Medicine*. London: Penguin Arkana, 1991.
17. Pertiaric L, Shaw D, Murray V. Toxic effects of herbal medicines and food supplements. *Lancet* 1993; **342**: 180–181.
18. Wong AHC, Smith M, Boon HS. Herbal remedies in psychiatric practice. Archives of General Psychiatry 1998; **55**: 1033–1044.
19. Aslam M, Davis SS. Heavy metal toxicity of some Asian medicines in the UK. *Journal of Pharmacy and Pharmacology* 1980; **32**: 83.
20. Homeopathy. *Effective Health Care Bulletin* 2002; 7: 1–12.

Further reading

Cooke B, Ernst E. Aromatherapy: a systematic review. *British Journal of General Practice* 2000; **455**: 444–445.
Ernst E, Rand JI, Stevinson C. Complementary therapies for depression. *Archives of General Psychiatry* 1998; **55**: 1026–1032.
Fugh-Berman A. Herb-drug interactions. *Lancet* 2000; **355**:134–138.
Walter G, Rey JM. The relevance of herbal treatments for psychiatric practice. *Australian & New Zealand Journal of Psychiatry* 2000; **33**: 482–489.

Driving and psychotropic drugs

Many factors have been shown to affect driving performance. These include age, personality, physical and mental state and being under the influence of alcohol, prescribed medicines, street drugs or 'over the counter' medicines[1]. Studying the effects of any of these factors in isolation is extremely difficult. Some studies have assessed the effect of medication on tests such as response-time and attention[2] but these tests do not directly measure ability or inability to drive.

It has been estimated that up to 10% of people killed or injured in road traffic accidents (RTAs) may be taking psychotropic medication[3]. Patients with personality disorders and alcoholism have the highest rates of motoring offences and are more likely to be involved in accidents[3]. Driving while unfit through taking prescribed or illicit drugs is an offence and may lead to prosecution. People whose driving ability may be impaired through their illness or prescribed medication should inform their insurance company. Failure to do so is considered to be 'witholding a material fact' and may render the insurance policy void.

Effects of psychiatric medicines

Many psychotropics can impair alertness, concentration and driving performance. Drugs that block H_1, α_1-adrenergic or cholinergic receptors may be particularly problematic. Effects are particularly marked at the start of treatment and after increasing the dose. It is important to stop driving during this time if adversely affected. The use of alcohol will further increase any impairment.

Table Psychotropics and driving (see www.dvla.gov.uk)	
Drug	**Effect**
Hypnotics & anxiolytics	Benzodiazepines cause sedation and impaired attention, information processing, memory and motor co-ordination. The impairment is dose-related and greater with longer half-life drugs. When used as anxiolytics, benzodiazepines have been associated with an increased risk of RTAs[4]. One study found that zopiclone (despite having a short half-life) dramatically increased the risk of RTAs[4].
Antipsychotics	Sedation and EPSEs can impair coordination and response-time[1]. A high proportion of patients treated with antipsychotics may have an impaired ability to drive[5,6]. Clinical assessment is required.
Antidepressants	TCAs have been associated with an increased risk of RTAs,[7] although negative studies also exist[4]. SSRIs[8] and MAOIs may be safer long term but probably not during the acute phase of the illness[9] (where impairments may be illness- rather than medication- related[10]).
Anticonvulsants	Initial, dose-related side-effects may affect driving ability (e.g. blurred vision, ataxia and sedation). There are strict rules regarding epilepsy and driving.
Lithium	Lithium may impair visual adaptation to the dark[1] but the implications for driving safety are unknown.
Alcohol	Alcohol causes sedation and impaired coordination, vision, attention and information-processing. Alcohol-dependent drivers are twice as likely to be involved in traffic accidents and offences than licensed drivers as a whole[3] and a third of all fatal RTAs involve alcohol-dependent drivers[3].

Drug-induced sedation

Many psychotropic drugs are sedative. The more sedative a drug is, the more likely it is to impair driving ability. Other medicines, either prescribed or bought over the counter, may also be sedative and/or affect driving ability (e.g. antihistamines[3]). One study found that 89% of patients taking other psychotropic drugs in addition to antidepressants failed a battery of 'fitness to drive' tests[9]. Since the degree of sedation any individual will experience is very difficult to predict, patients prescribed sedative drugs should be advised not to drive if they feel sedated.

DVLA regulations

Although the DVLA give quite specific guidelines regarding illness and ability to hold a driving licence (see summary of DVLA regulations on pages 258–259), the rules regarding taking medication and driving are rather more vague.

Note 6 of the 'At a Glance' guidelines for psychiatric disorders states that 'Driving while unfit through drugs ... is an offence', but what 'unfit through drugs' means appears to be at the discretion of the medical practitioner and individual concerned. The possible effects of various drugs are then listed, as in the table on the previous page.

DVLA – duty of the client

'If you have a medical condition which has become worse since your licence was issued, or you develop a new medical condition, you must write and inform the Drivers Medical Unit at the DVLA of the nature of your condition'. A list of the 'conditions' that interest the DVLA is provided but medication used to treat these conditions is not mentioned specifically. Insurance companies should also be informed.

DVLA – duty of the prescriber

Doctors must advise patients on the effects that their illness and prescribed medication may have on their 'fitness to drive'. See also below.

GMC guidance re confidentiality[11]

If a patient lacks the capacity to understand the advice given by the doctor about "fitness to drive" or drives contrary to that advice, it is the duty of the doctor to inform the DVLA. This duty is absolute. There is no room for discretion.

In order to persuade a patient to desist from driving, their next of kin may be directly informed of the patient's lack of 'fitness to drive'.

References

1. Metzner JL, Dentino AN, Goddard SL. Impairment in driving and psychiatric illness. *Journal of Neuropsychiatry* 1993; **5**: 211–220.
2. Ray WA, Thapa PB, Shorr RI. Medications and the older driver. *Clinics in Geriatric Medicine* 1993; **9**: 413–438.
3. Noyes R. Motor vehicle accidents related to psychiatric impairment. *Psychosomatics* 1985; **26**: 569–580.
4. Barbone F, McMahon AD, Davey PG *et al*. Association of road-traffic accidents with benzodiazepine use. *Lancet* 1998; **352**: 1331–1336.
5. Grabe HJ, Wolf T, Gratz S *et al*. The influence of clozapine and typical neuroleptics on information processing of the central nervous system under clinical conditions in schizophrenic disorders: implications for fitness to drive. *Neuropsychobiology* 1999; **40**: 196–201.
6. Wylie KR, Thompson DJ, Wildgust HJ. Effect of depot neuroleptics on driving performance in chronic schizophrenic patients. *Journal of Neurology, Neurosurgery and Psychiatry* 1993; **56**: 910–913.
7. Currie D, Hashemi K, Fothergill J *et al*. The use of anti-depressants and benzodiazepines in the perpetrators and victims of accidents. *Occupational Medicine* 1995; **45**: 323–325.

8. Hindmarsh I, Harrison C. The effects of paroxetine and other antidepressants in combination with alcohol on psychomotor activity related to car driving. *Acta Psychiatrica Scandinavica* 1989; **80**(Suppl. 350): 45.
9. Grabe HJ, Wolf T, Gratz S *et al.* The influence of polypharmacological antidepressive treatment on central nervous information processing of depressed patients: implications for fitness to drive. *Neuropsychobiology* 1998; **37**: 200–204.
10. Gerhard U, Hobi V. Cognitive-psychomotor functions with regard to fitness for driving of psychiatric patients treated with neuroleptics and antidepressants. *Neuropsychobiology* 1984; **12**: 39–47.
11. Morgan JF. DVLA and GMC guidelines on 'fitness to drive' and psychiatric disorders: knowledge following an educational campaign. *Medicine, Science and the Law* 1998; **38**: 28–31.

Further reading

Niveau G, Kelley-Puskas M. Psychiatric disorders and fitness to drive. *Journal of Medical Ethics* 2001; **27**: 36–39.

Table Summary of DVLA regulations

Diagnosis	Group 1 Entitlement (Cars and Motorcycles)		Group 2 Entitlement (Heavy Goods or Public Service Vehicles)	
	Notify DVLA?	Notes	Notify DVLA?	Notes
Uncomplicated Anxiety or Depression	No	Consider effects of medication (see page 255).	No	Very minor short-lived illnesses need not be notified to DVLA. Consider effects of medication (see page 255).
Severe Anxiety States or Depressive Illnesses	Yes	Driving should cease pending the outcome of medical enquiry. A period of stability will be required before driving can be resumed.	Yes	Licence revoked for minimum of 6 months. Driving usually permitted if illness long-standing but controlled on medication that does not impair driving.
Acute Psychotic Episodes of any type or cause	Yes	Patient should inform the DVLA (see guidance overleaf). Medical report requested by DVLA. Licence usually revoked for at least 12 months. DVLA consider mania/hypomania to be high risk.	Yes	Licence revoked for at least 3 years. Driving will only be permitted again if medication is minimal and does not interfere with driving ability and there is no significant likelihood of relapse.
Chronic Schizophrenia	Yes	Driving usually permitted in those who have not had a relapse in the past year (even if they continue to have symptoms & limited insight); conditional upon compliance with medication & stable behaviour.	Yes	
Dementia or any Organic Brain Syndrome	Yes	Patient should inform DVLA (see guidance overleaf) Decision regarding fitness to drive based on medical reports. In early dementia, licence may be issued subject to annual review.	Yes	Licence revoked.
Learning Disability	Yes	Severe LD – licence application will be refused. Mild LD – must be declared by patient on licence application form. Provisional licence may be issued: liaise with DVLA.	Yes	Only persons with minor degrees of learning disability will be considered for a licence.

Diagnosis	Group 1 Entitlement (Cars and Motorcycles)		Group 2 Entitlement (Heavy Goods or Public Service Vehicles)	
	Notify DVLA?	Notes	Notify DVLA?	Notes
Persistent Behaviour Disorder (e.g. violent behaviour)	Yes	Court or patient should inform DVLA. Licence revoked. Licence reissued only after behaviour has been satisfactorily controlled. Medical report. required	Yes	Licence refused/revoked. Possibility of licence if person matures and psychiatric reports confirm stability.
Alcohol Misuse 'Persistent misuse of alcohol confirmed by medical enquiry'	Yes	Licence refused/revoked for confirmed, persistent alcohol misuse until minimum of 6 months' controlled drinking or abstinence attained. Medical reports required.	Yes	Same as Group I except one year's controlled drinking or abstinence required.
Alcohol Dependency	Yes	Licence refused/revoked until a 1-year period free from alcohol problems attained. Abstinence usually required. Additional restrictions if seizures occur.	Yes	Licence not granted if there is a history of alcohol dependency in the past 3 years. Additional restrictions if seizures occur.
Alcohol-Related Disorders (e.g. psychosis)	Yes	Patient should inform DVLA. Medical reports required. Licence usually refused/revoked until satisfactory recovery.	Yes	Licence refused/revoked.
Drug Misuse and Dependency NB: Benzodiazepines prescribed above BNF limits for any reason constitute misuse/dependency for DVLA purposes	Yes	Licence revoked until drug free period shown below is attained. Assessment and urine screen arranged by DVLA may be required. 6-month drug-free period for cannabis, amphetamines, ecstasy & other psychoactive substances. I year drug free period for heroin, morphine, methadone (there are exceptions for those on a supervised maintenance programme), cocaine & benzodiazepines. Additional restrictions if seizures occur.	Yes	Licence revocation until drug-free period attained. Assessment and urine screen arranged by DVLA will normally be required. I-year drug-free period for cannabis, amphetamines, ecstasy & other psychoactive substances. 3-year drug-free, period for heroin, morphine, methadone cocaine & benzodiazepines. Additional restrictions if seizures occur.

Full information can be found at: www.dvla.gov.uk.

Communication with patients/service users

Follow the CAAT system.

Consultative

Those being prescribed medication should be consulted about their preferences with regard to adverse effects and likely outcomes with different medication. Patients' informed preferences should influence drug choice. Ideally, patients themselves should choose which medication they are prescribed. When patients are too ill to be consulted about drug choice, the opportunity for informative discussion should be provided as soon as it is appropriate

Accurate

Patients have the right to factually accurate information about medicines and prescribing choices. Health care workers should recognise the limits of their knowledge and refer for expert advice when necessary. Consider, also, the provision of written information and patient telephone helplines.

Appropriate

Information should be presented in such a way that it can be readily understood. It is more important to tell patients how medication affects symptoms than to try to explain complex theories of drug action. It is rarely necessary to discuss, for instance, receptor theory, but likely outcomes should certainly be discussed. Everyone should be afforded the opportunity to be given more information having first reflected on the information initially provided or after having gained first-hand experience of medication prescribed.

True

Patients have the right to be told the truth about medicines. It is morally right to impart all *relevant* information to those prescribed medication. Being 'economical with the truth' is unethical and likely to damage relationships and perhaps lead to litigation. Clearly, it is impossible to tell patients everything that is known about a particular medication, but it is possible to direct patients to more comprehensive, well-grounded sources of information.

Index

261

267

MAUDSLEY DISCUSSION PAPERS

The Maudsley Discussion Papers are a series of pamphlets on important contemporary issues in psychiatry and mental health. The titles currently available in the series include:

1. **The General Practitioner, the Psychiatrist and the Burden of Mental Health Care**
   (Prof Goldberg & Prof Gournay, 1997)

2. **Hard to Swallow: Compulsory Treatment in Eating Disorders**
   (Janet Treasure & Rosalind Ramsay, 1997)

3. **Has Community Care Failed?**
   (Graham Thornicroft & David Goldberg, 1998)

4. **Should the English Special Hospitals be Closed?**
   (John Gunn & Anthony Maden, 1998)

5. **Should Psychiatrists Treat Personality Disorders?**
   (Paul Moran, 1999)

6. **Specialist Services for Minority Ethnic Groups?**
   (Kamaldeep Bhui, Dinesh Bhugra & Kwame McKenzie, 2000)

7. **Adoption as a Placement Choice: Arguments and Evidence**
   (Alan Rushton, 2000)

8. **Should Mental Health Nurses Prescribe?**
   (Kevin Gournay & Richard Gray, 2001)

9. **Does Schizophrenia Exist?**
   (Jim Van Os & Peter McKenna, 2003)

All titles are £4 per copy (incl. p&p). Orders should be sent together with a cheque payable to *King's College London* to:

Mrs Sarah Smith
Division of Psychological Medicine
Institute of Psychiatry PO Box 63
De Crespigny Park
London SE5 8AF